Otosclerosis and Stapes Surgery

Editors

ADRIEN A. ESHRAGHI
FRED F. TELISCHI

OTOLARYNGOLOGIC CLINICS OF NORTH AMERICA

www.oto.theclinics.com

Consulting Editor
SUJANA S. CHANDRASEKHAR

April 2018 • Volume 51 • Number 2

ELSEVIER

1600 John F. Kennedy Boulevard • Suite 1800 • Philadelphia, Pennsylvania, 19103-2899

http://www.oto.theclinics.com

OTOLARYNGOLOGIC CLINICS OF NORTH AMERICA Volume 51, Number 2
April 2018 ISSN 0030-6665, ISBN-13: 978-0-323-56996-5

Editor: Jessica McCool
Developmental Editor: Sara Watkins

Otolaryngologic Clinics of North America (ISSN 0030-6665) is published bimonthly by Elsevier, Inc., 360 Park Avenue South, New York, NY 10010-1710. Months of issue are February, April, June, August, October, and December. Business and Editorial Offices: 1600 John F. Kennedy Blvd., Suite 1800, Philadelphia, PA 19103-2899. Customer Service Office: 6277 Sea Harbor Drive, Orlando, FL 32887-4800. Periodicals postage paid at New York, NY and additional mailing offices. Subscription prices are $396.00 per year (US individuals), $835.00 per year (US institutions), $100.00 per year (US student/resident), $519.00 per year (Canadian individuals), $1058.00 per year (Canadian institutions), $556.00 per year (international individuals), $1058.00 per year (international institutions), $270.00 per year (international & Canadian student/resident). Foreign air speed delivery is included in all *Clinics'* subscription prices. All prices are subject to change without notice. **POSTMASTER:** Send address changes to *Otolaryngologic Clinics of North America*, Elsevier Health Sciences Division, Subscription Customer Service, 3251 Riverport Lane, Maryland Heights, MO 63043. **Telephone: 1-800-654-2452 (U.S. and Canada); 314-447-8871 (outside U.S. and Canada). Fax: 314-447-8029. E-mail: journalscustomerservice-usa@elsevier.com (for print support); journalsonlinesupport-usa@elsevier.com (for online support).**

Reprints. For copies of 100 or more of articles in this publication, please contact the Commercial Reprints Department, Elsevier Inc., 360 Park Avenue South, New York, NY 10010-1710. Tel.: 212-633-3874; Fax: 212-633-3820; E-mail: reprints@elsevier.com.

Otolaryngologic Clinics of North America is also published in Spanish by McGraw-Hill Interamericana Editores S.A., P.O. Box 5-237, 06500 Mexico D.F., Mexico.

Otolaryngologic Clinics of North America is covered in *MEDLINE/PubMed (Index Medicus), Current Contents/Clinical Medicine, Excerpta Medica, BIOSIS, Science Citation Index,* and *ISI/BIOMED.*

PROGRAM OBJECTIVE

The goal of the *Otolaryngologic Clinics of North America* is to provide information on the latest trends in patient management, the newest advances; and provide a sound basis for choosing treatment options in the field of otolaryngology.

LEARNING OBJECTIVES

Upon completion of this activity, participants will be able to:
1. Review the audiology of and medical management of otosclerosis
2. Discuss special anatomical considerations, as well as, complication prevention and management in otosclerosis surgery
3. Recognize current and recent advances in otosclerosis surgery

ACCREDITATION

The Elsevier Office of Continuing Medical Education (EOCME) is accredited by the Accreditation Council for Continuing Medical Education (ACCME) to provide continuing medical education for physicians.

The EOCME designates this enduring material for a maximum of 15 *AMA PRA Category 1 Credit*(s)™. Physicians should claim only the credit commensurate with the extent of their participation in the activity.

All other health care professionals requesting continuing education credit for this enduring material will be issued a certificate of participation.

DISCLOSURE OF CONFLICTS OF INTEREST

The EOCME assesses conflict of interest with its instructors, faculty, planners, and other individuals who are in a position to control the content of CME activities. All relevant conflicts of interest that are identified are thoroughly vetted by EOCME for fair balance, scientific objectivity, and patient care recommendations. EOCME is committed to providing its learners with CME activities that promote improvements or quality in healthcare and not a specific proprietary business or a commercial interest.

The planning committee, staff, authors and editors listed below have identified no financial relationships or relationships to products or devices they or their spouse/life partner have with commercial interest related to the content of this CME activity:

Sumit K. Agrawal, MD, FRCSC; Patrick J. Antonelli, MD; Moises Arriaga, MD, MBA, FACS; Thomas A. Babcock, MD; Kestutis Paul Boyev, MD; Sujana S. Chandrasekhar, MD; Horace C.S. Cheng, MD, MASc; Ali A. Danesh, MS, PhD, FAAA, CCC-A; Norma de Oliveira Penido, MD, PhD; Andy de Oliveira Vicente, MD, PhD; Adrien A. Eshraghi, MD, MSc, FACS; Michael F. Foster, DO; James W. Hall III, PhD; Kristen Helm; Jacob B. Hunter, MD; Kadri Ila, MD; Reuven Ishai, MD; Alison Kemp; J. Walter Kutz Jr, MD, FACS; Fred Linthicum, MD; Xue Zhong Liu, MD, PhD, FACS; Michal Luntz, MD; Lawrence R. Lustig, MD; Jessica McCool; John T. McElveen Jr, MD; Michael J. McKenna, MD; Ronen Nazarian, MD; Emre Ocak, MD; Lorne S. Parnes, MD, FRCSC; Alicia M. Quesnel, MD; Apoorva T. Ramaswamy, MD; Helge Rask-Andersen, MD, PhD; Nadine Schart-Morén, PhD; Alexander Sevy, MD; Navid Shahnaz, PhD; Karin Strömbäck, MD, PhD, Fred F. Telischi, MEE, MD, FACS; Subhalakshmi Vaidyanathan; Amit Wolfovitz, MD.

The planning committee, staff, authors and editors listed below have identified financial relationships or relationships to products or devices they or their spouse/life partner have with commercial interest related to the content of this CME activity:

Douglas D. Backous, MD: has received honoraria for consulting with Medtronic and Stryker

Daniele Bernardeschi, MD, PhD: receives royalties or holds a patent with Collins Medical Equipment, French National Institute of Health, Medical Research, and University Pierre et Marie Curie

Brandon Isaacson, MD, FACS: is on the Advisory Board of Advanced Bionics and MED-EL, and is also a consultant for Stryker, Olympus, Storz, Advanced Bionics, and Medtronic

Hao Li, PhD: receives royalties or holds a patent with Collins Medical Equipment, French National Institute of Health, Medical Research, and University Pierre et Marie Curie

Yann Nguyen, MD, PhD: receives royalties or holds a patent with Collins Medical Equipment, French National Institute of Health, Medical Research, and University Pierre et Marie Curie

Alejandro Rivas, MD: is associated with the Cochlear Corporation, Advanced Bionics, MED-EL, Olympus, and Grace Medical

Olivier Sterkers, MD, PhD: receives royalties or holds a patent with Collins Medical Equipment, French National Institute of Health, Medical Research, and University Pierre et Marie Curie

UNAPPROVED/OFF-LABEL USE DISCLOSURE

The EOCME requires CME faculty to disclose to the participants:

1. When products or procedures being discussed are off-label, unlabelled, experimental, and/or investigational (not US Food and Drug Administration (FDA) approved; and
2. Any limitations on the information presented, such as data that are preliminary or that represent ongoing research, interim analyses, and/or unsupported opinions. Faculty may discuss information about pharmaceutical agents that is outside of FDA-approved labelling. This information is intended solely for CME and is not intended to promote off-label use of these medications. If you have any questions, contact the medical affairs department of the manufacturer for the most recent prescribing information.

TO ENROLL

To enroll in the *Otolaryngologic Clinics of North America* Continuing Medical Education program, call customer service at 1-800-654-2452 or sign up online at http://www.theclinics.com/home/cme. The CME program is available to subscribers for an additional annual fee of USD 260.

METHOD OF PARTICIPATION

In order to claim credit, participants must complete the following:

1. Complete enrolment as indicated above.
2. Read the activity.
3. Complete the CME Test and Evaluation. Participants must achieve a score of 70% on the test. All CME Tests and Evaluations must be completed online.

CME INQUIRIES/SPECIAL NEEDS

For all CME inquiries or special needs, please contact elsevierCME@elsevier.com.

Contributors

CONSULTING EDITOR

SUJANA S. CHANDRASEKHAR, MD
Director, New York Otology, Clinical Professor, Department of Otolaryngology–Head and Neck Surgery, Zucker School of Medicine at Hofstra-Northwell, Hempstead, New York, USA; Clinical Associate Professor, Department of Otolaryngology–Head and Neck Surgery, Icahn School of Medicine at Mount Sinai, New York, New York, USA

EDITORS

ADRIEN A. ESHRAGHI, MD, MSc, FACS
Professor of Otolaryngology, Otology, Neurotology and Skull Base Surgery, Director, Hearing Research Laboratory, Co-Director, University of Miami Ear Institute, University of Miami Miller School of Medicine, Miami, Florida, USA

FRED F. TELISCHI, MEE, MD, FACS
Chairman of Otolaryngology and Professor, Neurological Surgery and Biomedical Engineering, University of Miami Miller School of Medicine, Miami, Florida, USA

AUTHORS

SUMIT K. AGRAWAL, MD, FRCSC
Department of Otolaryngology–Head and Neck Surgery, Schulich School of Medicine & Dentistry, Western University, London, Ontario, Canada

PATRICK J. ANTONELLI, MD
Professor and Chair, Department of Otolaryngology, University of Florida, Gainesville, Florida, USA

MOISES ARRIAGA, MD, MBA, FACS
Clinical Professor, Department of Otolaryngology–Head and Neck Surgery, Louisiana State University School of Medicine, New Orleans, Louisiana, USA; Hearing and Balance Center, Our Lady of the Lake, Baton Rouge, Louisiana, USA

THOMAS A. BABCOCK, MD
Neurotology Fellow, Department of Otolaryngology, University of Miami Miller School of Medicine, Miami, Florida, USA

DOUGLAS D. BACKOUS, MD
Medical Director, Center for Hearing and Skull Base Surgery, Swedish Neuroscience Institute, Seattle, Washington, USA

DANIELE BERNARDESCHI, MD, PhD
Sorbonne Université, Inserm, UMR-S 1159 "Minimally Invasive Robot-based Hearing Rehabilitation," Otolaryngology Department, Unit of Otology, Auditory Implants and Skull Base Surgery, AP-HP, GHU Pitié-Salpêtrière, Paris, France

KESTUTIS PAUL BOYEV, MD
Associate Professor, Director, Division of Otology/Neurotology, Department of
Otolaryngology–Head and Neck Surgery, University of South Florida Morsani College
of Medicine, Tampa, Florida, USA

HORACE C.S. CHENG, MD, MASc
Department of Otolaryngology–Head and Neck Surgery, Schulich School of Medicine &
Dentistry, Western University, London, Ontario, Canada

ALI A. DANESH, MS, PhD, FAAA, CCC-A
Departments of Communication Sciences and Disorders and Clinical Biomedical
Sciences, Charles E. Schmidt College of Medicine, Florida Atlantic University, Boca
Raton, Florida, USA

NORMA DE OLIVEIRA PENIDO, MD, PhD
Professor, Department of Otorhinolaryngology–Head and Neck Surgery, Universidade
Federal de São Paulo, Escola Paulista de Medicina, São Paulo, São Paulo, Brazil

ANDY DE OLIVEIRA VICENTE, MD, PhD
Otorhinolaryngology Department, Hospital Especializado CEMA, São Paulo,
São Paulo, Brazil

ADRIEN A. ESHRAGHI, MD, MSc, FACS
Professor of Otolaryngology, Otology, Neurotology and Skull Base Surgery, Director,
Hearing Research Laboratory, Co-Director, University of Miami Ear Institute, University
of Miami Miller School of Medicine, Miami, Florida, USA

MICHAEL F. FOSTER, DO
Otology Fellow, Center for Hearing and Skull Base Surgery, Swedish Neuroscience
Institute, Seattle, Washington, USA

JAMES W. HALL III, PhD
Osborne College of Audiology, Salus University, Elkins Park, Pennsylvania, USA;
Department of Communicative Disorders, University of Hawaii, Honolulu, Hawaii, USA

JACOB B. HUNTER, MD
Department of Otolaryngology–Head and Neck Surgery, The University of Texas
Southwestern Medical Center, Dallas, Texas, USA

KADRI ILA, MD
Department of Otolaryngology, University of Miami Miller School of Medicine, Miami,
Florida, USA

BRANDON ISAACSON, MD, FACS
Department of Otolaryngology–Head and Neck Surgery, The University of Texas
Southwestern Medical Center, Dallas, Texas, USA

REUVEN ISHAI, MD
Research Fellow, Massachusetts Eye and Ear Otopathology Laboratory, Harvard Medical
School, Boston, Massachusetts, USA

J. WALTER KUTZ Jr, MD, FACS
Associate Professor, Department of Otolaryngology, The University of Texas
Southwestern Medical Center, Dallas, Texas, USA

HAO LI, PhD
Department of Surgical Sciences, Head and Neck Surgery, Section of Otolaryngology,
Uppsala University Hospital, Uppsala, Sweden

FRED LINTHICUM, MD
Department of Head and Neck Surgery, David Geffen School of Medicine, University of California, Los Angeles, Los Angeles, California, USA

XUE ZHONG LIU, MD, PhD, FACS
Professor, Department of Otolaryngology, University of Miami Miller School of Medicine, Miami, Florida, USA

MICHAL LUNTZ, MD
Director of Ear and Hearing Program, Chair, Department of Otolaryngology–Head and Neck Surgery, Bnai Zion Medical Center, The Ruth and Bruce Rappaport Faculty of Medicine, Technion – Israeli School of Technology, Haifa, Israel

LAWRENCE R. LUSTIG, MD
Chair, Department of Otolaryngology–Head and Neck Surgery, Columbia University Medical Center, New York, New York, USA

JOHN T. McELVEEN Jr, MD
President, Carolina Ear & Hearing Clinic, PC, Director, Carolina Ear Research Institute, Raleigh, North Carolina, USA

MICHAEL J. McKENNA, MD
Professor, Department of Otolaryngology, Director of Otology and Neurotology, Joseph B. Nadol Jr. Endowed Chair, Massachusetts Eye and Ear, Co-Director, Massachusetts Eye and Ear Otopathology Laboratory, Harvard Medical School, Boston, Massachusetts, USA

RONEN NAZARIAN, MD
Osborne Head & Neck Institute, Los Angeles, California, USA

YANN NGUYEN, MD, PhD
Sorbonne Université, Inserm, UMR-S 1159 "Minimally Invasive Robot-based Hearing Rehabilitation," Otolaryngology Department, Unit of Otology, Auditory Implants and Skull Base Surgery, AP-HP, GHU Pitié-Salpêtrière, Paris, France

EMRE OCAK, MD
Department of Otolaryngology, University of Miami Miller School of Medicine, Miami, Florida, USA

LORNE S. PARNES, MD, FRCSC
Departments of Otolaryngology–Head and Neck Surgery and Clinical Neurological Sciences, Schulich School of Medicine & Dentistry, Western University, London, Ontario, Canada

ALICIA M. QUESNEL, MD
Assistant Professor, Department of Otolaryngology, Division of Otology and Neurotology, Massachusetts Eye and Ear, Investigator, Massachusetts Eye and Ear Otopathology Laboratory, Harvard Medical School, Boston, Massachusetts, USA

APOORVA T. RAMASWAMY, MD
Resident, Department of Otolaryngology–Head and Neck Surgery, Columbia University Medical Center, New York, New York, USA

HELGE RASK-ANDERSEN, MD, PhD
Professor, Department of Surgical Sciences, Head and Neck Surgery, Section of Otolaryngology, Uppsala University Hospital, Uppsala, Sweden

ALEJANDRO RIVAS, MD
Department of Otolaryngology–Head and Neck Surgery, Vanderbilt University Medical Center, Nashville, Tennessee, USA

NADINE SCHART-MORÉN, MD
Department of Otolaryngology–Head and Neck Surgery, Uppsala University Hospital, Uppsala, Sweden

ALEXANDER SEVY, MD
Assistant Professor, Department of Otolaryngology–Head and Neck Surgery, Louisiana State University School of Medicine, New Orleans, Louisiana, USA; Hearing and Balance Center, Our Lady of the Lake, Baton Rouge, Louisiana, USA

NAVID SHAHNAZ, PhD
School of Audiology and Speech Sciences, Faculty of Medicine, The University of British Columbia, Vancouver, British Columbia, Canada

OLIVIER STERKERS, MD, PhD
Sorbonne Université, Inserm, UMR-S 1159 "Minimally Invasive Robot-based Hearing Rehabilitation," Otolaryngology Department, Unit of Otology, Auditory Implants and Skull Base Surgery, AP-HP, GHU Pitié-Salpêtrière, Paris, France

KARIN STRÖMBÄCK, MD, PhD
Department of Otolaryngology–Head and Neck Surgery, Uppsala University Hospital, Uppsala, Sweden

FRED F. TELISCHI, MEE, MD, FACS
Chairman of Otolaryngology and Professor, Neurological Surgery and Biomedical Engineering, University of Miami Miller School of Medicine, Miami, Florida, USA

AMIT WOLFOVITZ, MD
Department of Otolaryngology–Head and Neck Surgery, University of Miami Miller School of Medicine, Miami, Florida, USA

Contents

> The current advancements in otosclerosis therapy cannot be fully appreciated without studying the history, rediscovery, and modification of a once-forgotten procedure. The evolution of stapes surgery can be best summarized into 4 noteworthy eras: the preantibiotic era (which was forgotten and then rediscovered), the fenestration era (mainstreamed by Julius Lempert), the mobilization era (led by Samuel Rosen), and the modern stapedectomy era (revived and revolutionized by John Shea). Each era is unique with its own challenges and ingenious techniques to overcome what used to be among the leading causes of deafness.

> Otosclerosis is pathologically characterized by abnormal bony remodeling, which includes bone resorption, new bone deposition, and vascular proliferation in the temporal bone. Sensorineural hearing loss in otosclerosis is associated with extension of otosclerosis to the cochlear endosteum and deposition of collagen throughout the spiral ligament. Persistent or recurrent conductive hearing loss after stapedectomy has been associated with incomplete footplate fenestration, poor incus-prosthesis connection, and incus resorption in temporal bone specimens. Human temporal bone pathology has helped to define the role of computed tomography imaging for otosclerosis, confirming that computed tomography is highly sensitive for diagnosis yet limited in assessing cochlear endosteal involvement.

> Over the past several years, with the evolution of genetic and molecular research, several etiologic factors have been implicated in the pathogenesis of otosclerosis. Overall, current evidence suggests that otosclerosis is a complex disease with a variety of potential pathways contributing to the development of abnormal bone remodeling in the otic capsule. These pathways involved in the pathogenesis of otosclerosis are influenced by both genetic and environmental factors.

history, audiologic results, and physical findings, is discussed, and the causes of failure of primary surgery are reviewed. A discussion of evidence-based surgical technique and postoperative care then follows.

Yann Nguyen, Daniele Bernardeschi, and Olivier Sterkers

 Video content accompanies this article at http://www.oto.theclinics. com.

Otosclerosis surgery is performed through a transcanal approach and requires long, thin instruments with submillimetric precision and precise amplitude of motion. The functional outcomes and complications of otosclerosis surgery depend on the experience of the surgeon. Thus, any technologic assistance that can enhance the surgeon's dexterity and rapidly reduce the learning curve could yield an even safer surgical procedure. One of the options is to use robotic assistance to achieve this goal. An overview of different robots designed for otosclerosis surgery is presented, focusing on the RobOtol system that we have designed as a multitask platform for ear surgery.

John T. McElveen Jr and J. Walter Kutz Jr

Controversies have been associated with the etiology, diagnosis, evaluation, and management of otosclerosis since Valsalva first described stapes fixation as a cause of hearing loss. Although the exact mechanism of the bone remodeling associated with otosclerosis remains uncertain, stapedotomy has been accepted as the surgical treatment of most patients with stapedial otosclerosis. There remains a disparity of opinion, however, regarding the role of preoperative imaging, surgical technique, implant selection, and medical therapy for cochlear otosclerosis. In addition, opinions vary regarding the optimal postoperative care of patients undergoing stapedotomy and a patient's ability to participate in activities that may result in barotrauma.

OTOLARYNGOLOGIC CLINICS
OF NORTH AMERICA

THE CLINICS ARE AVAILABLE ONLINE!
Access your subscription at:
www.theclinics.com

Foreword

A Significant Treatable Cause of Hearing Loss in Our Time

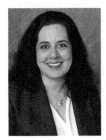

Sujana S. Chandrasekhar, MD
Consulting Editor

Otosclerosis is often called the disease in which the patient hears nothing and the physician sees nothing. This alludes to the often significant degree of hearing loss experienced by the patient and the regular lack of visible physical findings in this disorder.

Stapedotomy or stapedectomy surgery is likewise referred to as the easiest but most complicated surgery performed by otolaryngologists. In this circumstance, every step must be perfect, and every movement must be deliberate. There is a very short distance between a perfectly closed air-bone gap and a profound sensorineural hearing loss.

Nevertheless, there is no better feeling as an otolaryngologist when the prosthesis enters the opening in the oval window and the patient reports, "I can hear!" Or when the patient comes in for their postoperative visit complaining that the world around them is too loud. I had one patient who greeted me in the recovery room with a big smile and said, "It's so quiet!" She meant that, not only was her hearing better, but her tinnitus was gone. I pointed out to her that no ear doctor ever wants to hear that it is quiet!

Drs Eshraghi and Telischi have compiled a complete reference guide on otosclerosis. The story of this disease and interventions is told from history to pathology and molecular biology, to imaging and audiometric assessment, through the nuances of medical and surgical intervention.

Pathophysiologically, it begins as otospongiosis, a softening of the bone at the fissula ante fenestram and/or fossula post fenestram. Sometimes this is visible on physical examination as a promontory blush, also known as Schwartze sign. Drs Penido and Vicente explain how this can be imaged with state-of-the-art modalities and treated, which may result in prevention of progression of hearing loss and may even result in less need for surgery in certain individuals.

The anatomy of the middle ear is exquisitely complex. My residents have heard me raise a tympanomeatal flap and immediately exclaim a welcome to the most beautiful

Otolaryngol Clin N Am 51 (2018) xv–xvi
https://doi.org/10.1016/j.otc.2017.12.002
0030-6665/18/© 2017 Published by Elsevier Inc.

place on Earth, the middle ear. Ossicles, chorda tympani and facial nerves, round window niche, and air spaces all determine surgical outcomes. Drs Rask-Andersen and colleagues explore this in detail. It behooves every otolaryngologist, whether performing ear surgery or not, to understand this intricate three-dimensional anatomy from every conceivable angle. Dr Antonelli looks at this from the perspective of complications in otosclerosis surgery: how to avoid them, how to identify them, and how to approach them once they occur.

There are numerous ways to perform surgery for fenestral otosclerosis. In the beginning, there was lateral semicircular canal fenestration, then stapes mobilization, then stapedectomy, and now stapedotomy. The ear may be approached using a microscope or an endoscope, and robotics is just around the corner. The fenestra may be made with a pick, with a drill, or with a laser. The oval window may be sealed with blood, perichondrium, fascia, vein or fat. The prosthesis may be crimped on to the incus mechanically, by laser heat, or of its own "memory." The authors of the surgery technique articles have delved into their subjects and provide thorough resources for why, why not, how, and when.

Necessity for revision surgery is not common, but Drs Ramaswamy and Lustig provide an excellent reference article for how this is to be approached, and what the patient and the surgeon may expect as the outcome. Similarly, our understanding of far advanced otosclerosis has evolved in the past 20 years or so. We now understand the benefits of either stapes surgery or, more often, cochlear implantation in these patients. This is detailed well by the Guest Editors and Drs Ila and Ocak.

Otosclerosis is a disorder that affects a significant percentage of people and results in the loss or detriment to a major sense, that of hearing. It may be ameliorated reasonably or very well with nonsurgical interventions such as hearing aids. There are many possibilities for different types of interventions. All of this lends to a number of controversies. These are discussed by Drs McElveen and Kutz, and their subject matter is one with which every Otolaryngologist should be fully familiar.

That the smallest bone in the body can lead to such dramatic degree of hearing and quality-of-life impairment is in itself astonishing. I congratulate Drs Eshraghi and Telischi for their organization of this issue of *Otolaryngologic Clinics of North America*, and I urge you to take the time and energy to read these beautifully written and collated articles, and look at the extra materials provided on-line.

Sujana S. Chandrasekhar, MD
New York Otology
210 East 64th Street
New York, NY 10065, USA

Department of Otolaryngology–Head and Neck Surgery
Zucker School of Medicine at
Hofstra-Northwell
Hempstead, NY, USA

Department of Otolaryngology–Head and Neck Surgery
Icahn School of Medicine at Mount Sinai
New York, NY, USA

E-mail address:
ssc@nyotology.com

Website:
http://www.ears.nyc

Preface

Otosclerosis and Stapes Surgery

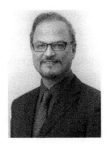 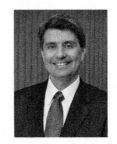

Adrien A. Eshraghi, MD, MSc, FACS   Fred F. Telischi, MEE, MD, FACS
Editors

The roots of our knowledge about otosclerosis go back to the early eighteenth century. Since then, countless numbers of scientists have studied the pathogenesis and therapy of the disease. The articles in this issue of Otolaryngologic Clinics of North America flow from history to pathophysiology, clinical evaluation, surgical and medical management to future perspectives. As concepts are constantly progressing, timely topics such as genetics and molecular biology, endoscopic ear surgery and robotic surgery are also included in this issue. Every article begins with key points and ends with the most relevant citations. Figures and supplementary videos are also included to enrich the content. We think that as the stable incidence makes otosclerosis a public health problem, every otolaryngologist and audiologist must be up-to-date in their knowledge in order to manage their patients properly. In this manner, this issue may be considered a reference guide to otosclerosis.

Historical aspects of otosclerosis and stapes surgery are presented within four distinctive eras, including pre-antibiotic, fenestration, mobilization, and modern stapedotomy. Understanding both the evolution of the surgery and the stories of innovative surgeons are important to fully appreciating the current advancements in the field.

As understanding the consequences of surgery provides insights into how to optimize surgical techniques, we believe that pathologic findings in otosclerosis, with particular attention to clinical relevance, will provide useful information for clinicians. The surgeon must keep in mind that although computed tomography is highly sensitive for the diagnosis of otosclerosis, it has only moderate sensitivity for identification of cochlear endosteal involvement.

With the evolution of genetic and molecular research, pathways involved in the pathogenesis of otosclerosis influenced by genetic and epigenetic factors are reviewed. These factors have been demonstrated to play a role in the development of several molecular pathways, including bone remodeling, immunologic, inflammatory, and

Otolaryngol Clin N Am 51 (2018) xvii–xix
https://doi.org/10.1016/j.otc.2017.12.001
0030-6665/18/© 2017 Published by Elsevier Inc.

endocrine. We believe these recent findings will stimulate new ideas about the complex molecular pathways of the disease and therefore, further research on the subject.

Despite its prevalent nature, one can easily misdiagnose otosclerosis, leading to unnecessary treatments. Clinical evaluation of the patient with otosclerosis provides valuable information in the differential diagnosis and a general overview of the disease.

The audiology of otosclerosis is undeniably one of the most important issues on the subject, as almost all the patients have a normal otoscopy on physical examination. The audiologist perspective and standard audiometric measurements, as well as newly practiced techniques like Wideband Acoustic Immittance, are included. The article, "Audiology of Otosclerosis," provides valuable information regarding the management of otosclerosis through amplification with hearing aids. The management of tinnitus in the otosclerotic population, including the use of sound and cognitive behavioral therapies, is also included.

Although the diagnosis is predominately clinical, it is beyond doubt that imaging has an important role for difficult cases in terms of differential diagnosis and perioperative planning. It can avoid complications in some cases.

We would like to thank Dr Rask-Andersen, who performed special anatomical dissections at our request, presented in the article, "Special Anatomical Considerations in Otosclerosis Surgery." The relationship between the otolith organs and the oval window based on freshly frozen human temporal bones with micro-CT using 3D rendering algorithms was illustrated beautifully.

Stapedotomy has lower complication rates when compared to stapedectomy, and because of its minimally invasive approaches, may represent the next major development in stapes surgery in selected patients. Valuable videos about the surgical procedures are available in this issue, presenting various techniques.

Choice of prosthesis is important in the surgical treatment of otosclerosis. A wide array of biomaterial availability has influenced stapes surgery techniques, especially methods for incus attachment. This issue emphasizes the importance of the stapes prostheses in terms of shape, size, and the biomaterial used.

It was controversial when Rodney Perkins first introduced laser surgery in otosclerosis, but the laser is now a popular surgical tool for stapes surgery. Though there is no clear advantage among the various available systems, many prefer handheld lasers for safety and ergonomic reasons.

There is a progressive trend in the use of endoscopes in otology. The advantages and disadvantages of transcanal endoscopic approach to stapes surgery are presented with beautiful endoscopic surgical illustrations.

Diagnosis of far advanced otosclerosis can be challenging. It requires a careful history, combined with an audiologic evaluation and/or imaging. Obtaining optimal results depends on proper selection among the treatment options. The choice between stapes surgery/hearing aid and cochlear implantation can, in many cases, be controversial. The stapedotomy, or hearing aids, appear to be the first step of treatment. Cochlear implantation should be the next step if hearing outcome is not satisfactory. Electrode insertion might be difficult and require special surgical technique.

As most clinicians and patients prefer surgery for the treatment of conductive hearing loss related to otosclerosis, much of the literature lacks information about medical treatment, so medical management of otosclerosis, focusing on the use of sodium fluoride and bisphosphonates to limit progression of the disease, is presented in this issue.

Revision stapes surgery must be approached cautiously. The importance of initial evaluation, preoperative planning, intraoperative techniques, and postoperative care in revision surgery for otosclerosis are discussed in the article, "Revision Surgery for Otosclerosis."

As with all surgical procedures, understanding the management of complications is essential, as they may occur even in the most experienced hands. Most early post-operative complications usually can be managed medically, while revision surgery may be necessary to achieve optimal long-term outcomes. Furthermore, patients must have comprehensive explanations of the potential negative effects of the elective operation during the informed consent process.

Technological assistance that can enhance the surgeon's dexterity and rapidly reduce the learning curve could yield safer surgical procedures for the disease. Robot-based devices have the potential to improve accuracy of the surgical gesture and might have the potential of making a similar influence as laser in stapes surgery. Otosclerosis and stapes surgery are not without controversy; from cause to medical and surgical treatment, which is further explored in the article "Controversies in Otosclerosis," in this issue.

Special thanks to all contributors for their outstanding articles. We would also like to thank Dr Emre Ocak and Dr Kadri Ila for their valuable input in preparation of this issue.

Adrien A. Eshraghi, MD, MSc, FACS
University of Miami Ear Institute
Department of Otolaryngology
Miller School of Medicine
1120 Northwest, 14th Street
Miami, FL 33136, USA

Fred F. Telischi, MEE, MD, FACS
University of Miami Ear Institute
Department of Otolaryngology
Miller School of Medicine
1120 Northwest, 14th Street
Miami, FL 33136, USA

E-mail addresses:
aeshraghi@med.miami.edu (A.A. Eshraghi)
ftelischi@med.miami.edu (F.F. Telischi)

History of Otosclerosis and Stapes Surgery

Ronen Nazarian, MD[a],*, John T. McElveen Jr, MD[b], Adrien A. Eshraghi, MD, MSc[c]

KEYWORDS

- Stapes • Otosclerosis • Stapedectomy • Stapedotomy • Fenestration • Lempert
- Rosen • Shea

KEY POINTS

- The study of otosclerosis dates back to as early as 1704 with the research of Antonio Maria Valsalva.
- Stapes surgery was first described by Johannes Kessel in 1876, but fell into disrepute in 1899 due to concerns of patient safety at the time.
- Julius Lempert's ingenious single-stage fenestration operation became the mainstream method to indirectly treat Otosclerosis in the 1930s to 1950s.
- John Shea rediscovered and modernized the stapedectomy procedure in 1956.
- Modern stapes surgery is still evolving, but studying the history, rediscovery, and modification of otosclerosis therapy is essential for appreciating advances in medicine today and in the future.

INTRODUCTION

The current advancements in otosclerosis therapy cannot be fully appreciated without studying the history, rediscovery, and modification of a once-forgotten procedure.

The study of otosclerosis dates back to as early as 1704 with the research of Antonio Maria Valsalva[1] (**Fig. 1**). Valsalva, who was Professor of Anatomy in Bologna, is credited with first describing stapes fixation as a cause of hearing loss. His meticulous postmortem dissections of a deaf patient in 1704 revealed fixation of the stapes as the cause of hearing loss. The dissections were performed in the Anatomical Theater of the Archiginnasio in Bologna, Italy (**Fig. 2**). In 1841, Toynbee's publication firmly established the link between deafness and stapes fixation. He dissected 1659 temporal bones and found stapes fixation in 39. He concluded that "osseous ankylosis of the stapes to the fenestra ovalis was one of the common causes of deafness."

Disclosure: The authors have nothing to disclose.
[a] Osborne Head and Neck Institute, 8631 West 3rd Street, Suite 945E, Los Angeles, CA 90048, USA; [b] Carolina Ear Institute, Carolina Ear and Hearing Clinic, Raleigh, NC, USA; [c] University of Miami Ear Institute
* Corresponding author.
E-mail address: Nazarian@ohni.org

oto.theclinics.com

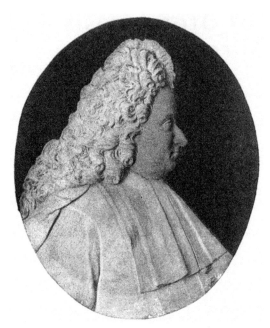

Fig. 1. Antonio Maria Valsalva. (*Data from* https://wellcomecollection.org/works/yhyxsfk3 under a Creative Commons Attribution 4.0 international license.)

In 1873, Schwartze described a reddish hue on the cochlear promontory of patients with active otosclerosis (Schwartze sign).[2] This active hyperemic stage with increased vascularity was later named otospongiosis by Siebenmann. It was assumed by Toynbee and others that chronic inflammatory mucosal changes in the middle ear resulted in secondary ankylosis of the stapes.[3] However, in December, 1893, some 52 years later, Adam Politzer (**Fig. 3**) described the histologic findings in 16 cases of stapes fixation. His findings indicated that the deafness, which had been attributed to chronic interstitial middle ear catarrh with secondary stapes fixation, was really due to a primary disorder of the labyrinthine capsule.[4] He referred to this pathology as otosclerosis. His findings were initially published in 1894 in Zeitschrift Für Ohrenheilkunde

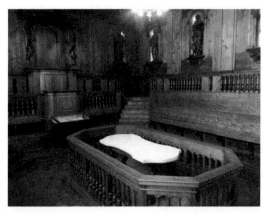

Fig. 2. The dissections of Valsalva were performed at the Anatomical Theater of The Archiginnasio in Bologna, Italy.

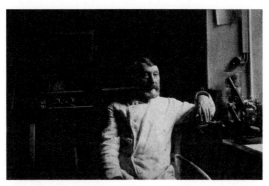

Fig. 3. Adam Politzer. (*Data from* https://wellcomeimages.org/indexplus/image/V0027026. html under a Creative Commons Attribution 4.0 international license.)

and then translated into English and published a few months later in the *Archives of Otology*. Despite both of these publications, Politzer's views, although histologically verified, were slow to catch on. It took almost half a century for Politzer's principles to gain universal acceptance.

It is not known exactly when the first attempts to mobilize the stapes were carried out; however, in 1842, Prospere Ménière reported the case of a patient who was able to temporarily improve his own hearing by tapping the stapes directly with a small gold rod.[5] Some cite this as the first attempt at stapes mobilization.

The ensuing evolution of stapes surgery can be best summarized into 4 noteworthy eras: the pre-antibiotic era (which was forgotten and then rediscovered), the fenestration era (mainstreamed by Julius Lempert), the mobilization era (led by Samuel Rosen), and the modern stapedectomy era (revived and revolutionized by John Shea).

Each era is unique with its own challenges and ingenious techniques to overcome what used to be a leading cause of deafness (**Fig. 4**). It is extremely worthwhile,

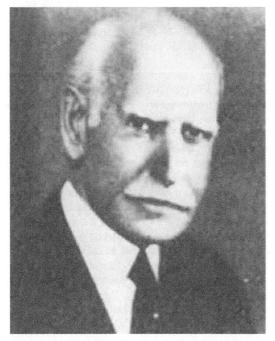

Fig. 4. Frederick L. Jack. (*From* Tange RA, The history of otosclerosis treatment. Amsterdam: Kugler Publications; 2014; with permission.)

educational, and entertaining to study all 4 of these eras as they bear timeless lessons for any physician with an interest in expanding and advancing medicine.

THE PRE-ANTIBIOTIC ERA

The first era of stapes surgery entailed some of the boldest surgical advancements, which were soon abandoned due to concerns of long-term efficacy and patient safety. Johannes Kessel[6] is considered the first to describe stapes surgery in 1876. He was under the mistaken opinion that the hearing loss associated with otosclerosis was caused by increased pressure in the inner ear fluids. He theorized that by removing the stapes, he could relieve that pressure. Before testing his hypothesis on humans, he removed the columella (stapes equivalent) from 2 pigeons. He was able to demonstrate that opening of the oval window did not necessarily result in destructive damage to the inner ear as was generally feared. Based on this experimental investigation in pigeons, he performed stapes mobilizations and also stapes removal in humans.

In 1878, Kessel[7] reported on the procedure in which he would incise the posterior part of the tympanic membrane, separate the incus from the stapes, and then attempt to mobilize the stapes by applying pressure to its head in various directions. When this was not successful, he would remove the stapes. He continued to publish similar reports throughout his career, demonstrating that transtympanic stapes mobilization and stapedectomy is an effective method for the improvement of hearing in stapes ankylosis.[8]

The German otologists Schwartze[9] and Lucae,[10] also carried out stapes mobilization and removal of the stapes. In 1890 and 1888, the French otologists Miot[11] and Boucheron[12] reported their experience with patients who had undergone a similar procedure, respectively. Hearing improvement was achieved in 74 cases out of 126 stapes mobilizations. In 1890, Miot[11] reported his successful results with 200 stapes mobilizations in a series of 5 articles. These results and techniques were very similar to the ones that Samuel Rosen would publish more than 60 years later.

In the United States, at the Massachusetts Eye and Ear Infirmary, C.J. Blake[13] (1892) and Frederick L. Jack[14] (1893) performed mobilization and removal of the stapes. The usual method of treatment was to approach the middle ear cavity via tympanic membrane incision rather than a reflection of a tympanomeatal flap. Illumination was poor and it is unlikely that any proper magnification was used. They reported that patients experienced improved hearing as the tympanic membrane healed over the oval window niche. At that time, no attempts were made to seal the oval window or to reconstruct the ossicular chain. Jack[15] also reported a particularly interesting case in which a patient who had a double stapedectomy maintained good hearing 10 years later. He described how the tympanic membrane had retracted in the healing process and created a moveable membrane over the oval window. This description became lost in the literature only to be found again over a century later by John Shea, convincing him that stapes surgery should be revisited.

In many of the patients who were operated on in Europe and the United States, hearing improvement was often temporary, sometimes lasting only for a period of days to weeks. Although not widely published, there is speculation that some patients experienced grave complications, which included labyrinthitis, meningitis, and even death.[16] The discovery of penicillin did not occur until 1928, and it is likely that these complications arose due to the absence of antibiotics as a prophylactic measure during and after surgery.

Because of its short-term hearing improvement and probable morbidity, this early form of stapes surgery fell into disrepute. In 1899, it was heatedly criticized by some of the leading otologists of the time, Politzer, Siebenmann, and Moure, at the 6th International Otology Congress in London. During this meeting, stapes surgery was declared "useless, often mutilating, and dangerous." They went on to say, "The question of surgical therapy for otosclerosis was interred with great pomp at the 1894 International Conference in Rome. There is no reason to revive it."[16] In 1900, Johannes Kessel was publicly censured for unscrupulousness. He resigned from his position in Jena in disgrace. Embittered, he retired from all scientific work.

The eager and bold first steps for stapes surgery had come to a sudden end. A movement to indirectly treat otosclerosis without manipulating the stapes was soon to begin, and surgery on the stapes would not be attempted again for more than half a century.

THE FENESTRATION ERA

Because surgical operations on the actual fixed stapes were considered too dangerous, surgeons began to use detour approaches to the inner ear using "third-window" fenestration techniques.

Passov (1897) and Floderus (1899) both proposed the idea of a fenestration along the promontory or vestibular labyrinth,[16] but it did not become fully established until 1913 when Jenkins[17] described a "fenestration of the lateral semicircular canal."

In the early 1920s, Gunnar Holmgren[18,19] (**Fig. 5**) inadvertently made an opening in the lateral semicircular canal while removing infection from the mastoid. He covered

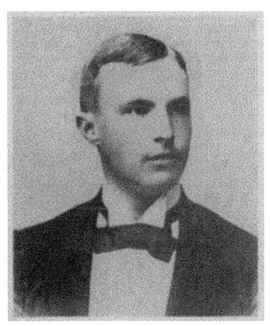

Fig. 5. Gunnar Holmgren. (*From* Hamberger C. Gunnar Holmgren (1875–1954). Arch Otolaryngol 1968;87(2):214–8; with permission.)

the area with mucoperiosteum and, to his surprise, the patient was able to hear better for a short while. With the new use of the operating microscope, Holmgren devised a three-staged "closed" fenestration operation on the lateral semicircular canal through a postauricular incision. The 3 stages would take place over a period of a few months, and he was able to achieve modest and limited results mainly because of infection or early closure of the fenestration due to bony regrowth.

In 1924, Maurice Sourdille[20] (**Fig. 6**) of Nantes, France visited Holmgren and observed a "closed fenestration" operation and realized the shortcoming of Holmgren's "closed" technique. Sourdille modified this operation and was the first to develop the fenestration of the lateral semicircular canal toward the outside in a three-stage "open" operation in which the fenestra would remain exteriorized instead of buried in a postauricular incision.[16] In 1937 he was able to produce a long-lasting hearing improvement in 64% of 109 operated patients with his tympanolabyrinthopexie. Sourdille would teach his operation to many otologists, including Juan Tato, who returned to Buenos Aires and performed the first fenestration operation in the new world in 1934.[21]

In 1937, Sourdille was invited to address the Otolaryngology Section of the New York Academy of Medicine. Julius Lempert (**Fig. 7**) was in the audience and, after Sourdille's presentation, he invited Professor Sourdille to dinner. Sourdille would later recall that during the dinner Lempert plied him with questions on details of the operative procedure. By combining what he had learned from Sourdille's three-stage postauricular operation with his own endaural techniques, Lempert was able to develop a new "single-stage" endaural fenestration operation just 3 months after the fateful dinner meeting. Lempert's single-stage operation quickly supplanted Sourdille's three-stage procedure worldwide.

Lempert's Legacy

In 1938, Julius Lempert[22] finally published his ingenious modification of the fenestration operation that made the procedure into a single-staged surgery. The story of Julius Lempert is worth special attention because it teaches lessons in facing adversity, perseverance, and the consequences of not adapting to change.

Lempert was born in a Jewish ghetto in Poland, where his parents escaped a deadly sweep by a Cossack troop when he was just 4 years old. In search of a better life, the Lemperts fled their village and eventually relocated to the Lower East Side of New York City.[23] Lempert worked several street jobs starting at a young age but eventually finished high school and applied to medical school. Due to family finances and Jewish

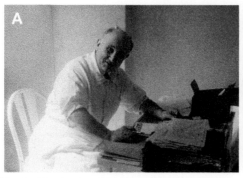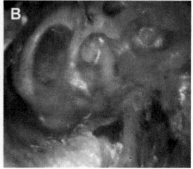

Fig. 6. (*A*) Maurice Sourdille. (*B*) Post-operative photo of a patient who underwent the fenestration operation by Sourdille in 1929. (*Courtesy of* F. Legent, France.)

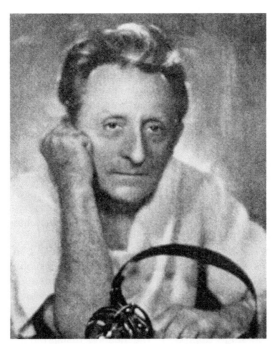

Fig. 7. Julius Lempert. (*From* Lustig L. Anesthesia, antisepsis, microscope: the confluence of neurotology. Otolaryngol Clin North Am 2007;40(3):415–37, with permission; and Shambaugh GE, Glasscock ME. Surgery of the ear. 3rd edition. Philadelphia: W.B. Saunders; 1980, with permission.)

quota systems[24] among first-tier medical schools at that time, Lempert was admitted to Long Island Medical College, which was considered a third-rate medical school.[23]

Lempert developed a strong interest in otolaryngology; however, chances of acceptance into this field from a third-tier medical school at that time were nearly impossible. Lempert decided to continue his pursuit of otolaryngology training by shadowing otolaryngology surgeons across New York. He visited operating rooms at Bellevue Hospital, Columbia, Cornell, Manhattan Eye and Ear, and New York Eye and Ear. Lempert would overstay his visits at these hospitals, eventually being asked to leave each and to never return.[23]

Lempert opened his own office and mailed announcements to all doctors in New York, stating boldly that he would return 50% of all his fees for any referrals of otolaryngology surgical cases.[23] Although facing scorn from other surgeons, Lempert quickly became one of the busiest otolaryngology surgeons in the city. By 1927, Lempert performed more than 1500 mastoid operations and hundreds of other otolaryngology surgeries. In 1928, Lempert published his first article in the *Archives of Otolaryngology* describing his new technique for performing the endaural mastoidectomy in contrast to the traditional postauricular approach.

Lempert was inspired by both Sourdille and Holmgren to develop his famous single-stage endaural fenestration operation. Sourdille's famous talk at the Otolaryngology Section of the New York Academy of Medicine and Lempert's visit to Holmgren at the Karolinska Institute in Stockholm both played vital roles in the development of his new procedure. Just like Sourdille, Holmgren received Lempert's visit to Stockholm in a generous, unguarded way, showing him all the details and unresolved obstacles of the fenestration procedure.[23] Holmgren encouraged Lempert to continue his research in Vienna, where autopsies were mandatory, thus giving Lempert an ample supply of cadavers to explore the fenestration technique. In Vienna, Lempert devised a method to convert Holmgren's three-stage procedure into a single-stage operation. He called this new operation the fenestration nov-ovalis.[23]

Lempert returned to New York and began performing his single-stage fenestration operation for advanced otosclerosis. The results of the operation were well-received by his patients but not by most surgeons at the time, who did not believe that Lempert was qualified or credible in performing such an operation.

Lempert's surgical tools also were not conventional. He was the first surgeon to use the dental drill instead of the chisel and mallet to dissect the mastoid. Other ingenious techniques included the use of magnifying loops and a customized headlight for illumination. Although ahead of his time, his unusual surgical techniques raised many eyebrows, and he was even asked to relinquish his privileges at a hospital where he operated. With the success of his current practice and increasing antipathy from his counterparts, Lempert ended up opening his own surgical institution, which he named the Endaural Hospital.[23]

Because he was never formally trained in otolaryngology, Lempert could not present at, or even be a member of, any otologic societies or professional organizations. In 1938, he was given the opportunity to publish his novel procedure in the *Archives of Otolaryngology*.[22] Most of his sample of 23 patients demonstrated successful results, and his article would later be recognized as a landmark paper for fenestration surgery. The single-stage endaural approach to fenestration was a significant improvement over Sordille's three-stage approach. The hearing results were consistent: more than 50% of patients noted hearing gains to 20 to 25 dB. However, at the time of publication, Lempert's work continued to draw skepticism from most ear surgeons.

Samuel Kopetzky, an ear surgeon and former president of the American Otological Society (AOS), realized the revolutionary nature of Lempert's single-stage fenestration operation and approached Lempert to see if he can observe, present, and acknowledge Lempert's work at the AOS upcoming meeting in Atlantic City that was to be held on May 6th, 1938. Meetings of the AOS were open to all doctors, but membership was by invitation only and limited to those considered to be among the professional elite of otologic surgeons. Lempert was thrilled by the prospect that his work would be finally legitimized by a leading ear authority and in the presence of the elite among otologists.[25]

Lempert spent many hours trying to teach Kopetzky every step of the procedure so that he could present it at the upcoming meeting. Kopetzky submitted his request to present at the upcoming AOS meeting, but members of the AOS council had heard rumors that Kopetzky may not be the actual surgeon behind the subject of the proposed presentation. Dr Harris Mosher, who was president of the AOS and an outspoken critic of Lempert's work, asked Dr Hoople to investigate this before the meeting.

Hoople made arrangements to observe Kopetzky perform the procedure. In the first case, Kopetzky was the surgeon on record and Julius Lempert was the young assistant. Kopetzky was just about to make the initial incision when he received an emergency phone call, requiring his services at another hospital. He informed Hoople that his assistant, Dr Lempert would complete the operative procedure. A few weeks later, Hoople again made arrangement to observe Kopetzky but similar events occurred, with Lempert performing most of the procedure. Hoople reported his findings to Dr Mosher and the AOS council.

Kopetzky presented his paper on May 6, 1938 to the AOS. To Lempert's disappointment, Kopetzky never mentioned Lempert's name throughout the presentation. Dr Mosher presided over the meeting and, armed with the data provided by Hoople, allowed no discussion. He immediately rose and pounded his gavel. An emergency meeting of the AOS council was held in Mosher's suite and Kopetzky was interrogated. Despite his disapproval of Lempert, Mosher was more bothered that Kopetzky broke his professional code of ethics. At the emergency meeting, the council voted to expel Kopetzky from membership in the AOS.[26] Lempert's professional career was finally vindicated. Lempert was given sole credit for the paper, "Improvement of Hearing in Cases of Otosclerosis," published in the *Archives of Otolaryngology* in 1938.

Lempert's single-stage fenestration technique became the mainstream operation for otosclerosis. He organized temporal bone courses twice a year to teach his operation to other surgeons. There was no way to know that, soon, an accidental rediscovery of a once forgotten procedure would reemerge and render Lempert's fenestration surgery obsolete. Lempert could never allow himself to transition from his fenestration procedure to stapes mobilization or stapedectomy, and lost everything as the fenestration operation gave way to these procedures. Lempert would eventually die alone, feeble-minded in a nursing home in 1968.

THE MOBILIZATION ERA

Samuel Rosen (**Fig. 8**) was the first to describe stapes mobilization after nearly half a century. Rosen was the fourth of 5 children of a peddler. He lived in a poor section of Syracuse, NY. His brothers and sisters paid his tuition at Syracuse University.[27] Originally, he

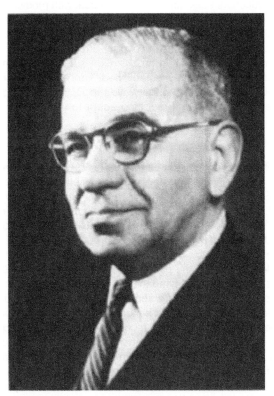

Fig. 8. Samuel Rosen. (*From* House HP. The evolution of otosclerosis surgery. Otolaryngol Clin North Am 1993;26(3):330; with permission.)

studied law but switched to medicine. After his training, he decided to meet Lempert to learn the fenestration technique and eventually became a successful otolaryngologist.

Rosen performed Lempert's fenestration operation; however, his modification to the surgery was that he would check for the mobility of the stapes to ensure it was fixed before proceeding to a semicircular canal fenestration.[28] In 1952, Rosen developed, almost by accident, the operation that would make him famous around the world.

During a routine procedure, Rosen accidentally mobilized the stapes while tapping on it to check for fixation. The patient, who was awake during the procedure, began to notice sound coming from the operating room next door.[28] Astonished, Rosen practiced the procedure on cadavers several times before trying it again on an actual patient. His surgery began to gain global attention but, similar to Lempert's early struggles, wide skepticism ensued.

Rosen's procedure was performed under local anesthesia and involved a transcanal approach. Patients had immediate results on the operating room table and the recovery period was quick. The surgery was relatively simple when compared with Lempert's fenestration operation and was easy to teach.

In 1955, the AOS invited both Lempert and Rosen to present their work in the same session. During the discussion, it became obvious that Lempert did not approve of his former student's new mobilization technique. Howard House was in the audience and, as recorded in his biography, recalled how Lempert's attack on Rosen was similar to the blind hostility that Lempert himself had experienced earlier in his own career: "The brilliant innovator seemed unable to accept the inexorable nature of progress in science that comes as practitioners seek different ways to deal with medical problems."[29]

Similar to Holmgren and Lempert, Rosen continued to perform his own invented operation throughout his career. The shortcoming of the mobilization procedure was that many patients would refixate shortly after the operation. Rosen would often take patients back for revision mobilization surgery. After more than half a century, stapes surgery was finally reestablished. A movement to fine-tune and preserve stapes mobility was already underway, and Rosen was soon to experience the consequences of failing to embrace and adapt to change.

THE STAPEDECTOMY ERA

John Shea (**Fig. 9**) was only in his thirties when he first described the stapedectomy procedure. Shea was trained in the techniques of both Lempert and Rosen in the 1950s. In 1953, Shea visited Rosen who recommended that he to go to Vienna to study at the First Ear Clinic to practice mobilization of the stapes on the abundant cadaver material available there.[21] While serving as a clinical fellow in Vienna, he stumbled across the early literature of stapes surgery from the late 1800s, including the report by Frederick L. Jack of a double stapedectomy patient in 1892. Jack's long-lost report described how the patient was still hearing, even 10 years after stapedectomy, most likely due to the tympanic membrane healing over the oval window and creating a mobile membrane. After reading the paper, Shea had realized the significance of Jack's procedure, and that it must be possible to remove and replace an otosclerotic stapes with a prosthesis.[21] In collaboration with the engineer Treace, he created a stapes prosthesis made of the then newly discovered biocompatible material Teflon (**Fig. 10**). In a female patient with otosclerosis, after removal of the stapes and covering of the oval window with subcutaneous tissue, he used this Teflon stapes prosthesis for the first time on May 1, 1956, with complete success.[30,31]

At the time of Shea's discovery, the complete removal of the stapes was still considered very dangerous and was forbidden. Many surgeons were still

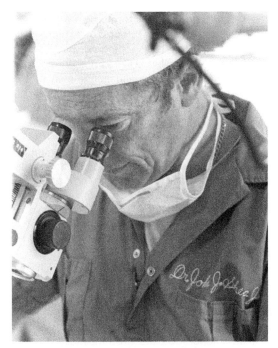

Fig. 9. John Shea. (*Courtesy of* Shea Ear Clinic; Memphis, TN.)

critical of the stapes mobilization technique. Nevertheless, Shea collaborated with Howard House to discuss his newly discovered procedure during a question-and-answer session at the First Symposium on Stapes Mobilization at the annual Triological Society meeting in May 1956. Howard House was to be

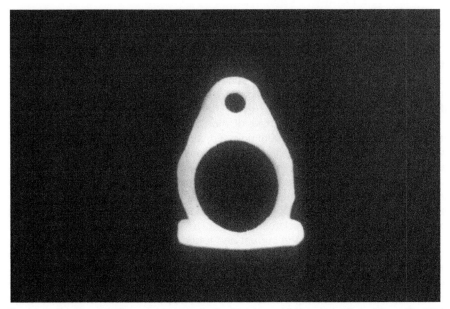

Fig. 10. John Shea's Teflon stapes prosthesis. (*Courtesy of* Shea Ear Clinic; Memphis, TN.)

the moderator of the session, and so they formulated a plan. Knowing the trouble that both Lempert and Rosen had gone through to overcome their critics, House decided that Shea would be the last person to be called for questions on that day.[28] As planned, Shea was called last and presented the results of his technique. At the end of Shea's comments, House immediately hit the gavel, indicating that time was up and there was no time for further questions.[28] Members from the audience were furiously rising to criticize Shea's comments; however, the plan worked and Shea's presentation was included in the published transcripts of the meeting.

Shea formally presented another 89 stapedectomy cases the following year at the Second Symposium on Stapes Mobilization in 1958. Within a decade, Shea's stapedectomy procedure became the standard operation for the treatment of otosclerosis. In the 1960s, thousands of hearing-impaired patients with otosclerosis were treated with great success. After the Teflon stapes, Shea used a hollow polyethylene tube and then a piston made entirely of Teflon.[16] In 1960, Schuknecht[32] developed a steel wire-adipose tissue prosthesis to address both the need to seal the vestibule and to reconstruct the ossicular chain.

The complete removal of the footplate is now reserved for only select cases. As the stapedectomy procedure evolved, various methods to remove just a portion of the footplate were devised. Eventually, the procedure was modified so that only a small fenestration was created through the footplate. An even less invasive, implantless procedure was described by Silverstein[33] for select patients who may benefit from removal of only the fixed anterior footplate while maintaining ossicular continuity via the posterior crus.

Modern stapes surgery is still evolving, and the laser has become the tool of choice to create an opening in the footplate that is small enough to fit a piston prosthesis and reduce injury to the vestibule. The footplate fenestration of the stapedotomy procedure is now a distant reminder of the days of Holmgren's and Lempert's semicircular canal fenestration (**Fig. 11**).

DISCUSSION

Otosclerosis is among the most fascinating diseases in otology. The evolution of its treatment so far, the revival of a once forbidden and forgotten surgery, its intellectual challenges, and the ingenious techniques for improving its surgical treatment make otosclerosis a subject for continuous clinical research and an inspiration to all (**Fig. 12**).

The path to the current treatment of otosclerosis with stapedotomy has been tortuous. Many of the pioneers were ridiculed, and some, such as Johannes Kessel, were forced to resign their positions. Other pioneers, such as Holmgren, Lempert, and Rosen, could not accept change and became obsolete. These histories bear lessons in overcoming professional adversity, but also the consequences of unremitting triumph. In the end, a young man, Dr John Shea, who, with the help of a politically savvy older man, Dr Howard House, enabled stapes surgery to return to its rightful place in the treatment of otosclerosis.

As we continue to review the current and future trends of medicine and surgery, we must also remember the past, as old and forgotten knowledge may serve as the candle to enlighten the dark mysteries we face today. In the same context, scientists, clinicians, and surgeons must embrace change. As Howard House once told Julius Lempert, "Change is constant, and happy are those that can change with it."

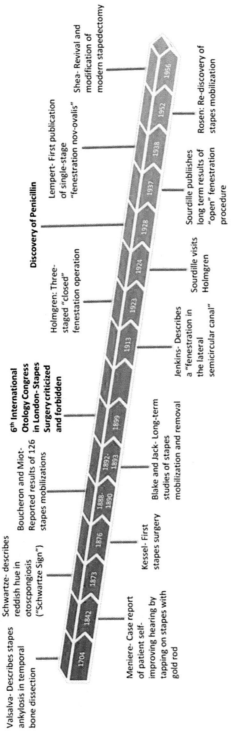

Fig. 11. A timeline of advancements in otosclerosis therapy.

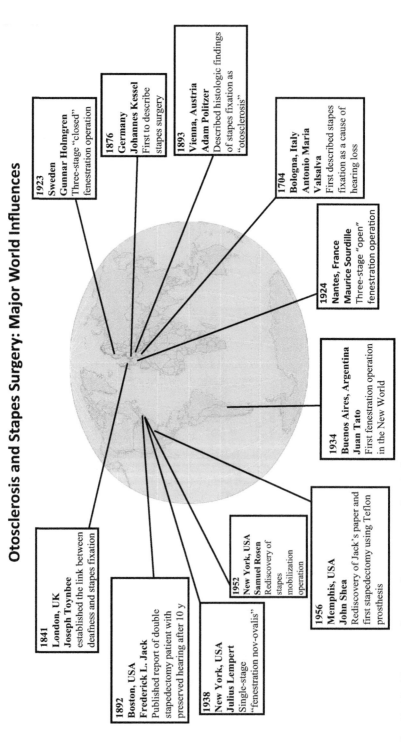

Otosclerosis and Stapes Surgery: Major World Influences

1923
Sweden
Gunnar Holmgren
Three-stage "closed" fenestration operation

1876
Germany
Johannes Kessel
First to describe stapes surgery

1893
Vienna, Austria
Adam Politzer
Described histologic findings of stapes fixation as "otosclerosis"

1704
Bologna, Italy
Antonio Maria Valsalva
First described stapes fixation as a cause of hearing loss

1924
Nantes, France
Maurice Sourdille
Three-stage "open" fenestration operation

1934
Buenos Aires, Argentina
Juan Tato
First fenestration operation in the New World

1841
London, UK
Joseph Toynbee
established the link between deafness and stapes fixation

1892
Boston, USA
Frederick L. Jack
Published report of double stapedectomy patient with preserved hearing after 10 y

1938
New York, USA
Julius Lempert
Single-stage "fenestration nov-ovalis"

1952
New York, USA
Samuel Rosen
Rediscovery of stapes mobilization operation

1956
Memphis, USA
John Shea
Rediscovery of Jack's paper and first stapedectomy using Teflon prosthesis

Fig. 12. World map: major contributors to otosclerosis therapy.

REFERENCES

1. Valsalva AM. The human ear (Latin). Bononiae (Italy): C. Pisarri; 1704.
2. Isaacson B, Kutz JW, Roland PS. Otosclerosis. In: Johnson J, Rosen C, editors. Bailey's head and neck surgery otolaryngology. 5th edition. Baltimore (MD): Lippincott Williams & Wilkins; 2014. p. 2487.
3. Handzel O, McKenna M. Surgery for otosclerosis. In: Gulya A, Minor L, Poe D, editors. Glasscock-Shambaugh surgery of the ear. 6th edition. Shelton (CT): People's Medical Publishing House; 2010. p. 529–30.
4. Mudry A. Adam Politzer (1835-1920) and the description of otosclerosis. Otol Neurotol 2006;27:276–81.
5. Menière P. De l'exploration de l'appareil auditif, ou recherches sur les moyens prospres à conduir au diagnostic des maladies de l'oreille. Gaz Med Paris 1842;10:114–7.
6. Kessel J. Über die Durchschneidung des Steigbügelmuskels beim Menschen und über die Extraction des Steigbügels resp. der Columella bei Thieren. Arch Ohrenheilkd 1876;11:199–217.
7. Kessel J. Über das mobilisieren des Steigbügels durch ausschneiden des Trommelfelles, Hammers und amboss bei Undurchgängigkeit der Tuba. Arch Ohrenh 1878;13:69.
8. Kessel J. Über die vordere Tenotomie, Mobilisierung und Extraction des Steigbügels; zitiert in Grunert C: Wissenschaftliche Rundschau. Arch Ohrenheilkd 1897; 42:57–8.
9. Schwartze HHR. Lehrbuch der chirurgischen Krankheiten des Ohres. Stuttgart (Germany): Enke; 1885.
10. Lucae A. Über operative Entfernung des Trommelfells und der beiden grösseren Gehörknöchelchen bei Sklerose der Paukenschleimhaut. Arch Ohrenh 1885;22: 233–42.
11. Miot C. De la mobilisation de l'etrier. Rev Laryngol Otol Rhinol 1890;10:113–30.
12. Boucheron E. La mobilisation de l'étrier et son procédé opératoire. Union Med Paris 1888;46:412–3.
13. Blake CJ. Operation for removal of the stapes. Box M S J 1892;127:469.
14. Jack F. Remarkable improvement in hearing by removal of the stapes. Trans Am Otol Soc 1893;5:284–305.
15. Jack FL. Further observations on removal of the stapes. Trans Am Otol Soc 1893; 5:474.
16. Häusler R. General history of stapedectomy. In: Arnold W, Häusler R, editors. Otosclerosis and stapes surgery. Advances in oto-rhino-laryngology, vol. 65. Basel (Switzerland): S. Karger AG; 2007. p. 1–5.
17. Jenkins GJ. Otosclerosis: certain clinical features and experimental operative procedures. Trans XVIIth Inter Congr Med London 1913;16:609–18.
18. Holmgren G. The surgery of otosclerosis. Ann Otol Rhinol Laryngol 1937;46:3–12.
19. Holmgren G. Some experiences in the surgery of otosclerosis. Acta Otolaryngol 1923;5:460–6.
20. Sourdille M. New technique in the surgical treatment of severe and progressive deafness from otosclerosis. Bull N Y Acad Med 1937;13:673–91.
21. Shea JJ, Shea PF, McKenna MJ. Stapedectomy for otosclerosis. In: Surgery of ear, Glasscock-Shambaugh. 5th edition. 2003. p. 547–75.
22. Lempert J. Improvement of hearing in cases of otosclerosis: a new one stage surgical technique. Arch Otolaryngol 1938;28:42–97.

23. Hyman S. Between Mosher and Lempert. In: For the world to hear: a biography of Howard P. House. Pasadena (CA): Hope Publishing House; 1990. p. 116–25.

24. Lerner B. In a time of quotas, a quiet pose in defiance. The New York Times 2009. Available at: http://www.nytimes.com/2009/05/26/health/26quot.html. Accessed April 15, 2017.

25. Hyman S. Moral test at Harvard. In: For the world to hear: a biography of Howard P. House. Pasadena (CA): Hope Publishing House; 1990. p. 144–52.

26. Hyman S. The faces of ambiguity. In: For the world to hear: a biography of Howard P. House. Pasadena (CA): Hope Publishing House; 1990. p. 171–4.

27. Fowler G. Dr. Samuel Rosen, ear surgery pioneer, dies at 84. The New York Times 1981. Available at: http://www.nytimes.com/1981/11/06/obituaries/dr-samuel-rosen-ear-surgery-pioneer-dies-at-84.html. Accessed April 15, 2017.

28. House H, Rosen S, Shea J. Interview: otosclerosis surgery: the stapes era. House Ear Institute Archives. 2014. Available at: https://www.youtube.com/watch?v=jh2qOWMFXkY. Accessed April 15, 2017.

29. Hyman S. The setting and the rising sun. In: For the world to hear: a biography of Howard P. House. Pasadena (CA): Hope Publishing House; 1990. p. 246–51.

30. Shea JJ. A personal history of stapedectomy. Am J Otol 1998;19:2–12.

31. Shea JJ. Fenestration of the oval window. Ann Otol Rhinol Laryngol 1958;67: 932–51.

32. Schuknecht HF. Stapedotomy and graft-prosthesis operation. Acta Otolaryngol 1960;51:241–3.

33. Silverstein H. Laser stapedotomy minus prosthesis (laser STAMP): a minimally invasive procedure. Am J Otol 1998;19:277–82.

Otosclerosis
Temporal Bone Pathology

Alicia M. Quesnel, MD[a,b,c,]*, Reuven Ishai, MD[b,c], Michael J. McKenna, MD[a,b,c]

KEYWORDS

- Temporal bone pathology • Otopathology • Otosclerosis

KEY POINTS

- The pathologic hallmark of otosclerosis is abnormal bony remodeling, which includes bone resorption, new bone deposition, and vascular proliferation in the temporal bone.
- Otosclerosis involves more than one site in the otic capsule in 49% to 60% of temporal bone specimens.
- Sensorineural hearing loss in otosclerosis is associated with extension of otosclerosis to the cochlear endosteum and deposition of collagen throughout the spiral ligament (ie, hyalinization).
- Persistent or recurrent conductive hearing loss after stapedectomy has been associated with incomplete footplate fenestration, poor incus-prosthesis connection, and incus resorption in temporal bone specimens.
- Among temporal bone specimens, computed tomography is highly sensitive for the diagnosis of otosclerosis but has only moderate sensitivity for identification of cochlear endosteal involvement.

INTRODUCTION

Otosclerosis is a multifactorial bone disorder with genetic and environmental causes that occurs solely in the otic capsule bone.[1] The disease results in a progressive conductive hearing loss, although up to one-third of patients ultimately develop a mixed hearing loss.[2] The pathologic hallmark of the disease is abnormal bony remodeling, which includes bone resorption, new bone deposition, and vascular proliferation in the temporal bone (**Fig. 1**). This article reviews the pathologic findings in otosclerosis, with particular attention to clinical relevance. It also includes postsurgical pathology, because understanding the consequences of surgery provides insight into how to optimize surgical techniques.

Disclosure Statement: The authors have nothing to disclose.
[a] Division of Otology and Neurotology, Department of Otolaryngology, Massachusetts Eye and Ear, 243 Charles Street, Boston, MA 02114, USA; [b] Massachusetts Eye and Ear Otopathology Laboratory, 243 Charles Street, Boston, MA 02114, USA; [c] Department of Otolaryngology, Harvard Medical School, 25 Shattuck Street, Boston MA 02115, USA
* Corresponding author.
E-mail address: alicia_quesnel@meei.harvard.edu

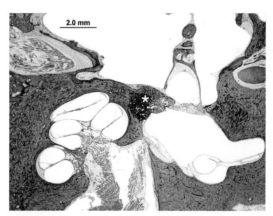

Fig. 1. Low-power, hematoxylin and eosin (H&E)-stained section (original magnification ×1.25) from the right temporal bone of an 83-year-old woman with bilateral progressive mixed hearing loss and clinical diagnosis of otosclerosis during life. There is a focus of otosclerosis (*asterisk*) at the anterior margin of the stapes footplate that has fixed the footplate. The stapes footplate bone has also been replaced by otosclerotic bone, and the footplate is therefore abnormally thickened.

PATHOLOGY OF OTOSCLEROSIS
Historical Perspective

Because otosclerosis is a primary disease of the otic capsule, the postmortem pathologic evaluation of temporal bone specimens has been particularly important in understanding the pathophysiology of the disease. Although Valsalva first reported stapes ankylosis as a cause of hearing loss in 1704, the ankylosis was thought to be caused by an inflammatory reaction in the middle ear (called a "dry catarrh" of the middle ear) for nearly two more centuries.[3] In 1893, Adam Politzer asserted that the stapes ankylosis was caused by "new bone, overgrowing the oval window and stapes" based on his postmortem pathologic studies. By 1901, he had introduced the term "otosclerosis" to describe this distinct pathologic entity. In the modern era, temporal bone pathologic studies continue to inform clinical management of patients with otosclerosis by deepening the understanding of pathophysiology of the disease. Specifically, pathologic studies have helped further define the mechanism of sensorineural hearing loss in otosclerosis,[4–6] depicted the causes of persistent hearing loss after stapedectomy,[7] highlighted some potential pitfalls for cochlear implantation in far advanced otosclerosis,[8] and investigated the accuracy of computed tomography (CT) in otosclerosis.[9] Some of these findings are reviewed in this article.

Definitions

Clinical otosclerosis is defined as otosclerosis that results in a conductive (or mixed) hearing loss caused by fixation of the stapes, and thus is diagnosed during life. Histologic otosclerosis refers to the diagnosis of otosclerosis based on the postmortem histopathologic evaluation of temporal bone sections, in patients who did not have stapes fixation. Although the clinical prevalence is estimated to be 0.3% to 0.4%[10,11] of the population, the prevalence of histologic otosclerosis is significantly higher. This ranges from 2.5% among temporal bones from consecutive deceased patients initially screened by gross observation and microradiology of the temporal bone slices[12] to 12% among temporal bone specimens procured by a temporal bone laboratory and studied by light microscopy.[13]

Light Microscopy Description of Otosclerosis

Many authors have described the light microscopy findings in otosclerosis, which are summarized here.[13–15] Otosclerosis begins with an "otospongiotic" phase in which the normal lamellar otic capsule bone around vessels is resorbed, creating perivascular (or pseudovascular) spaces[16] (**Fig. 2**). These areas are often highly cellular, with increased numbers of osteoclasts that appear as large multinucleated cells (**Fig. 3**). On hematoxylin and eosin staining, these areas are often highly acidophilic, and create a circumscribed front at which there is a clear demarcation between normal/unaffected bone and the otosclerotic focus. Ultimately, new woven bone is deposited, which may be larger in volume than the bone that was resorbed, and sometimes results in thickening of the involved area (eg, the stapes footplate). Presumably, the new bone is converted to lamellar bone, which is dense, and results in a "sclerotic" focus that is highly eosinophilic and relatively acellular. Active resorption and bone deposition are often juxtaposed in the same focus of otosclerosis (see **Fig. 2**B).

Sites of Involvement and Clinical Implications

The most commonly involved area of the otic capsule is the area anterior to the oval window, with 96% of temporal bones demonstrating a focus of otosclerosis in this location.[15] Because this area is nearly always involved, the fissula ante fenestrum, which is an embryologic remnant containing a tract of fibrous tissue anterior to the oval window, was postulated to be involved in the cause of otosclerosis. However, the existence of cases in which there is an otosclerotic focus anterior to the oval window that is distinct from the fissula ante fenestrum does not support this hypothesis.[17] Because the remodeled otosclerotic bone is often larger in volume than the resorbed bone, a focus of otosclerosis anterior to the oval window may result in "jamming" of

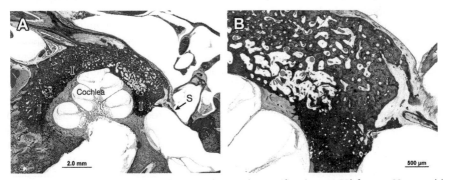

Fig. 2. (A) Low-power, H&E-stained section (original magnification ×1.25) from a 68-year-old woman who reported her hearing loss began at age 17 and progressed rapidly. An audiogram at age 32 showed a right severe sensorineural hearing loss and left profound hearing loss. The section illustrates extensive otosclerosis surrounding the cochlea, and anterior and posterior otosclerotic foci that fix the stapes footplate (S). There are areas of active (A) and inactive (I) otosclerosis around the cochlea. (B) High-power (×4) image of an area of the otic capsule showing active otosclerosis with large pseudovascular spaces (*top half of the image*) juxtaposed to an area of inactive otosclerosis (*bottom half of the image*) with dense bone, small pseudovascular spaces, and more intense eosinophilic staining.

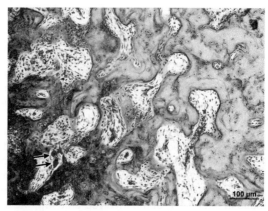

Fig. 3. High-power H&E section (original magnification ×20) through a focus of active otosclerosis (also called "otospongiosis") in the right temporal bone from a 73-year-old woman with bilateral mixed hearing loss, with approximately 50-dB conductive component. She wore a hearing aid on the right for 20 years before her death. This high-power image is notable for large pseudovascular spaces, immature woven bone deposition, and the presence of osteoclasts. Osteoclasts are the large multinucleated cells within the pseudovascular space noted by the arrows.

the stapes footplate (**Fig. 4**A). This displaces the stapes posteriorly, closes the posterior stapedovestibular joint (SVJ) space, and results in a conductive loss, even without actual fixation of the stapes (**Fig. 4**B, C). Cherukupally and colleagues[18] found a correlation between the degree of narrowing of the posterior SVJ space and the amount of the hearing loss. Furthermore, they found that true bony fixation of the footplate was associated with air-bone gaps greater than 30 dB. The clinical implication of this work is that the surgeon may consider waiting until the air-bone gap progresses to greater than 30 dB before recommending stapedectomy, to potentially avoid a floating footplate during stapedectomy surgery. A floating footplate may be challenging to fenestrate, particularly if there is no laser available, and removal may carry a significant risk of sensorineural hearing loss.

Otosclerosis involves more than one site in the otic capsule in 49% to 60% of temporal bone specimens.[15,19] Merchant and colleagues[19] examined the prevalence of otosclerosis at the posterior SVJ in 140 temporal bone specimens with otosclerosis and found that 41% had otosclerosis involving the posterior SVJ with bony ankylosis and an additional 21% had otosclerosis at the posterior SVJ but no bony otosclerosis. These findings have clinical implications for the stapedotomy minus prosthesis (STAMP) procedure.[20] STAMP enables successful correction of the air-bone gap in otosclerosis with minimal surgical trauma at the oval window, and better long-term high-frequency hearing results than conventional stapedotomy in properly selected patients.[21] In the STAMP procedure, the anterior crus of the stapes is transected and footplate is transected linearly in the mid-portion to allow mobilization of the posterior half. Because this procedure relies on mobilizing the posterior half of the footplate, surgeons should be aware that 62% of patients might not be good candidates because of otosclerosis at the posterior SVJ with current fixation or risk of future fixation.

Otosclerosis involves the round window niche in 30% of temporal bones,[15] but rarely completely obliterates the round window niche. **Fig. 5** illustrates a case where it would have been difficult to determine intraoperatively whether the round window niche was completely obliterated. With even a small portion of the round window

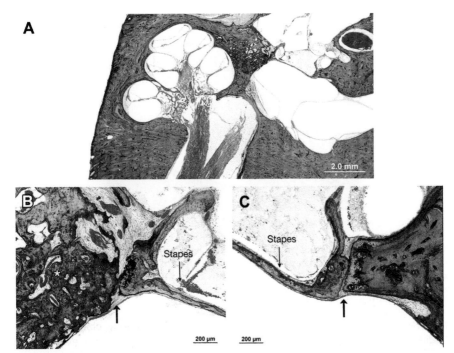

Fig. 4. (A) Low-power H&E section (original magnification ×1.25) from the right temporal bone of a 69-year-old woman who was found to have bilateral conductive hearing loss on an audiogram at age 41. There is a focus of otosclerosis anterior to the stapes footplate (*asterisk*). High-power images (×10) through the anterior (*B*) and posterior (*C*) oval window illustrate the concept of "jamming." In B, the otosclerotic focus has contacted the stapes footplate but does not fix it. Arrow indicates the anterior stapedo-vestibular joint. Rather, the footplate is displaced posteriorly so that movement is limited because of impingement on the bone at the posterior margin of the oval window (*C*). Arrow indicates the posterior stapedo-vestibular joint space.

membrane exposed, a stapedectomy surgery would be expected to successfully correct the air-bone gap. Therefore, the clinical implication is that the surgeon should proceed with a primary stapedectomy even if the round window area was involved with otosclerosis; however, if the air-bone gap failed to improve, it would not likely be worth attempting a revision surgery.

The stapes footplate is involved in 12% to 15% of temporal bones.[15] Rarely, significant thickening of the stapes footplate with a minor fixation across the SVJ (called a "biscuit footplate") occurs when there is a primary focus of otosclerosis within the footplate (**Fig. 6**). This remarkably thickened footplate cannot be penetrated with a laser for stapedotomy and great care must be taken not to displace the footplate into the vestibule if an otologic drill is used for the fenestra.

Otosclerosis may cause intracochlear deposition of bone, particularly in cases of far advanced otosclerosis.[22,23] Unlike patients with neo-ossification of the cochlea caused by meningitis, patients with intracochlear involvement to otosclerosis rarely have new bone deposition beyond the first half of the basal turn.[24] When cochlear implantation is considered in these patients, the bone filling the scala tympani of the basal turn usually can be gently removed with microinstruments or drilled to allow placement of the electrode array.[25,26]

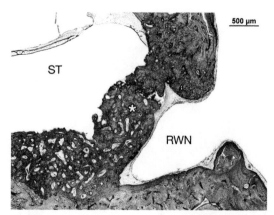

Fig. 5. High-power H&E image (original magnification ×4) through the round window niche (RWN) and cochlea in a 60-year-old woman who had bilateral conductive hearing loss. There is extensive otosclerotic bone that involves the cochlea at the round window, including bone that has been deposited inside the cochlea in the scala tympani (ST) adjacent to the round window membrane (*asterisk*). In this case, it would not be possible to intraoperatively assess whether there was complete round window obliteration.

Sensorineural Hearing Loss in Otosclerosis and Associated Histopathologic Findings

Although most patients with otosclerosis present with conductive hearing loss, a minority develop a mixed hearing loss caused by otosclerosis.[27–30] In one retrospective study of 357 ears with otosclerosis, 34% developed a clinically significant (>10 dB) bone conduction threshold shift over 10 years of follow-up that was greater than

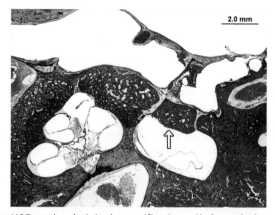

Fig. 6. Low-power H&E section (original magnification ×2) through the cochlea, vestibule, stapes, and middle ear in a 65-year-old woman who had developed progressive mixed hearing loss beginning at age 12. She underwent bilateral fenestration operations and revisions in her 40s. This case is notable for the markedly thickened stapes footplate with minimal surrounding fixation (although fixation was seen on another section), called a "biscuit" footplate (*arrow*). Stapedectomy in this patient would have been challenging, because laser stapedotomy would not be possible given the thickness of the footplate, and use of the drill risks dislodging the footplate into the vestibule.

expected for age-related changes.[2] Based on review of human temporal bones with otosclerosis, pure sensorineural hearing loss caused by otosclerosis without stapes fixation is exceedingly rare.[31]

The major histopathologic correlates of the sensorineural component of hearing loss in otosclerosis are involvement of the cochlear endosteum by otosclerosis and deposition of collagen throughout the spiral ligament, called hyalinization[5,32–34] (**Fig. 7**). Hyalinization occurs adjacent to active foci of otosclerosis (ie, otospongiosis), and only occurs when the otosclerotic focus invades the cochlear endosteum[32] (see **Fig. 7**). Immunohistochemical staining of human temporal bones has demonstrated the hyalin material is composed primarily of type I collagen, chrondroitin sulfate, and keratin sulfate.[35] In a study of 37 temporal bones with otosclerosis, the mean bone conduction threshold was significantly worse in cases when there were two or more foci of endosteal involvement. Spiral ganglion cell counts were not significantly reduced in these cases; however, total outer hair cell counts were modestly reduced compared with otosclerotic temporal bones with fewer than two sites of endosteal involvement and compared with temporal bones with typical age-related hearing loss.[5] Nelson and Hinojosa[36] found a variable amount of degeneration of inner and outer hair cells and spiral ganglion neurons in temporal bones with otosclerosis, and did not find an association of hair cell or spiral ganglion neuron degeneration with the extent of endosteal involvement by otosclerosis. Thus, reductions in the hair cell or spiral ganglion neuron populations are not likely the major cause of the sensorineural component of hearing loss in otosclerosis.

Spiral ligament hyalinization and endosteal involvement by otosclerosis has been associated with atrophy of the adjacent stria vascularis.[4,5] In a study using immunohistochemical staining on human temporal bone specimens, Doherty and Linthicum[4] found a reduced expression of carbonic anhydrase I and sodium-potassium ATPase in regions of the cochlea with hyalinization of the spiral ligament. Disruption of the potassium ion recycling mechanism and the endocochlear potential may contribute to the sensorineural hearing loss seen in otosclerosis.

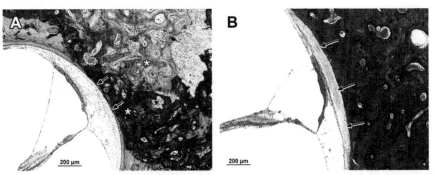

Fig. 7. (A) High-power image (H&E section, original magnification ×10) of otic capsule bone adjacent to the basal turn of the cochlea in a 73-year-old woman with otosclerosis. There is an active focus (*asterisks*) that extends close to the cochlear endosteum but does not invade through the endosteum (*arrows*). The spiral ligament is paucicellular, but there is no hyalin deposition. (B) High-power H&E image (×10) of otic capsule bone adjacent to the basal turn of the cochlea in a 65-year-old woman with otosclerosis. The pink acellular material in the spiral ligament is hyalin that has been deposited adjacent to an area where the otosclerotic focus completely erodes through the cochlear endosteum (*arrows*). This finding is associated with sensorineural hearing loss in otosclerosis.

HUMAN TEMPORAL BONE PATHOLOGY AFTER SURGERY FOR OTOSCLEROSIS
Post-stapedectomy Pathology

The etiologies of persistent or recurrent conductive hearing loss after stapedectomy surgery are delineated through the study of temporal bone specimens from patients who underwent stapedectomy during life. Given the limitations of in vivo imaging of the temporal bone, the cause of a failed or only partly successful correction of the air-bone gap after stapedectomy may not be readily apparent. Ideally, the stapes prosthesis should be freely mobile within the fenestra or the oval window, extend 0.25 mm into the vestibule, and have a secure connection to the long process of the incus (**Fig. 8**A). The etiologies of persistent conductive hearing loss include (1) incomplete fenestration of the footplate (**Fig. 8**B), (2) poor connection between the prosthesis and the incus, (3) complete obliteration of the round window (see **Fig. 5**), (4) middle ear effusion (not common because these patients typically do not have eustachian tube dysfunction), and (5) alternative diagnoses including third window syndromes (eg, superior semicircular canal dehiscence) or other types of ossicular fixation (eg, malleus fixation; **Fig. 9**).

Another post-stapedectomy pathologic finding is the increased incidence of endolymphatic hydrops in patients who underwent a stapedectomy during life. In a study comparing 93 operated temporal bones with otosclerosis, 156 nonoperated temporal bones with otosclerosis, and 253 temporal bones with presbycusis (control subjects), the respective percentage of specimens with endolymphatic hydrops was 11.8%, 1.9%, and 3.5% (**Fig. 10**).[37] Furthermore, an increasing number of revision surgeries was strongly correlated with an increasing likelihood of endolymphatic hydrops.[37] This suggests that the low-frequency bone conduction threshold shift seen in some patients post-stapedectomy may be related to endolymphatic hydrops. The increased risk of sensorineural hearing loss with revision surgery may be related to an increased incidence of a severely hydropic saccular membrane that may be predisposed to rupture on removal or replacement of a prosthesis (**Fig. 11**).

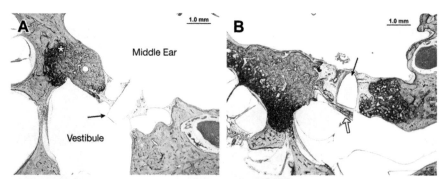

Fig. 8. (*A*) High-power image (H&E, original magnification ×2) through the oval window area in a patient who had undergone total stapedectomy during life with successful correction of the air-bone gap. The prosthesis was removed just before sectioning, and a silhouette of the piston is shown by a thin membranous layer that once surrounded the prosthesis (*arrow*). The ideal prosthesis position is depicted in this case, with a freely mobile prosthesis and sealed oval window. An asterisk marks a focus of otosclerosis anterior to the footplate. (*B*) High-power H&E image (×2) through the oval window in a patient who underwent unsuccessful stapedectomy during life. The reason for failure is incomplete fenestration into the vestibule and a residual piece of the stapes footplate (*open arrow*) on top of which the prosthesis rested. The silhouette of the piston is indicated by the black arrow.

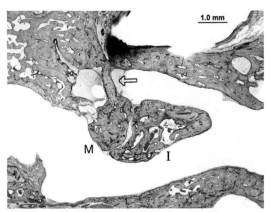

Fig. 9. High-power image (H&E, original magnification ×2) through the epitympanum showing a bony bar (*arrow*) fixing the malleus head (M) to the lateral epitympanic wall. The incudomalleolar joint appears normal and the incus short process (I) is normally formed. Malleus head fixation represents an alternative cause to otosclerosis in patients who undergo exploratory tympanotomy for conductive hearing loss. It may also occur concurrently with otosclerosis.

Pathology After Cochlear Implantation in Far Advanced Otosclerosis

Temporal bone specimens from patients who underwent cochlear implantation during life for far advanced otosclerosis demonstrate an intracochlear granulomatous foreign body reaction to the electrodes,[38] development of a fibrous capsule around the electrode array, and new intracochlear bone formation.[24,39] These findings are the same as in patients who underwent cochlear implantation for other causes of deafness.[38,39] Facial nerve stimulation is a rare complication of cochlear implantation, which occurs more commonly in patients implanted for far advanced otosclerosis.[40] Seyyedi and colleagues[8] reported on 13 temporal bones from 11 patients with otosclerosis who had undergone cochlear implantation during life. Among those who had received

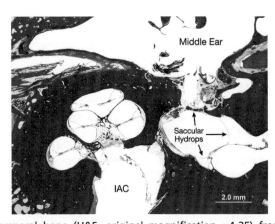

Fig. 10. Right temporal bone (H&E, original magnification ×1.25) from an 83-year-old woman with otosclerosis who underwent a stapes mobilization at age 29, and a fat wire stapedectomy at age 34, both of which were unsuccessful. After the stapedectomy, she had progressive worsening of bone thresholds in the right ear. She reported some vertigo in her 40s but was not diagnosed with Meniere disease. There is marked saccular hydrops with adherence of the membrane to the undersurface of the stapes footplate remnant.

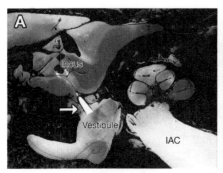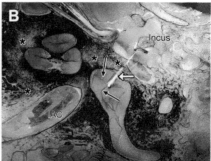

Fig. 11. (*A*) Low-power image showing the stapes prosthesis (*arrow*) in situ after toluidine blue application and horizontal sectioning of the specimen up to the point of the prosthesis (original magnification ×1.25). This patient underwent successful stapedectomy with a piston prosthesis, and ideal prosthesis position is shown with no obstructing surrounding bone and fibrous membrane seal of the oval window. (*B*) Low-power (×2), toluidine blue, image of the temporal bone specimen from a different patient who underwent stapedectomy during life for otosclerosis (*asterisks*). In this case, there is saccular hydrops, with adherence of the saccular membrane (*black arrows*) to the vestibular surface of the prosthesis (*white arrow*).

straight/lateral wall electrodes (n = 10), there was a significant correlation between facial nerve stimulation during life and the presence of otosclerosis involving the labyrinthine facial nerve canal, cochlear endosteum of the adjacent portion of the lower basal turn, and the intervening otic capsule bone. In the three temporal bones from patients who had perimodiolar electrodes, there was no facial nerve stimulation during life even though two of these three temporal bones had otosclerosis involving the previously noted areas between the labyrinthine facial and the cochlear endosteum of the basal turn. Computational modeling suggests that increased conductivity of the otosclerotic bone allows current to leak outside of the cochlea, particularly in lateral wall electrode arrays.[41] These findings, in conjunction with the temporal bone pathology, help explain the pathophysiologic mechanism of increased risk of facial nerve stimulation in implanted patients with otosclerosis.

COMPUTED TOMOGRAPHY AND HISTOLOGY CORRELATION IN OTOSCLEROSIS

Although the diagnosis of otosclerosis is usually made based on history, otologic examination, and audiologic findings, radiologic confirmation of the diagnosis and evaluation of the extent of otosclerosis may help inform clinical management of these patients.[9,42–44] Pathologic confirmation of the diagnosis may not be possible during life, because many surgeons use a small fenestra technique in which there is no stapes footplate specimen and a total stapedectomy specimen may not contain a diagnostic focus of otosclerosis.[45] Multiple clinical studies comparing a radiologic diagnosis of otosclerosis based on high-resolution temporal bone CT with the diagnosis based on history, examination, audiology, and sometimes intraoperative findings have shown good sensitivity, ranging from 80% to 91% in selected studies.[42,43,46] Direct comparison within the same temporal bone specimen of pathology and CT imaging enables a comparison with the gold standard for diagnosis of otosclerosis (ie, pathology). In a blinded, controlled study of 46 human temporal bone specimens with (n = 10) and without (n = 36) otosclerosis that underwent CT imaging (using the same collimation and parameters as clinical high-resolution temporal bone CT imaging), the sensitivity and specificity for the diagnosis of otosclerosis was 80% and 92%, respectively[9] (**Fig. 12**). The sensitivity of CT

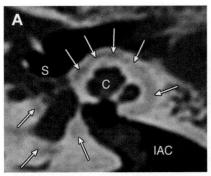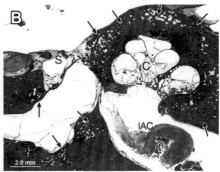

Fig. 12. (*A*) High-resolution computed tomography image taken of a temporal bone specimen before histologic processing. The arrows depict extensive hypodense areas surrounding the cochlea (C), the internal auditory canal (IAC), and anterior and posterior to the stapes (S). (*B*) The matched histologic section (H&E, original magnification ×1.25) shows these hypodense areas correspond to otosclerotic bone (*arrows*).

for identification of cochlear endosteal involvement by otosclerosis, which is associated with elevated bone thresholds (ie, mixed hearing loss rather than purely conductive hearing loss), was 63%; however, the specificity was 100%.[9] In addition, a study comparing CT densitometry of otosclerotic foci (as measured in Hounsfield units on the CT image) with the matched histologic slide from specimens that had undergone imaging before histologic processing demonstrated that CT densitometry can distinguish normal otic capsule bone from otosclerotic bone.[47]

SUMMARY

Otosclerosis is pathologically characterized by resorption of otic capsule bone, and deposition of abnormal otosclerotic or otospongiotic bone with varying proportions of pseudovascular spaces, woven bone, and lamellar bone. Active otosclerotic foci are typically characterized by large pseudovascular spaces, and high cellular density, including multinucleated osteoclasts. Inactive foci are characterized by dense lamellar bone that has replaced normal otic capsule bone. The area anterior to the oval window is involved in nearly all cases; however, many cases have multisite involvement around the otic capsule. Human temporal bone pathology has been paramount in determining the pathophysiology of otosclerosis, including mechanisms for conductive and sensorineural hearing loss. Human temporal bone pathology has also enabled evaluation of the effects and potential complications of surgery for otosclerosis, and has helped to define the role of CT imaging for otosclerosis.

REFERENCES

1. Wang PC, Merchant SN, McKenna MJ, et al. Does otosclerosis occur only in the temporal bone? Am J Otol 1999;20:162–5.
2. Ishai R, Halpin CF, Shin JJ, et al. Long-term incidence and degree of sensorineural hearing loss in otosclerosis. Otol Neurotol 2016;37:1489–96.
3. Mudry A. First descriptions of the ankylosis of the stapes. Otol Neurotol 2010;31: 1177.
4. Doherty JK, Linthicum FH Jr. Spiral ligament and stria vascularis changes in cochlear otosclerosis: effect on hearing level. Otol Neurotol 2004;25:457–64.

5. Kwok OT, Nadol JB Jr. Correlation of otosclerotic foci and degenerative changes in the organ of Corti and spiral ganglion. Am J Otolaryngol 1989;10:1–12.
6. Richard C, Doherty JK, Fayad JN, et al. Identification of target proteins involved in cochlear otosclerosis. Otol Neurotol 2015;36:923–31.
7. Nadol JB Jr. Histopathology of residual and recurrent conductive hearing loss after stapedectomy. Otol Neurotol 2001;22:162–9.
8. Seyyedi M, Herrmann BS, Eddington DK, et al. The pathologic basis of facial nerve stimulation in otosclerosis and multi-channel cochlear implantation. Otol Neurotol 2013;34:1603–9.
9. Quesnel AM, Moonis G, Appel J, et al. Correlation of computed tomography with histopathology in otosclerosis. Otol Neurotol 2013;34:22–8.
10. Hall JG. Otosclerosis in Norway, a geographical and genetical study. Acta Otolaryngol Suppl 1974;324:1–20.
11. Pearson RD, Kurland LT, Cody DT. Incidence of diagnosed clinical otosclerosis. Arch Otolaryngol 1974;99:288–91.
12. Declau F, Van Spaendonck M, Timmermans JP, et al. Prevalence of otosclerosis in an unselected series of temporal bones. Otol Neurotol 2001;22:596–602.
13. Guild SR. Histologic otosclerosis. Ann Otol Rhinol Laryngol 1944;31:1045–71.
14. Kelemen G, Linthicum FH Jr. Labyrinthine otosclerosis. Acta Otolaryngol Suppl 1969;253:1–68.
15. Schuknecht HF, Barber W. Histologic variants in otosclerosis. Laryngoscope 1985;95:1307–17.
16. Linthicum FH Jr. Histopathology of otosclerosis. Otolaryngol Clin North Am 1993; 26:335–52.
17. Bretlau P. Relation of the otosclerotic focus to the fissula ante-fenestram. J Laryngol Otol 1969;83:1185–93.
18. Cherukupally SR, Merchant SN, Rosowski JJ. Correlations between pathologic changes in the stapes and conductive hearing loss in otosclerosis. Ann Otol Rhinol Laryngol 1998;107:319–26.
19. Merchant SN, Incesulu A, Glynn RJ, et al. Histologic studies of the posterior stapediovestibular joint in otosclerosis. Otol Neurotol 2001;22:305–10.
20. Silverstein H. Laser stapedotomy minus prosthesis (laser STAMP): a minimally invasive procedure. Am J Otol 1998;19:277–82.
21. Silverstein H, Hoffmann KK, Thompson JH Jr, et al. Hearing outcome of laser stapedotomy minus prosthesis (STAMP) versus conventional laser stapedotomy. Otol Neurotol 2004;25:106–11.
22. Silveira AR, Linthicum FH Jr. New bone formation in patients with cochlear implants and otosclerosis. Otol Neurotol 2011;32:e38.
23. Gildener-Leapman N, Linthicum FH Jr. Histopathology of cochlear otosclerosis: implications for cochlear implantation. Otol Neurotol 2011;32:e56–7.
24. Fayad J, Moloy P, Linthicum FH Jr. Cochlear otosclerosis: does bone formation affect cochlear implant surgery? Am J Otol 1990;11:196–200.
25. Marshall AH, Fanning N, Symons S, et al. Cochlear implantation in cochlear otosclerosis. The Laryngoscope 2005;115:1728–33.
26. Semaan MT, Gehani NC, Tummala N, et al. Cochlear implantation outcomes in patients with far advanced otosclerosis. Am J Otolaryngol 2012;33:608–14.
27. Sataloff J, Farb S, Menduke H, et al. Sensori-neural hearing loss in otosclerosis. Trans Am Acad Ophthalmol Otolaryngol 1964;68:243–8.
28. Shambaugh GE Jr. The course of clinical otosclerosis. Arch Otolaryngol 1963;78: 509–14.

29. Browning GG, Gatehouse S. Sensorineural hearing loss in stapedial otosclerosis. Ann Otol Rhinol Laryngol 1984;93:13–6.
30. Ramsay HA, Linthicum FH Jr. Mixed hearing loss in otosclerosis: indication for long-term follow-up. Am J Otol 1994;15:536–9.
31. Schuknecht HF. Cochlear otosclerosis. An intractable absurdity. J Laryngol Otol 1983;8:81–3.
32. Parahy C, Linthicum FH Jr. Otosclerosis: relationship of spiral ligament hyalinization to sensorineural hearing loss. Laryngoscope 1983;93:717–20.
33. Lindsay JR, Beal DD. Sensorineural deafness in otosclerosis. Observations on histopathology. Ann Otol Rhinol Laryngol 1966;75:436–57.
34. Elonka DR, Applebaum EL. Otosclerotic involvement of the cochlea: a histologic and audiologic study. Otolaryngol Head Neck Surg 1981;89:343–51.
35. Nelson EG, Hinojosa R. Analysis of the hyalinization reaction in otosclerosis. JAMA Otolaryngol Head Neck Surg 2014;140:555–9.
36. Nelson EG, Hinojosa R. Questioning the relationship between cochlear otosclerosis and sensorineural hearing loss: a quantitative evaluation of cochlear structures in cases of otosclerosis and review of the literature. Laryngoscope 2004; 114:1214–30.
37. Ishai R, Halpin CF, McKenna MJ, et al. How often does stapedectomy for otosclerosis result in endolymphatic hydrops? Otol Neurotol 2016;37:984–90.
38. Seyyedi M, Nadol JB Jr. Intracochlear inflammatory response to cochlear implant electrodes in humans. Otol Neurotol 2014;35:1545–51.
39. Kamakura T, Nadol JB Jr. Correlation between word recognition score and intracochlear new bone and fibrous tissue after cochlear implantation in the human. Hear Res 2016;339:132–41.
40. Broomfield S, Mawman D, Woolford TJ, et al. Non-auditory stimulation in adult cochlear implant users. Cochlear Implants Int 2000;1:55–66.
41. Frijns JH, Kalkman RK, Briaire JJ. Stimulation of the facial nerve by intracochlear electrodes in otosclerosis: a computer modeling study. Otol Neurotol 2009;30: 1168–74.
42. Lagleyre S, Sorrentino T, Calmels MN, et al. Reliability of high-resolution CT scan in diagnosis of otosclerosis. Otol Neurotol 2009;30:1152–9.
43. Shin YJ, Fraysse B, Deguine O, et al. Sensorineural hearing loss and otosclerosis: a clinical and radiologic survey of 437 cases. Acta Otolaryngol 2001;121:200–4.
44. Valvassori GE. Imaging of otosclerosis. Otolaryngol Clin North Am 1993;26: 359–71.
45. Quesnel AM, Ishai R, Cureoglu S, et al. Lack of evidence for nonotosclerotic stapes fixation in human temporal bone histopathology. Otol Neurotol 2016;37: 316–20.
46. Redfors YD, Grondahl HG, Hellgren J, et al. Otosclerosis: anatomy and pathology in the temporal bone assessed by multi-slice and cone-beam CT. Otol Neurotol 2012;33:922–7.
47. Quesnel AM, Ishai R, Meehan T, et al. Histologic grade of otosclerosis correlates with computed tomography densitometry measurements in human temporal bone specimens. Paper presented at: American Otological Society Spring Meeting. San Diego, CA, USA, April 30, 2017.

Otosclerosis
From Genetics to Molecular Biology

Thomas A. Babcock, MD*, Xue Zhong Liu, MD, PhD

KEYWORDS

- Otosclerosis • Otic capsule • Genetics • Gene • Pathophysiology

KEY POINTS

- Otosclerosis is considered an autosomal dominant disease with reduced penetrance but approximately 40% to 50% of all clinical cases have been reported to be sporadic with a lack of positive family history.
- Many studies propose that otosclerosis is a complex genetic disease, caused by a combination of genetic and environmental factors.
- The genetic factors demonstrated to play a role in the development of otosclerosis are involved in several molecular pathways, including bone remodeling, immunologic pathways, inflammation, and endocrine pathways.

INTRODUCTION

Hereditary forms of conductive hearing loss consistent with clinical otosclerosis were first described in the late nineteenth century.[1,2] An understanding of the inheritance of otosclerosis was subsequently refined over the course of several years, with later studies demonstrating an autosomal dominant mode of inheritance with incomplete penetrance between 25% and 40%.[3–10] To date, although there are cases of familial clinical otosclerosis with autosomal dominant inheritance, a majority of cases do not follow a clear mendelian autosomal dominant pattern of inheritance, and approximately 40% to 50% of all clinical cases have been reported to be sporadic with a lack of positive family history.[11,12] It has been proposed that this may be due to reduced penetrance, other models of inheritance besides autosomal dominant, new mutations, phenocopies, or complex or multifactorial forms of otosclerosis caused by a combination of environmental and genetic factors.[12,13] Perhaps the most commonly accepted explanation for the development of disease in a majority of cases

Disclosure Statement: X.Z. Liu's research is supported by R01 DC05575, R01 DC01246, and R01 DC012115 (National Institutes of Health/National Institute on Deafness and Other Communication Disorders). T.A. Babcock has nothing to disclose.
Department of Otolaryngology, University of Miami Miller School of Medicine, 1120 NorthWest 14th Street, 5th Floor, Miami, FL 33136, USA
* Corresponding author.
E-mail address: thomas.babcock@bhcpns.org

Otolaryngol Clin N Am 51 (2018) 305–318
https://doi.org/10.1016/j.otc.2017.11.002
0030-6665/18/© 2017 Elsevier Inc. All rights reserved.

oto.theclinics.com

is contribution from a combination of various environmental and genetic factors. The concept of a complex disease caused by a spectrum of combined environmental and genetic factors is not unique to otosclerosis; several chronic diseases, such as age-related hearing loss, Alzheimer disease, and coronary artery disease, are believed to develop in a similar fashion.[13] To this effect, over the past several years, extensive research has implicated various environmental and genetic factors in the pathophysiology of otosclerosis (**Fig. 1**). The genetic factors dmonstrated to play a role in the development of otosclerosis are involved in several molecular pathways, including bone remodeling, immunologic pathways, inflammation, and endocrine pathways. This article discusses several environmental and genetic factors that have been demonstrated to contribute to the development of otosclerosis. Chromosomal loci with disease-causing mutations that have been identified using linkage studies in familial cases of otosclerosis with clear mendelian segregation are reviewed.

EPIDEMIOLOGY

Otosclerosis is most prevalent in white populations of European descent, with a prevalence of approximately 0.3% to 0.4%, although it is rare among African blacks.[11] Ethnic disparities in prevalence of clinical otosclerosis may be a reflection of differences in environmental and genetic factors. There has been a reported decline in the incidence of clinical otosclerosis among white populations over the past several years.[14] Perhaps further genetic and epidemiologic studies will help elucidate the ethnic disparities in disease prevalence and the pathogenesis of otosclerosis.

BONE REMODELING IN THE OTIC CAPSULE AND OTOSCLEROSIS

The otic capsule has several unique characteristics that may be important features in the context of development of otosclerosis. It consists of an of inner endosteal layer, intermediate endochondral layer, and outer periosteal layer and arises through a process called endochondral ossification during fetal development, a process consisting of initial formation of a cartilaginous structure, which is subsequently replaced by bone.[11] After endochondral ossification, small foci of embryonic remnant called globuli interossei persist in the intermediate endochondral layer and contain quiescent

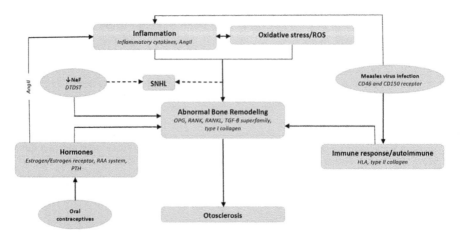

Fig. 1. Correlation of various environmental and molecular etiologic factors implicated in the pathogenesis of otosclerosis. AngII, angiotensin II; NaF, sodium fluoride; RAA, renin-angiotensin-aldosterone; ROS, reactive oxygen species; SNHL, sensorineural hearing loss.

osteocytes and chondrocytes.[11,15] Furthermore, the otic capsule undergoes little bone remodeling or turnover in comparison to other parts of the human skeleton.[16,17] Bone remodeling, consisting of a balanced process of bone resorption by osteoclasts and bone deposition by osteoblasts, is tightly regulated by a group of cytokines, including osteoprotegrin (OPG), receptor activator of nuclear factor κB (RANK), and RANK ligand (RANKL) as well as transforming growth factor β (TGF-β)1.[11,18] In the otic capsule, research has demonstrated high concentrations of OPG are produced by the spiral ligament of the cochlea and secreted into perilymph, playing an important role in shifting the balance of bone remodeling to favor inhibition of bone turnover.[17,19] In the setting of otosclerosis, there is dysregulation of bone remodeling that occurs solely within the otic capsule, giving rise to otosclerotic foci. Areas of the otic capsule with a propensity for development of otosclerotic foci include the fissula ante fenestrum and oval window, round window, and adjacent to the cochlea.[17] Although significant research has been aimed to determine factors that trigger dysregulation of bone turnover within the otic capsule, the process remains poorly understood. Perhaps improved understanding of otic capsule embryogenesis as well as normal bone remodeling within the otic capsule will provide additional clues regarding the pathogenesis of otosclerosis.

ENVIRONMENTAL FACTORS
Measles Virus Infection

Over approximately the past 30 years, several investigators have investigated the potential role of measles virus infection in the pathogenesis of otosclerosis. In 1986, McKenna and colleagues[20] were the first were the first to implicate persistent measles infection in the development of otosclerosis after identifying the presence of filamentous structures resembling measles virus nucleocapsid in osteoblast-like cells of 2 otospongiotic tissue specimens. Subsequently, several studies supported this hypothesis using various investigative techniques, including identification of measles virus structures on electron microscopy, identification of measles virus proteins using immunohistochemistry, identification of measles virus RNA in otosclerotic tissue using reverse transcriptase–polymerase chain reaction, and demonstration of a high concentration of anti-measles virus immunoglobulin G in the perilymph and serum of patients with otosclerosis.[21–24] Furthermore, the measles virus demonstrates a high affinity for the otic capsule, possibly explaining why otosclerotic changes occur solely in this location.[25,26]

Only humans and primates are hosts of the measles virus due to complementary cell surface receptors CD46 and CD150.[25,26] Given the potential role of measles virus in the pathogenesis of otosclerosis, it has been suggested that this may be a contributing factor to difficulty developing an animal model for otosclerosis.[11] A recent study demonstrated novel splice variants in the CD46 receptor gene in otosclerotic stapes footplates, demonstrating a potential association between measles virus infection, the CD46 receptor, and otosclerosis.[27]

Despite evidence implicating chronic measles virus infection in the pathogenesis of otosclerosis, the role of the measles virus in disease development remains subject of debate. Many studies could not find evidence of measles virus infection in all otosclerotic bone and, in addition, there has been difficulty confirming or replicating previously published findings with subsequent studies.[28] Furthermore, the mechanism by which persistent measles virus infection contributes to the pathogenesis of otosclerosis is not well established.

From an epidemiologic perspective, it has been proposed that the decrease in otosclerosis incidence may be due to the introduction of the measles vaccine in the

1970s.[14] It was also reported that the incidence of otosclerosis was lower in patients who were vaccinated against the measles virus, implying a direct causal relationship between measles and otosclerosis. In developing countries where measles is highly endemic, however, the prevalence of otosclerosis is low, such as in African countries. Conversely, in developed countries with populations of primarily European descent, children have been immunized against measles since the 1960s and 1970s, yet the prevalence of otosclerosis remains relatively high in comparison.[13]

Sodium Fluoride

Several studies spanning back to the 1960s have investigated the effects of drinking water fluoridation on the prevalence of otosclerosis and progression of associated hearing loss, with some studies demonstrating an association between clinical otosclerosis, deterioration in hearing, and low fluoride content in the drinking water.[29–31] Furthermore, several investigators have investigated the use of sodium fluoride oral supplementation in the treatment of otosclerosis to prevent hearing deterioration with beneficial effect.[32,33] Sodium fluoride is thought to inhibit proteolytic enzymes and stabilize pathologically increased bone turnover.[34] A more recent study also demonstrated that sodium fluoride inhibits diastrophic dysplasia sulfate transporter (DTDST), which plays a major role in bone turnover by participating in the sulfation of bone matrix glycosaminogycans and was found to have increased activity in otosclerotic stapes.[34] The increased activity of DTDST was correlated with sensorineural hearing loss; thus, its inhibition may prevent hearing deterioration. Although an association between otosclerosis and drinking water fluoridation has been demonstrated, as well as the beneficial effects of treatment with sodium fluoride supplementation, these findings have not been consistent across studies. A recent systematic review evaluating the effect of sodium fluoride on hearing deterioration in otosclerosis concluded that there was limited evidence for the effectiveness of sodium fluoride in patients with otosclerosis.[35]

Oral Contraception

The potential involvement of hormones, such as estrogen, in the development of otosclerosis has been proposed; thus, the potential role of oral contraception use in the development of the disease has also been suggested. These hypotheses are based on, at least in part, the difference in disease prevalence between men and women, the observation that otosclerosis often manifests around the time of pregnancy, and the established role of estrogen in bone metabolism. Although there are case reports of hearing loss with oral contraceptive and hormone replacement therapy, in a large cohort study of approximately 17,000 women followed for periods up to 26 years, no association between oral contraceptive use and the development of otosclerosis was identified.[36,37]

THE GENETICS OF OTOSCLEROSIS
Complex Forms of Otosclerosis

Recent studies suggest otosclerosis is predominantly a complex or multifactorial disease with variable genetic and environmental factors contributing to the development of a similar pathology.[11,13,38] Over the past several years, approaches to investigate complex genetic diseases have evolved significantly, with genetic association studies commonly used to identify a genetic variant associated with a complex diseases or trait.[11] In a case-control genetic association study, a commonly used form of genetic association study, genetic variants are compared between large groups of cases and controls to identify genetic susceptibility factors that influence the development of complex diseases. Case-control studies can be performed via candidate gene–based association study if specific causal genetic variants are suspected or as a genome-wide association study. When a significant association is found in case-control genetic association studies, it is important to replicate the results in an independent population to minimize false-positive results. A well-designed replication study confirming the original finding strongly increases the evidence in favor of a genetic association. Nonreplication, however, does not necessarily rule out a genuine association and may be indicative of inadequate sample size or different disease-causing variants predominating in different populations.[11]

An alternative to genetic association studies for identification of molecular contributors to a disease is to perform a microarray of gene expression in diseased tissue and compare with that of a control. Using gene expression analysis on bone cell cultures obtained from otosclerotic and control stapes, several genes and molecular pathways have been implicated in otosclerosis pathophysiology, several of which overlap with those identified in genetic association studies. Herein, several genes and molecular pathways that have been investigated using gene association studies and gene expression analysis are reviewed. These genes and molecular pathways have roles in bone metabolism, the immune system, inflammation, and the endocrine system. To date, several genetic association and gene expression studies have been performed to determine genetic variants and molecular pathways involved in the development of otosclerosis.

Altered bone metabolism

Type I collagens Mutations of type I collagen genes have been established as the underlying cause of osteogenesis imperfecta type I. Given the common histopathology and clinical manifestations of this milder form of osteogenesis imperfecta and otosclerosis, McKenna and colleagues[39] hypothesized that there was a common genetic basis for the disease of altered bone metabolism and performed the first case-control genetic association study to investigate the genetic basis of otosclerosis. The investigators demonstrated a significant association between clinical otosclerosis and the type I collagen COL1A1 gene in a small population of individuals of European descent living in Massachusetts. McKenna and colleagues[40] subsequently demonstrated a significant association between clinical otosclerosis and the Sp1 binding site polymorphism in the first intron of COL1A1 in a comparison of 100 otosclerosis patients and unmatched controls. In 2007, Chen and colleagues[41] further confirmed the association of COL1A1 expression and the Sp1 binding site polymorphism with otosclerosis in the same population from Massachusetts as well as in a small German population. Furthermore, they demonstrated that some of the associated polymorphisms alter binding of transcription factors that regulate transcription of COL1A2, leading to an increased production of COL1A1 homotrimers. In normal conditions, COL1A1 and COL1A2 associate in a 2:1 ratio to form a collagen type I triple helix.[41] This abnormal gene expression and formation of COL1A1 homotrimers has been implicated in abnormal bone deposition in the otic capsule and development of otosclerosis. Although associations between genetic variants of COL1A1 and otosclerosis have been demonstrated, this could not be replicated in a case-control study performed by Rodriguez and colleagues,[42] consisting of 100 cases and 100 matched controls in a Spanish population.

Transforming growth factor-β superfamily Molecular pathways involving the TGF-β superfamily of cytokines play an important role in bone remodeling. In the context of otosclerosis, in a gene expression analysis performed by Ealy and colleagues,[43] several of the genes with differences in expression between otosclerotic stapes footplates and controls were related to TGF-β signaling. TGF-β1 is a member of the TGF-β superfamily and plays an important role in the embryonic development of the otic capsule as well as in the maintenance and turnover of the bone of the otic capsule in conjunction with other cytokines, including OPG, RANK, and RANKL.[44] In human otosclerotic bone cell cultures, TGF-β1 has been demonstrated to modify expression of glycosaminoglycans, fibronectin, and collagen of the extracellular matrix.[45] TGF-β1 has been associated with otosclerosis in 2 large independent population studies consisting of Belgian-Dutch and French populations.[46,47] Recently, a de novo mutation $-832>A$ was identified in the promoter of TGF-β1 in an otosclerosis patient and was associated with a decreased level of TGF-β1 transcript, which could affect the susceptibility to otosclerosis development.[48]

With the identification of an association between TGF-β1 and otosclerosis in Belgian-Dutch and French populations, Schrauwen and colleagues[49] performed a large candidate gene–based association study on the same populations using 13 new candidate genes. The genes were selected based on their interaction with TGF-β1, function in metabolism of the otic capsule, involvement in syndromic and nonsyndromic forms of stapes fixation, and other hypotheses regarding the cause for otosclerosis. Bone morphogenetic proteins 2 and 4 (BMP2 and BMP4) were the only 2 genes with a significant association in both populations. BMP2 and BMP4 are also member of the TGF-β cytokine superfamily, suggesting that alterations in this pathway involved in bone remodeling may be important in otosclerosis disease susceptibility.

The Role of the immune system

HLA system HLA represents the major histocompatibility complex in humans and plays an important role in the immunologic response by presenting antigenic peptides to T cells. HLA has been implicated in several diseases, in particular those with an immunologic component. Although a correlation between otosclerosis and certain HLA antigens has been reported, this association has not been consistent or reproducible on various studies.[50] Nonetheless, those studies demonstrating a significant association between HLA and otosclerosis suggest a possible immunologic pathology, and certain HLA determinants may affect disease susceptibly in select populations. Further studies are needed to confirm a true association between HLA antigens and otosclerosis.

Autoimmunity The role of the immune system and autoimmune reaction against the otic capsule has been suggested as a potential contributing factor in otosclerosis. Immune cells and immune modulating factors have been demonstrated in otosclerotic foci.[51] Early studies proposed an autoimmune reaction to type II collagen and minor collagens as a possible etiology for otosclerosis.[52] The type II collagen gene COL2A1 was first analyzed due to the abundance of type II collagen in the globuli interossei. Furthermore, type II collagen has been associated with other localized chondrodysplastic lesions.[53] Although early studies supported this hypothesis, subsequent genetic association studies, histologic analysis, and immunohistochemical analysis did not support autoreactivity to collagen as a cause of otosclerosis.[54] It has also been proposed that an autoimmune reaction due to an ongoing immune response to chronic measles virus infection is a critical factor in the development of otosclerosis. Overall, the role of autoimmunity in the pathogenesis of otosclerosis remains unclear.

Inflammation

Inflammatory cytokines Several studies have implicated inflammatory cytokines in the pathogenesis of otosclerosis. Among the inflammatory cytokines investigated, expression of tumor necrosis factor α (TNF-α), and TNF-α receptor have been correlated with the histologic activity of otosclerosis, with increased expression during active otosclerosis.[55] TNF-α has been demonstrated to promote bone resorption and potentially is a catalyst for dysregulation of bone metabolism in otosclerosis. Increased TNF-α expression is also a potential contributing factor for sensorineural hearing loss in otosclerosis. In addition to TNF-α, angiotensin II, which regulates the production of proinflammatory cytokines, has been implicated as key factor in inflammatory pathways and abnormal bone remodeling in otosclerosis.[56–58] The potential role of angiotensin II is discussed later.

Oxidative stress Oxidative stress and reactive oxygen species have the potential to effect several cell signaling pathways and may play an important role in the pathophysiology of otosclerosis. A recent study investigated the possible involvement of oxidative stress in the development of otosclerosis through immunohistochemistry for 4-hydroxynonenal (HNE)-protein adducts in otosclerotic and control stapedial bones.[58] HNE is a major bioactive marker of lipid peroxidation and acts as a second messenger of free radicals. The study demonstrated that although HNE-protein adducts were present in both samples, there was a significant difference in distribution with multifocal areas of irregular HNE-protein adduct positivity in pathologic bone formation regions of otosclerotic samples. HNE-protein adducts were present only in the periosteal region of control samples. The study also demonstrated the effect of HNE and angiotensin II on the regulation of bone cell proliferation, differentiation, and apoptosis, further supporting their potential role in the pathogenesis of otosclerosis. In addition to inflammatory cytokines, oxidative stress and reactive oxygen species have been linked to other forms of hearing loss and may play a role in sensorineural hearing loss associated with otosclerosis.

The role of the endocrine system

Estrogen Many investigators have implicated sex hormones, namely estrogen, in the development of otosclerosis, given that women are affected more frequently than men and otosclerosis often manifests or progresses during or shortly after pregnancy. Although otosclerosis has been reported to manifest or progress during pregnancy, a correlation between development of otosclerosis and pregnancy is still debated. A retrospective study comparing the progression of hearing loss between female patients with and without children did not demonstrate a significant difference between the 2 groups.[59] Furthermore, there was no deleterious impact on hearing with increased number of pregnancies. In an attempt to explain the molecular basis for the affect of estrogen on the otic capsule in otosclerosis, investigators have proposed that a variant of expressed receptor type in otosclerotic tissue may mediate the potential affect of estrogen on the development otosclerosis and abnormal bone remodeling. It has also been demonstrated that estrogen promotes prolactin release. Recent data show that prolactin decreases OPG and increases RANKL, influencing bone metabolism.[36]

Renin-angiotensin-aldosterone system Angiotensin II has been implicated in the key events of inflammation and bone remodeling through interaction with various growth factors and cytokines.[56–58] Interest in the renin-angiotensin-aldosterone system contributing to the development of otosclerosis was likely prompted, at least in part, by demonstrated stimulation of the pathway during pregnancy and the commonly accepted notion that otosclerosis can manifest during or shortly after pregnancy.[60] In 2008, a candidate gene–based association study investigating the role of the renin-angiotensin-aldosterone system in otosclerosis in a French white population was performed and demonstrated that genetic polymorphisms in the angiotensinogen and angiotensinogen converting enzyme genes were linked to higher plasma concentrations of angiotensin II and were also associated with a higher relative risk of otosclerosis occurrence.[61] Furthermore, it has been demonstrated that angiotensin II increases the in vitro secretion of interleukin 6 and decreases alkaline phosphatase activity in only otosclerotic cells, suggesting a role of angiotensin II in dysregulation of bone remodeling and development of otosclerosis.[61] Although there is evidence to support the role of the renin-angiotensin-aldosterone system in otosclerosis pathophysiology, a replicate candidate gene–based association study performed in a large Belgian-Dutch population was unable to confirm this association.[62]

Parathyroid hormone and parathyroid hormone–related receptor expression Considering the major role parathyroid hormone (PTH) plays in the physiology of bone turnover, PTH has been implicated in the pathogenesis of otosclerosis. Although an early study demonstrated normal levels of calcium, phosphorus, and alkaline phosphatase in patients with otosclerosis, a more recent study has demonstrated elevated alkaline phosphatase in patients that have had otosclerosis for many years.[63,64] Other studies have showed that higher PTH concentrations were required to stimulate adenylate cyclase activity as well as a lower PTH–PTH-related peptide receptor mRNA expression associated with a lower cyclic AMP response in otosclerotic stapes cell cultures.[65] These findings suggest that an abnormal response to PTH may be contributing to the abnormal bone turnover in otosclerosis.

Other potential contributing genes and molecular pathways

A recent genome-wide association study identified a significant association with the gene encoding reelin (RELN), an extracellular matrix protein that is known to function in brain development and synaptic plasticity.[66] This association was confirmed across multiple populations with allelic heterogeneity.[67,68] Expression studies have demonstrated that RELN is present in human stapes cell cultures and mouse inner ear, but its function in these tissues, as well as its role in the pathogenesis of otosclerosis, remains unclear.[66]

Monogenic Forms of Otosclerosis

Linkage analyses using families with clear mendelian segregation of autosomal dominant clinical otosclerosis have identified several genetic loci for disease-causing mutations (**Table 1**). Linkage analysis can be used to identify chromosomal locations and genetic factors responsible for mendelian segregation of a monogenic disease within a family. Typically, hundreds to several thousand genetic markers are segregated together with the disease of interest within a family. Once the chromosomal region for the responsible gene is identified, the locus can be further refined through additional markers and genetic databases describing which genes reside within the linked region. Subsequently, suspected candidate genes within the linked interval, such as genes involved in bone metabolism and remodeling in the setting of otosclerosis, are subjected to a mutation analysis to identify the underlying genetic mutation. Identification of genetic factors contributing to an autosomal dominant disease with reduced penetrance and genetic heterogeneity using family linkage studies can prove a challenging task, as in the setting of clinical otosclerosis. To date, 8 known

Table 1
Genetic loci contributing to familial cases of otosclerosis with mendelian segregation identified using family linkage studies

Locus	Position	Family Countries of Origin
OTSC1	15q25–26	South India, Tunisia
OTSC2	7q34–36	Belgium, England
OTSC3	6p21.3–22.3	Cyprus, Tunisia
OTSC4	16q21–23.2	Israel
OTSC5	3q22–24	Netherlands
OTSC6[a]	—	—
OTSC7	6q13–16.1	Greece, Netherlands
OTSC8	9p13.1–q21.11	Tunisia
OTSC9[a]	—	—
OTSC10	1q41–44	Netherlands

[a] Loci names OTSC6 and OTSC9 have been reserved by the Human Genome Organisation Gene Nomenclature Committee but have yet to be published.
   Data from Refs.[11,38,76]

chromosomal loci have been identified (OTSC1–5, OTSC7, OTSC8, and OTSC10) in familial cases of monogenic otosclerosis.[69–76] Although several genetic loci have been localized in familial otosclerosis using linkage analysis and, within these regions, several good candidate genes have been identified, none of the otosclerosis-causing genetic mutations within these chromosomal locations has been identified. A recent study implicated the T-cell receptor β locus as the causative agent in the OTSC2 region, causing alterations in T-cell development and aging, but the mechanisms for these alterations, as well as their contribution to dysregulation of bone remodeling, have not been well described.[77]

FUTURE DIRECTIONS

In recent years, next-generation sequencing has revolutionized genomics and molecular biology with more readily available, advanced sequencing technologies that can be performed quickly. With these recent advances, there have been numerous reports of novel genetic mutations identified, including the identification of genetic mutations involved in rare mendelian disorders and common complex traits. A recent study used techniques, including next-generation sequencing, to identify causal genetic mutations in 4 families exhibiting autosomal dominant inheritance of familial clinical otosclerosis.[78] Multiple missense mutations were identified in the serpin peptidase inhibitor, clade F (SERPINF1) gene. Other variants were located in the 5′-untranslated region of an alternative spliced transcript SERPINF1-012, the major SERPINF1 transcript in human stapes bone. These mutations in the 5′-untranslated region were determined to cause reduced expression of SERPINF1-012. SERPINF1 encodes pigment epithelium–derived growth factor, a potent inhibitor of angiogenesis and known regulator of bone remodeling. Angiogenesis has previously been proposed as a key feature of clinical otosclerosis due to associated Schwartze sign and elevated promontory blood flow on doppler flowmetry in patients with clinical otosclerosis.[18] Furthermore, mutations in SERPINF1 have recently been show to result in a rare form of osteogenesis imperfecta, type VI, another disorder of bone remodeling and metabolism.[79] The recent study utilizing next generation sequencing to identify causal genetic mutations in autosomal dominant, familial clinical otosclerosis highlights the potential future utility of advanced sequencing techniques in identifying additional disease-associated genetic mutations in otosclerosis, even in the setting of variable penetrance and heterogeneity.

SUMMARY

Despite advances in knowledge of environmental and genetic factors that may contribute the development of otosclerosis, an understanding of development of the disease remains unclear. Overall, studies suggest a heterogenous etiology for otosclerosis with variable environmental and genetic factors contributing to the development of a similar pathology. The genetic factors involved in disease development represent a variety of molecular pathways including bone remodeling, immunologic pathways, inflammation, and endocrine pathways. An understanding of the interplay between environmental factors, genetic factors, and implicated molecular pathways will likely continue to evolve with advances in molecular genetics.

REFERENCES

1. Toynbee J. Pathological and surgical observations on the diseases of the ear. Med Chir Trans 1861;24:190–205.
2. Magnus A. Über Verlauf and Sectionsbefund eines Falles von hochgradiger and eigenthumlicher Gehörstörung. Arch Ohrenheilk 1876;11:244–51.
3. Albrecht W. Über der Verenbung der konstitutionell sporadischen Taubstummheit der hereditaren Labyrinthschwerhörigkeit und der Otosclerose. Arch Ohr Nas Kehlkopfheilk 1922;110:15–48.
4. Larsson A. Otosclerosis: a genetic and clinical study. Acta Otolaryngol Suppl 1960;154:1–86.
5. Bauer J, Stein C. Vererbung und Konstituion bei ohrenkrakheiten. Z Konstitutionslehre 1925;10:483–545.
6. Hernandez-Orozco F, Courtney GT. Genetic aspects of clinical otosclerosis. Ann Otol Rhinol Laryngol 1964;73:632–44.
7. Morrison AW. Genetic factors in otosclerosis. Ann R Coll Surg Engl 1967;41:202–37.
8. Morrison AW, Bundey SE. The inheritance of otosclerosis. J Laryngol Otol 1970;84:921–32.
9. Causse JR, Causse JB. Otospongiosis as a genetic disease: early detection, medical management, and prevention. Am J Otol 1984;5:211–23.
10. Gapany-Gapanavicus B. Otosclerosis: genetic and surgical rehabilitation. New York: Halstead Press; 1975.
11. Thys M, Van Camp G. Genetics of otosclerosis. Otol Neurotol 2009;30:1021–32.
12. Rudic M, Keogh I, Wagner R, et al. The pathophysiology of otosclerosis: review of current research. Hear Res 2015;330:51–6.
13. Schrauwen I, Van Camp G. The etiology of otosclerosis: a combination of genes and environment. Laryngoscope 2010;120:1195–202.
14. Arnold W, Busch R, Arnold A, et al. The influence of measles vaccination on the incidence of otosclerosis in Germany. Eur Arch Otorhinolaryngol 2007;264:741–8.
15. Schuknecht HF. Pathology of the ear. 2nd edition. Philadelphia: Lea and Febiger; 1993.

16. Frisch T, Sorensen MS, Overgaard S, et al. Estimation of volume referent bone turnover in the otic capsule after sequential point labeling. Ann Otol Rhinol Laryngol 2000;109:33–9.

17. Frisch T, Sorensen MS, Overgaard S, et al. Predilection of otosclerotic foci related to the bone turnover in the otic capsule. Acta Otolaryngol Suppl 2000;543:111–3.

18. Stankovic KM, McKenna MJ. Current research in otosclerosis. Curr Opin Otolaryngol Head Neck Surg 2006;14:347–51.

19. Zehnder AF, Kristiansen AG, Adams JC, et al. Osteoprotegerin in the inner ear may inhibit bone remodeling in the otic capsule. Laryngoscope 2005;24:43–9.

20. McKenna MJ, Mills BG, Galey FR, et al. Filamentous structures morphologically similar to viral nucleocapsids in otosclerotic lesions in two patients. Am J Otol 1986;7(1):25–8.

21. Arnold W, Friedmann I. Presence of viral specific antigens (measles, rubella) around the active otosclerotic focus. Ann Otol Rhinol Laryngol 1987;66:167–71.

22. McKenna MJ, Mills BG. Ultrastructural and immunohistochemical evidence of measles virus in active otosclerosis. Acta Otolaryngol Suppl 1990;470:130–9.

23. Niedermeyer H, Arnold W, Neubert WJ, et al. Evidence of measles virus RNA in otosclerotic tissue. ORL J Otorhinolaryngol Relat Spec 1994;56:130–2.

24. Arnold W, Niedermeyer HP, Lehn N, et al. Measles virus in otosclerosis and the specific immune response of the inner ear. Acta Otolaryngol Stoch 1996;116:705–9.

25. Dorig RE, Marcil A, Chopra A, et al. The human CD46 molecule is a receptor for measles virus (edmonston strain). Cell 1993;75:295–305.

26. Tatsuo H, Ono N, Tanaka K, et al. SLAM (CDw150) is a cellular receptor for measles virus. Nature 2000;406:893–7.

27. Karosi T, Szalmas A, Csomor P, et al. Disease-associated novel CD46 splicing variants and pathologic bone remodeling in otosclerosis. Laryngoscope 2008; 118:1669–79.

28. Grayeli AB, Palmer P, Tran Ba Huy P, et al. No evidence of measles virus in stapes samples from patients with otosclerosis. J Clin Microbiol 2000;38:2655–60.

29. Daniel HJ III. Stapedial otosclerosis and fluorine in the drinking water. Arch Otolaryngol 1969;90:585–9.

30. Vartiainen E, Vartiainen T. Effect of drinking water fluoridation on the prevalence of otosclerosis. J Laryngol Otol 1997;111:20–2.

31. Vartiainen E, Vartiainen J. The effect of drinking water fluoridation on the natural course of hearing in patients with otosclerosis. Acta Otolaryngol 1996;116: 747–50.

32. Bretlau P, Salomon G, Johnsen NJ. Otospongiosis and sodium fluoride. A clinical double-blinded, placebo-controlled study on sodium fluoride treatment in otospongiosis. Am J Otol 1989;10:20–2.

33. Bretlau P, Causse J, Causse JB, et al. Otospongiosis and sodium fluoride. A blind experimental and clinical evaluation of the effect of sodium fluoride treatment in patients with otospongiosis. Ann Otol Rhinol Laryngol 1985;94:102–7.

34. Grayeli AB, Escoubet B, Bichara M, et al. Increased activity of the diastrophic dysplasia sulfate transporter in otosclerosis and its inhibition by sodium fluoride. Otol Neurotol 2003;24:854–62.

35. Hentschel MA, Huizinga P, van der Velden DL, et al. Limited evidence for the effect of sodium fluoride on deterioration of hearing loss in patients with otosclerosis: a systematic review of the literature. Otol Neurotol 2014;35:1052–7.

36. Horner KC. The effect of sex hormones on bone metabolism of the otic capsule – an overview. Hear Res 2009;252:56–60.

37. Vessey M, Painter R. Oral contraception and ear disease: findings in a large cohort study. Contraception 2001;63:61–3.
38. Ealy M, Smith RJH. The genetics of otosclerosis. Hear Res 2010;252:70–4.
39. McKenna MJ, Kristiansen AG, Bartley ML, et al. Association of COL1A1 and otosclerosis: evidence for a shared genetic etiology with mild osteogenesis imperfect. Am J Otol 1998;19:604–10.
40. McKenna MJ, Nguyen-Huynth AT, Kristiansen AG. Association of otosclerosis with Sp1 binding site polymorphism in COL1A1 gene: evidence for shared genetic etiology with osteoporosis. Otol Neurotol 2004;25:447–50.
41. Chen W, Meyer NC, McKenna MJ, et al. Single-nucleotide polymorphism of the COL1A1 regulatory regions are associated with otosclerosis. Clin Genet 2007; 71:406–14.
42. Rodriguez L, Rodriguez S, Hermida J, et al. Proposed association between COL1A1 and COL1A2 genes and otosclerosis is not supported by a case-control study in Spain. Am J Med Genet 2004;128:19–22.
43. Ealy M, Chen W, Ryu GY, et al. Gene expression analysis of human otosclerotic stapedial footplates. Hear Res 2008;240:80–6.
44. Janssens K, ten Dijke P, Janssens S, et al. Transforming growth factor-beta1 to the bone. Endocr Rev 2005;26:743–74.
45. Bodo M, Venti S, Beavan SR, et al. Phenotype of in vitro human otosclerotic cells and its modulation by TGF beta. Cell Mol Biol 1995;41:1039–49.
46. Thys M, Schrauwen L, Vanderstraeten K, et al. The coding polymorphism T263I in TGF-beta1 is associated with otosclerosis in two independent populations. Hum Mol Genet 2007;16:2021–30.
47. Thys M, Schrauwen L, Vanderstraeten K, et al. Detection of rare nonsynonymous variants of TGFB1 in otosclerosis patients. Ann Hum Genet 2009;73:171–5.
48. Priyadarshi S, Hansdah K, Sundar Ray C, et al. Otosclerosis associated with de novo mutation -832G>A in the TGFB1 gene promoter causing a decreased expression level. Sci Rep 2016;6:29572.
49. Schrauwen L, Thys M, Vanderstraeten K, et al. Association of bone morphogenetic proteins with otosclerosis. J Bone Min Res 2008;23:507–16.
50. Moumoulidis I, Axon P, Baguley P, et al. A review on the genetics of otosclerosis. Clin Otolaryngol 2007;32:239–47.
51. Altermatt HJ, Gerber HA, Gaeng D, et al. Immunohistochemical findings in otosclerotic lesions [in German]. HNO 1992;40:476–9.
52. Yoo TJ. Etiopathogenesis of otosclerosis: a hypothesis. Ann Otol Rhinol Laryngol 1984;93:28–33.
53. McKenna MJ, Kristiansen AG. The role of measles virus and hereditary in the development of otosclerosis. In: Veldman JE, Passàli D, Lim DJ, editors. New frontiers in immunobiology. Monroe (NY): Library Research Associates, Inc.; 2000. p. 51–6.
54. Sorensen MS, Nielsen LP, Bretlau, et al. The role of type II collagen autoimmunity in otosclerosis revisited. Acta Otolaryngol 1988;105:242–7.
55. Csomor P, Sziklai I, Karosi T. TNF-α receptor expression correlates with histologic activity of otosclerosis. Otol Neurotol 2009;30:1131–7.
56. Lamparter S, Kling L, Schrader M, et al. Effects of angiotensin II on bone cells in vitro. J Cell Physiol 1998;175:89–98.
57. Rudic M, Nguyen C, Nguyen Y, et al. Effect of angiotensin II on inflammation pathways in human primary bone cell cultures in otosclerosis. Audiol Neurootol 2012; 17:169–78.

58. Rudic M, Milkovic L, Zarkovic K, et al. The effects of angiotensin II and the oxidative stress mediator 4-hydroxynonenal on human osteoblast-like cell growth: possible relevance to otosclerosis. Free Radic Biol Med 2013;57:22–8.

59. Lippy WH, Erenholz LP, Schuring AG, et al. Does pregnancy affect otosclerosis? Laryngoscope 2005;115:1833–6.

60. Schrier RW, Durr JA. Pregnancy: an overfill or underfill state. Am J Kidney Dis 1987;9:284–9.

61. Imauchi Y, Jeunemaitre X, Boussion M. Relation between renin-angiotensin-aldosterone system and otosclerosis: a genetic association and in vitro study. Otol Neurotol 2008;29:295–301.

62. Schrauwen I, Thys M, Vanderstraeten K, et al. No evidence for association between renin-angiotensin-aldosterone system and otosclerosis in a large Belgian-Dutch population. Otol Neurotol 2009;30:1079–83.

63. Jensen KJ, Nielsen HE, Eibrond O, et al. Mineral content of skeletal bones in otosclerosis. Clin Otolaryngol Allied Sci 1979;4:339–42.

64. Lolov SR, Edrev GE, Kyurkchiev SD, et al. Elevated autoantibodies in sera from otosclerotic patients are related to the disease duration. Acta Otolaryngol 1998; 118:375–80.

65. Grayeli AB, Sterkers O, Roulleau P, et al. Parathyroid hormone-parathyroid hormone-related peptide receptor expression and function in otosclerosis. Am J Physiol 1999;277:E1005–12.

66. Schrauwen I, Ealy M, Huentelman MJ, et al. A genome-wide analysis identifies genetic variants in the RELN gene associated with otosclerosis. Am J Hum Genet 2009;84:328–38.

67. Schrauwen I, Ealy M, Fransen E, et al. Genetic variants in the RELN gene are associated with otosclerosis in multiple European populations. Hum Genet 2010;127:155–62.

68. Khalfallah A, Schrauwen I, Mnaja M, et al. Genetic variants in RELN are associated with otosclerosis in a non-European population from Tunisia. Ann Hum Genet 2010;74:399–405.

69. Tomek MS, Brown MR, Mani SR, et al. Localization of a gene for otosclerosis to chromosome 15q25-q26. Hum Mol Genet 1998;7:285–90.

70. Van Den Bogaert K, Govaerts PJ, Schatteman I, et al. A second gene for otosclerosis, OTSC2, maps to chromosome 7q34-36. Am J Hum Genet 2001;68:495–500.

71. Chen W, Campbell CA, Green GE, et al. Linkage of otosclerosis to a third locus (OTSC3) on human chromosome 6p21.3-22-3. J Med Genet 2002;39:473–7.

72. Browenstein Z, Goldfarb A, Levi H, et al. Chromosomal mapping and phenotype characterization of hereditary otosclerosis linked to the OTSC4 locus. Arch Otolaryngol Head Neck Surg 2006;132:416–24.

73. Van Den Bogaert K, De Leenheer EM, Chen W, et al. A fifth locus for otosclerosis, OTSC5, maps to chromosome 3q22-24. J Med Genet 2004;41:450–3.

74. Thys M, Van Den Bogaert K, Iliadou V, et al. A seventh locus for otosclerosis, OTSC7, maps to chromosome 6q13-16.1. Eur J Hum Genet 2007;15:362–8.

75. Bel Hadji Ali I, Thys M, Beltaief N, et al. A new locus for otosclerosis, OTSC8, maps to the pericentometric region of chromosome 9. Hum Genet 2008;123:267–72.

76. Schrauwen I, Weegerink NJ, Fransen E, et al. A new locus for otosclerosis, OTSC10, maps to chromosome 1q41-44. Clin Genet 2011;79:495–7.

77. Schrauwen I, Venken K, Vanderstraeten K, et al. Involvement of T-cell receptor-beta alterations in the development of otosclerosis linked to OTSC2. Genes Immun 2010;11:246–53.

78. Ziff JL, Crompton M, Powell HR, et al. Mutations and altered expression of SERPINF1 in patients with familial otosclerosis. Hum Mol Genet 2016;25: 2393–403.

79. Wang JY, Liu Y, Song LJ, et al. Novel mutations in SERPINF1 result in rare osteogenesis imperfect type VI. Calcif Tissue Int 2017;100:55–66.

Clinical Evaluation of the Patient with Otosclerosis

Michael F. Foster, DO*, Douglas D. Backous, MD

KEYWORDS

- Otosclerosis • Conductive hearing loss • Mixed hearing loss • Carhartt's notch

KEY POINTS

- Otosclerosis classically presents in an adult with progressive unilateral conductive or mixed hearing loss, absent stapedial reflexes and normal otoscopy.
- An examination using a 512 Hz tuning fork is essential to diagnosis; if the examination does not correlate with the audiogram, repeat the audiogram.
- Radiologic evaluation is not essential in diagnosis but can identify other etiologies of conductive hearing loss in the setting of normal otoscopy, such as superior semicircular canal dehiscence or enlarged vestibular aqueduct.
- A computed tomography (CT) scan of the temporal bone should be performed to identify superior semicircular canal dehiscence in patients with a conductive hearing loss and symptoms of a third window phenomenon.
- A masking dilemma in bilateral far advanced otosclerosis creates a difficult clinical picture, so each case should be carefully assessed by the audiology team prior to surgical intervention.

INTRODUCTION

Otosclerosis, an autosomal dominant condition involving the otic capsule, is histologically characterized by abnormal resorption and reformation of labyrinthine bone. Otosclerosis most commonly manifests clinically as a conductive hearing loss. However, because of variable penetrance, a mixed (conductive-sensorineural) hearing loss and purely sensorineural hearing loss can occur.[1–5]

The condition is most common in the Caucasian population affecting approximately 1%. An average of 10% of Caucasians have been found to have histologic evidence of otosclerosis in 2 large cadaveric studies; however, only 12% of those with histologic findings exhibited clinical signs and symptoms of otosclerosis.[6,7] Japanese and South

Disclosure Statement: D.D. Backous has received honoraria for consulting with Medtronic, and Stryker. M.F. Foster has nothing to disclose.
Center for Hearing and Skull Base Surgery, Swedish Neuroscience Institute, 550 17th Avenue, Suite 540, Seattle, WA 98122, USA
* Corresponding author.
E-mail address: michaelfoster5@gmail.com

American populations exhibit an incidence of 0.5%, and the African American population have even fewer cases. Average prevalence is 0.3%.[8] Despite race, when 1 ear is effected the contralateral ear will show histologic signs of otosclerosis 80% of the time.

Average age of presentation is 15 to 45 years. Otosclerosis advances more rapidly in females than males. Hormonal factors have been implicated in progression of otosclerosis. Females have reported onset of hearing loss or worsening of symptoms during pregnancy. Estrogen receptors have been found on otosclerosis plaques. Despite this, Stankovic and colleagues minimized the association between pregnancy and progression of otosclerosis.[9] This correlation remains controversial.

Clayton showed a statistically significant likelihood of women with otosclerosis to have osteoporosis when compared to their counterparts with presbycusis only.[10]

Approximately 60% of patients with clinical otosclerosis report a family history of the condition. The remaining 40% are thought to represent autosomal-dominant inherited cases with failure of penetrance in other family members, new mutations, those with environmental etiology, and rare cases of alternate inheritance (ie, autosomal recessive).[11]

A patient's clinical presentation is directly affected by the location and extent of the sclerotic lesion. A lesion originating from the fissula ante fenestrum and advancing across the annular ligament of the stapes footplate will result in stapes footplate fixation and conductive hearing loss. Less commonly, the lesion progresses medially into the endosteum of the cochlea and results in a sensorineural hearing loss.

CLINICAL PRESENTATION – HISTORY

The classic presentation of otosclerosis is an adult-onset, progressive conductive hearing loss. Patients may describe improved hearing clarity in noisy environments. This phenomenon is known as Paracusis of Willis, wherein the conductive hearing loss subdues the background noise such that it improves the signal-to-noise ratio for the patient.

Vestibular symptoms have been reported in up to 40% of patients with otosclerosis. It is important to tease out the specifics of the vestibular complaint while obtaining the history, as misdiagnosis can have significant implications on treatment outcomes. For example, in the setting of Meniere disease, saccular distention due to endolymphatic hydrops can put the saccular membrane in contact with the underside of the stapes footplate. A stapedotomy here can lead to injury of the membrane and profound sensorineural hearing loss (SNHL), thus making Meniere disease is a relative contraindication to a stapedotomy. Furthermore, Mikulec reported 8 patients with unilateral conductive hearing loss, presumed otosclerosis, who failed to improve following an uncomplicated stapes procedure. These patients were found to have superior semicircular canal dehiscence (SSCD).[12–14] It is important to screen for third window symptoms such as autophony, pulsatile tinnitus, or pressure-induced vertigo in the setting of conductive hearing loss.

CLINICAL PRESENTATION – PHYSICAL EXAMINATION

A complete head and neck and otological examination is performed. Otosclerosis most commonly presents with normal otoscopy. A reddish blush may be noted on the promontory. In 1873, Schwartze described a reddish hue on the cochlear promontory observed through an intact tympanic membrane. Highly vascular areas of otospongiosis (early phase otosclerosis) have a reddish hue under otoscopic or microscopic examination. This finding is aptly named the Schwartze sign.[1]

Tuning Fork Examination

This examination confirms the audiometric findings and determines if the patient would benefit from surgical intervention.

The Weber test is performed by placing a tuning fork on the patient's forehead, bridge of nose, or upper incisors. The patient will perceive sound in the ear with a conductive hearing loss, and the ear with a greater conductive loss in the setting of bilateral disease.[15] The test is sensitive to a 5 dB difference between ears.

The Rinne test evaluates the patient's perceived loudness of air conduction compared with bone conduction. A 256 or 512 Hz tuning fork is first held 2 to 3 cm away from the external auditory canal (air conduction); then the base is placed firmly over the mastoid bone (bone conduction).[16]

Bone conduction perceived louder than air conduction is termed a negative Rinne test. This is diagnostic for a conductive hearing loss. 256 Hz tuning fork is indicative of a 10 to 15 dB air bone gap. 512 Hz tuning fork reveals a 20 to 25 dB air bone gap. A patient with a conductive hearing loss is considered a surgical candidate for stapedotomy when he or she shows a negative Rinne test at 512 Hz. Air conduction perceived louder that bone conduction is termed a positive Rinne test.

Audiometric Testing

A standard audiometric battery should be performed including pure tone thresholds with air conduction and bone conduction, speech reception thresholds, word recognition scores, and immitance testing (tympanometry and acoustic reflexes).

On an audiogram, otosclerosis is seen as a unilateral or bilateral air bone gap, usually greater in the low frequencies. Speech recognition scores are typically as expected for the degree of hearing loss noted. Bone conduction may show a depression at 2000 Hz without a coinciding depression in air conduction, narrowing the air bone gap at that frequency. This is known as a Carhart notch and is common but not exclusive to otosclerosis (**Fig. 1**). This apparent depression of bone conduction is a result of an impedance mismatch of the otic capsule from stapes fixation. Coinciding SNHL is

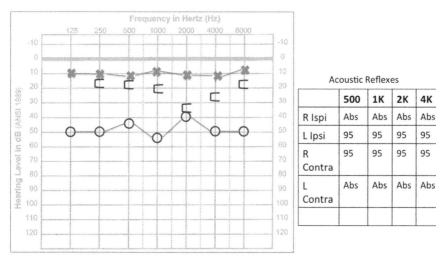

Fig. 1. Audiogram showing normal hearing of the left ear (X), a moderate conductive hearing loss in the right ear (O), and classic Carhartt's Notch at 2K Hz. Acoustic reflexes are absent ipsilateral when testing the right ear, and absent contralateral when testing the left.

variable. In a retrospective study of 290 patients with over 10 years of follow-up, Ishai and colleagues showed approximately one-third of patients with otosclerosis will have clinically significant progression of SNHL greater than age-matched controls with normal ears.[17]

Immitance testing of acoustic (stapedial) reflexes is an integral component of the audiometric workup. Ipsilateral acoustic reflexes are characteristically absent in the setting of stapedial fixation due to otosclerosis (see **Fig. 1**; **Fig. 2**). The on-off effect is indicative of early stapes fixation, shown by decreased impedance at the onset and the end of the stimulus. Intact acoustic reflexes can be indicative of early otosclerosis or direct the examiner toward another etiology of the conductive hearing loss such as SSCD or enlarged vestibular aqueduct (EVA). A recent retrospective study showed that of patients with conductive hearing loss and at least 1 detectable acoustic reflex, a nonossicular etiology was present in 52% of ears. They found that screening for third window symptoms (autophony, pulsatile tinnitus, or pressure-induced vertigo) in addition to acoustic reflexes carries a 94% positive predictive value of correctly diagnosing an ossicular etiology.[18,19] A patient with conductive hearing loss and suprathreshold bone conduction and/or an acoustic reflex in at least 1 frequency with or without complaints of third window symptoms should have a CT of the temporal bones to rule out SSCD or EVA prior to middle ear exploration (**Fig. 3**).

Radiologic Evaluation

Although the diagnosis of otosclerosis is primarily a diagnosis obtained by history and audiometric testing, there are certain cases where radiology can help clarify the clinical picture. A CT scan can confirm the diagnosis of otosclerosis. An active otosclerotic focus will project as a focus of hypolucency at the fissula ante fenestrum (**Fig. 4**), or lucency can completely encircle the cochlea in more advanced otosclerosis - this is termed a halo sign. (**Fig. 5**). A CT scan is especially helpful to identify superior canal dehiscence in a patient with a conductive hearing loss and symptoms of a third window phenomena (**Fig. 6**). Although a CT scan is useful to confirm the diagnosis of

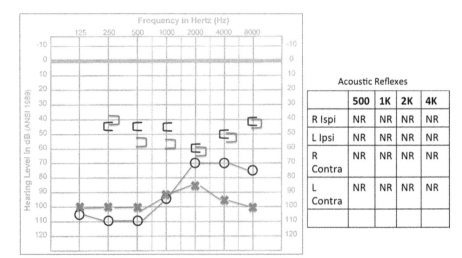

Fig. 2. Audiogram showing a bilateral profound mixed hearing loss and absent acoustic reflexes bilaterally.

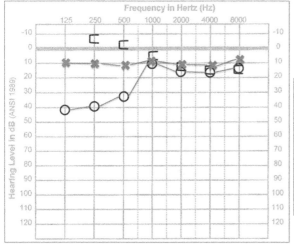

	500	1K	2K	4K
Acoustic Reflexes				
R Ispi	95	95	95	95
L Ipsi	95	95	95	95
R Contra	95	95	95	95
L Contra	95	95	95	95

Fig. 3. Audiogram showing normal hearing of the left ear (X) and a moderator low-frequency conductive hearing loss in the right ear (O). Suprathreshold right-sided bone conduction is suggestive of superior semicircular canal dehiscence. Acoustic reflexes are present bilaterally.

otosclerosis or direct the clinician toward other pathology, a normal CT scan of the temporal bones does not rule out otosclerosis.

Finally, the role of stapedotomy is unclear in far-advanced otosclerosis with significant sensorineural deficit and a superimposed conductive component (see **Fig. 3**). The masking dilemma in this situation makes a reliable audiometric diagnosis difficult; thus discussion of the case with the audiology team proves valuable. The role of stapedotomy in far advanced otosclerosis should be considered on a case-by-case basis.

In summary, the clinical evaluation of otosclerosis relies on a careful history and audiometric testing to guide the practitioner to a treatment plan beneficial for the patient (**Fig. 7**).

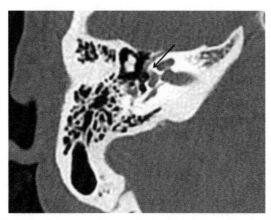

Fig. 4. Axial CT of the right temporal bone. Foci of lucency at the fissula ante fenestrum (*arrow*).

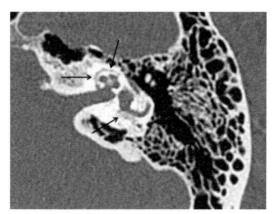

Fig. 5. Axial CT of the left temporal bone. Multiple foci of active otosclerosis surrounding the cochlea and labyrinth (*arrows*). Halo Sign.

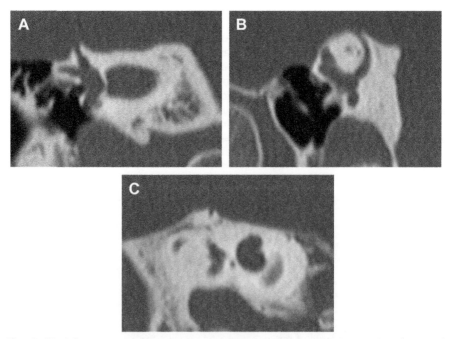

Fig. 6. CT right temporal bone without contrast showing superior semicrcular canal dehiscence in 3 planes. (*A*) Coronal view. (*B*) Pöschl view, Pöschl images are cut in a plane perpendicular to the long axis of the temporal bone. This plane is 45° offset from both the coronal and saggital plane. The superior semicircular canal will appear as a ring. (*C*) Stenver view; Stenver images are cut perpendicular to the Pöschl images and show a cross section of the superior bony cortex of the superior semicircular canal.

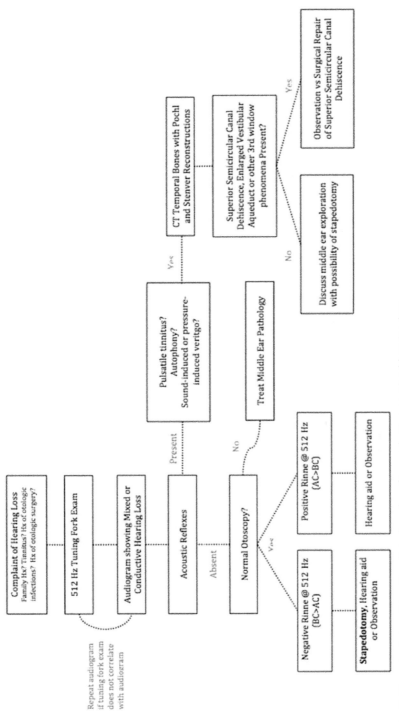

Fig. 7. Flow chart describing the clinical workup for conductive or mixed hearing loss.

REFERENCES

1. Isaacson B, Kutz JW Jr, Roland PS. Otosclerosis. In: Johnson JT, Rosen CA, editors. Bailey's head and neck surgery: otolaryngology. 5th edition. Philadelphia: Lippincott Williams & Wilkins; 2014. p. 2487–502.
2. House JW, Cunningham CD. Otosclerosis. In: NiParko JK, editor. Cummings otolaryngology head & neck surgery. 5th edition. Philadelphia: Mosby/Elsevier; 2010. p. 2028–35.
3. Mudry A. Adam Politzer (1835-1920) and the description of otosclerosis. Otol Neurotol 2006;27:276–81.
4. Chole RA, McKenna M. Basic science review; pathophysiology of otosclerosis. Otol Neurotol 2001;22:249–57.
5. Menger DJ, Tange RA. The aetiology of otosclerosis: a review of the literature. Clin Otolaryngol 2003;28:112–20.
6. Guild SR. Histologic otosclerosis. Ann Otol Rhinol Laryngol 1944;53:246–66.
7. Weber M. Otosklerose und Umbau der Labyrinthcapsel. Leipzig (Germany): Peoschel and Trepte; 1935.
8. Gordon MA. The genetics of otosclerosis: a review. Am J Otol 1989;10:426–38.
9. Stankovich KM, McKenna MJ. Current research in otosclerosis. Curr Opin Otolaryngol Head Neck Surg 2006;14:347–51.
10. Clayton AE, Mikulec AA, Mikulec KH, et al. Association between osteoporosis and otosclerosis in women. J Laryngol Otol 2004;118:617–21.
11. Morrison A, Bundey S. The inheritance of otosclerosis. J Laryngol Otol 1970;84: 921–32.
12. Mikulec AA, McKenna MJ, Ramsey MJ, et al. Superior semicircular canal dehiscence presenting as conductive hearing loss without vertigo. Otol Neurotol 2004; 25:121–9.
13. Kim SC, Lee W-S, Kim M, et al. Third windows as a cause of failure in hearing gain after exploratory tympanotomy. Otolaryngol Head Neck Surg 2011;145:303–8.
14. Li PMMC, Bergeron C, Monafred A, et al. Superior semicircular canal dehiscence diagnosed after failed stapedotomy for conductive hearing loss. Am J Otolaryngol 2011;32:441–4.
15. Blakeley BW, Siddique S. A qualitative explanation of the weber test. Otolaryngol Head Neck Surg 1999;120:1–4.
16. Chole RA, Cook GB. The Rinne test for conductive deafness. Arch Otolaryngol Head Neck Surg 1988;114:399–403.
17. Ishai R, Halpin CF, Shin JJ, et al. Long-term incidence and degree of sensorineural hearing loss in otosclerosis. Otol Neurotol 2016;37:1489–96.
18. Hong RS, Metz CM, Bojrab DJ, et al. Acoustic reflex screening of conductive hearing loss for third window disorders. Otolaryngol Head Neck Surg 2016; 154(2):343–8.
19. Moller AR. Acoustic reflex in man. J Acoust Soc Am 1962;34:1524–34.

The Audiology of Otosclerosis

Ali A. Danesh, MS, PhD[a,b,*], Navid Shahnaz, PhD[c],
James W. Hall III, PhD[d,e]

KEYWORDS

- Carhart notch • Immittance measurement and otosclerosis • Reflectance
- Wideband acoustic immittance and otosclerosis • Middle ear muscle reflex
- Power absorbance and otosclerosis • Hearing aids and otosclerosis
- Tinnitus and otosclerosis

KEY POINTS

- For most patients with otosclerosis, audiologic biomarkers include reduced middle ear compliance as revealed by tympanometry, and a 10- to 15-dB reduction in sound transmission via bone conduction most often in the vicinity of 2000 Hz (known as Carhart notch).
- Wideband acoustic immittance is an effective technique in identifying middle ear pathologies, such as otosclerosis; it can provide all the useful information that could be obtained from conventional and multifrequency tympanometry and additional information on the transfer of energy into the middle ear system across much wider range of frequencies.
- Middle ear resonance frequency shifts to higher frequency regions in most of the otosclerotic ears.
- In addition to middle ear ossicular surgery, hearing aids and implantable hearing devices are alternative approaches for the management of hearing loss in patients with otosclerosis.
- Tinnitus sound therapy and cognitive behavioral therapy are successfully used for the management of tinnitus in the otosclerotic population.

Disclosure: The authors have nothing to disclose.
[a] Department of Communication Sciences and Disorders, Florida Atlantic University, ED 434 777 Glades Road, Boca Raton, FL 33431, USA; [b] Department of Clinical Biomedical Sciences, Schmidt College of Medicine, Florida Atlantic University, ED 434 777 Glades Road, Boca Raton, FL 33431, USA; [c] School of Audiology and Speech Sciences, Faculty of Medicine, University of British Columbia, 2177 Wesbrook Mall, Friedman Building, Vancouver, British Columbia V6T 1Z3, Canada; [d] Osborne College of Audiology, Salus University, 8360 Old York Road, Elkins Park, PA 19027, USA; [e] Department of Communication Sciences and Disorders, University of Hawaii, 677 Ala Moana Boulevard, Honolulu, HI 96813, USA
* Corresponding author. ED 434 777 Glades Road, Boca Raton, FL 33431.
E-mail address: danesh@fau.edu

INTRODUCTION

For many otologists and audiologists, otosclerosis is not a puzzling condition anymore. Advances in diagnostic and therapeutic procedures have provided a vast number of patients with otosclerosis with proper management. This article is designed in a fashion that enables otologists in better diagnosis and management of otosclerosis with the use of audiologic procedures. The accuracy of audiometric air-bone gap, appropriate use of masking techniques, and immittance measurements can completely influence the decisions made by otologists for the surgical management of otosclerosis. Otologists rely on the precision of the audiologic results and determination of the degree of the conductive component. Therefore, a precise audiologic work-up is a crucial part of the diagnostic protocol for otosclerosis. This article reviews the audiologic diagnostic test battery and the audiologic management of auditory effects of otosclerosis.

AUDIOMETRIC PATTERNS

As with other middle ear disorders, otosclerosis reduces sound-related energy passing from the tympanic membrane to the inner ear. Fixation and resultant stiffening of the ossicular chain almost always produces a hearing loss, particularly for lower-frequency sounds. The characteristic pattern of hearing loss in otosclerosis is useful in diagnosing the disease.[1–3] The diagnostic value of hearing assessment is enhanced when such test procedures as pure tone audiometry, tympanometry, and acoustic reflexes are combined into a test battery. Indeed, for most patients with otosclerosis, a unique pattern of findings for an appropriate collection of auditory tests almost always contributes to early and accurate diagnosis. Basic hearing test findings in patients with otosclerosis are summarized in **Table 1**.

Table 1
Patterns of basic auditory findings in patients with the diagnosis of otosclerosis

Procedure	Findings
Pure tone audiometry	
Air conduction	Hearing loss greater for low frequencies.
Bone conduction	Apparent decrease in bone conduction thresholds sometimes with a notching deficit at 2000 Hz (Carhart notch). Actual bone conduction hearing is typically normal.
Audiometric Weber test	Perception of low-frequency pure tone stimuli in the ear with conductive hearing loss.
Sensorineural acuity level test	Presence of an air-bone gap and confirmation of normal bone conduction hearing.
Acoustic immittance measures	
Tympanometry	Shallow type A tympanogram reflecting increased stiffness of the ossicular chain (see immittance measurement section for further discussion).
Acoustic reflexes	Absence of stapedial acoustic reflex activity even in patients with minimal air-bone gap and conductive hearing loss. Atypical acoustic reflex pattern in patients with very early subclinical otosclerosis.
Otoacoustic emissions	Otoacoustic emissions cannot be detected in patients with otosclerosis and conductive hearing loss. Recovery of detectable otoacoustic emissions is possible in patients following microtraumatic stapedotomy.

Representative pure tone audiometry findings for one ear of a patient with otosclerosis are shown in **Fig. 1**. There is a conductive hearing loss with considerably poorer hearing sensitivity for air versus bone conduction hearing. Bone conduction hearing is generally normal with the exception of a distinct notch-like decrease in bone conduction thresholds in the audiogram region of the 2000 Hz. The horizontal dotted line indicates actual bone conduction hearing whereas the bone conduction thresholds reflect an apparent deficit in sensory function. "Mechanical modifications" and effects of middle ear resonant frequency in bone conduction hearing associated with stapes fixation in patients with otosclerosis have been appreciated since the 1940s (discussed later). Indeed, normal bone conduction hearing sensitivity is unusual for patients with otosclerosis. Multiple theories have been offered for the negative effect of middle ear abnormalities on the response to bone conduction stimulation. However, evidence and agreement in support of a single mechanism are lacking.

Named after the well-known audiologist who first described it in detail,[1,4] Carhart notch has for more than 60 years been one of the most recognizable audiometric features of otosclerosis. Carhart[1] described an average decrease in bone conduction thresholds of 5 dB at 500 Hz, 10 dB at 1000 Hz, 15 dB at 2000 Hz, and 5 dB at 4000 Hz, as illustrated in **Fig. 1**.

More recent studies raise three general questions about the diagnostic value and specificity of a notching deficit in bone conduction thresholds at 2000 Hz.[5–8] First, bone conduction hearing thresholds are often decreased also at other test frequencies in patients with the diagnosis of otosclerosis. Researchers have observed for patients with the diagnosis of otosclerosis the possibility of a notching deficit in bone conduction thresholds in the low-, mid-, and high-frequency region, not just at 2000 Hz.[9,10]

Second, Carhart notch at 2000 Hz is not invariably observed in patients with the diagnosis of otosclerosis or fixation of the ossicular chain. A group of scientists reported a 2000-Hz notch in bone conduction thresholds for only 31% of 102 patients

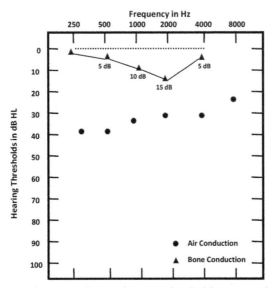

Fig. 1. Typical air and bone conduction hearing threshold patterns for a patient with otosclerosis. Notice the appearance of Carhart notch in bone conduction hearing at 2000 Hz. The *dotted line* indicates true bone conduction hearing or "cochlear reserve." (*Courtesy of* James W. Hall III, PhD, Salus University, Elkins Park, PA.)

with stapes fixation.[7] Finally, related to this second point, patients with etiologies for conductive hearing loss other than otosclerosis may show a notching deficit in bone conduction thresholds at 2000 Hz. Studies have reported the presence of Carhart notch in one-third of a series of 75 patients with congenital aural atresia.[8] Carhart notch pattern was shown only for 30% of patients with malleus or incus fixation and for 26% of 19 patients with detachment or discontinuity at the malleus and incus joint.[7] The resonant frequencies of the middle ear and particularly the ossicular chain seem to be in the vicinity of 2000 Hz, which is potentially why a reduction at 2000 Hz is seen in a good number of patients with stapes fixation as seen in otosclerosis.[4,7,8] In advanced cases of otosclerosis, conductive hearing loss develops into mixed hearing loss. Additionally, in cases with cochlear otosclerosis, moderate to profound sensorineural hearing losses are commonly observed in clinical practice.

Two additional pure tone hearing tests deserve mention because they sometimes contribute to the accurate assessment of auditory status in patients with otosclerosis. One is the audiometric Weber test and the other procedure is the sensorineural acuity level or sensorineural acuity level test.[2,3,11,12] The sensorineural acuity level technique provides valuable clinical information and plays a unique role in clinical audiology when performed with insert earphones and used as a supplement to conventional bone-conduction measurements for confirming ear-specific information on sensory hearing thresholds (see **Table 1**).

As summarized in **Table 1**, three other auditory findings are consistent with fixation of the ossicular chain and typical of patients with otosclerosis, in addition to the conductive hearing loss and Carhart notch. One is a shallow type A tympanogram, referred to as type As, which reflects abnormal restriction of the ossicular chain (discussed later).[3,13] A second typical finding is the absence of normal acoustic reflex activity, even for patients who have little evidence of conductive hearing loss with pure tone audiometry.[2,3] Indeed, the presence of acoustic reflex activity at expected intensity levels, that is, about 85 dB for pure tone stimuli, essentially rules out fixation of the ossicular chain and otosclerosis. Third, word recognition scores in quiet are good or excellent in most patients with otosclerosis, even in those with some apparent deficit in bone conduction hearing thresholds.

We conclude this discussion of auditory findings in otosclerosis with a few comments about the possible application of otoacoustic emissions (OAEs). There is a general consensus that OAEs are not recordable in patients with middle ear dysfunction including those with fixation of the ossicular chain and otosclerosis. However, several recent published papers describe a potential role for OAEs in the evaluation of auditory function following "microtraumatic stapedotomy."[14,15] Although results are inconsistent among studies and variable among patients, there are reports of the emergence of detectable OAEs in the frequency region of 1000 to 1500 Hz perhaps associated with normalization of the resonance frequency of the middle ear following microtraumatic stapedotomy.

MIDDLE EAR ANALYSIS IN OTOSCLEROTIC EARS

For clinicians, middle ear analysis is the most important diagnostic component of otosclerosis. Many have encountered cases with a conductive pathology and normally appearing tympanograms where the nature of underlying pathology is not clear. Simply put, not all of the ears with otosclerosis show a reduced tympanometric compliance and not all of the tympanograms with reduced compliance are caused by otosclerosis. The following section describes the science behind differentiation of the underlying middle ear pathologies with the use of immittance measurements.

Immittance Measurements

Immittance measurement has been used for several decades in the assessment of middle ear disorders. Immittance measurement consists of tympanometry and middle ear muscle reflex (MMR). Individuals with otosclerosis typically present a conductive hearing loss, sometimes type As or normal type A tympanograms,[16,17] absent MMRs, and normal otoscopic results. The normal otoscopy with conductive hearing loss is not distinctive to otosclerosis.[18] Similar patterns have been observed in cases of superior canal dehiscence and ossicular discontinuity.[19] However, MMRs are present in superior canal dehiscence and a type Ad tympanogram is observed in ossicular chain discontinuity. Differentiation of middle ear pathologies with the use of immittance measurements can sometimes be paradoxic.

Tympanometry

Tympanometry is a safe and quick method for assessing middle ear function. In this technique, a pliable probe is sealed in the external ear canal. Then a sound is presented while the air pressure is changed within the ear canal. The sound pressure level monitored at the probe tip provides an index of the ease with which acoustic energy flows into the middle ear system, which is referred to as acoustic admittance (Ya). Currently, tympanometry is mainly conducted at a conventional low probe tone frequency. Tympanometry performed at conventional low probe tone frequency (226 Hz) cannot identify most of the lesions that specifically affect the ossicular chain. For example, information provided by a conventional 226-Hz tympanogram is typically inadequate for distinguishing a normal middle ear from otosclerotic (stapes fixation) ears.[20–26]

Different parameters can be obtained from a conventional low probe tone frequency tympanogram. Two absolute parameters, static admittance (Y_{tm} – admittance at the level of the tympanic membrane) and tympanometric width in daPa, are most often derived from conventional low probe tone frequency tympanometry. Several studies have compared Y_{tm} in healthy and otosclerotic ears.[16,25–30] These studies have consistently shown that, on average, Y_{tm} tends to be lower in otosclerotic ears. However, the extensive overlap in the distributions of Y_{tm} for these two groups at conventional low probe tone frequency severely limits the diagnostic utility of this measure.

It has been shown that an abnormality is most obvious when the probe tone frequency approaches the frequency at which middle ear vibrates most readily.[26,31–33] This frequency is called the resonant frequency. Middle ear pathologies, such as otosclerosis, affect the resonant frequency of the middle ear system. The greatest impact of middle ear pathology on the Y_{tm} is at frequencies close to the resonant frequency.[26,34] Therefore, Y_{tm} measured in the vicinity of the resonant frequency may provide the most useful information regarding the differential diagnosis of middle ear pathologies. Several clinical and laboratory studies have reported prominent differences between healthy and otosclerotic ears[25,26,33,35–37] when Y_{tm} recorded using higher probe tone frequencies or resonant frequency were compared between healthy ears and otosclerotic ears.

Tympanometric shape has also been reported to be affected by otosclerosis. A measure that is, most commonly used to index the sharpness of the tympanometric peak at conventional low probe tone frequency is the tympanometric width. Some studies have reported narrower tympanometric peaks in otosclerotic ears than healthy ears.[25,38–40]

The appearance of multifrequency devices has made it possible to derive immittance subcomponents, susceptance (B) and conductance (G), and to perform tympanometry across a wide range of probe tone frequencies. Recent studies suggest that identification of otosclerosis (or stapes fixation) is improved using measures derived from multifrequency tympanometry or by combining tympanometric variables in specific ways.[25,26,31,33,41,42]

One potentially useful parameter that is derived from multifrequency tympanometry is an estimate of the middle ear resonant frequency. The resonant frequency of the middle ear system may be shifted higher or lower compared with healthy ears by various pathologies. One major effect of otosclerosis is to increase the stiffness of the middle ear system resulting in a shift of the middle ear resonant frequency to the higher values. In the case of otosclerosis, the resonant frequency has been shown to be significantly higher than healthy ears.[21,25,26,43–47]

Middle Ear Muscle Reflex

MMR is measured by monitoring the change of the immittance, either a decrease in admittance or an increase in impedance, in the ear canal in response to a sufficiently loud sound. Stapedial muscles contract in both ears simultaneously in response to a sufficiently loud sound presented to one or both ears. This contraction is recorded in either ear by monitoring the change of immittance, which is time-locked to the stimulus presentation. To elicit stapedial muscle contraction in response to a loud sound, middle ear (conductive system), cochlea, 8th cranial nerve, and stapedial branch of the 7th cranial nerve should be intact. MMR is an excellent tool in conjunction with tympanometry to detect the presence or absence of the middle ear disorders including otosclerosis.

Normally, MMR is absent in presence of a modest conductive hearing loss of only 20 dB.[48] Typically, in cases of unilateral otosclerosis, MMR is absent in the ipsilateral mode (stimulus and probe tone are presented to the affected side-probe ear). However, MMR is elevated or absent in contralateral mode depending on the severity of the conductive hearing loss. It should be noted that contralateral MMR in the unaffected side is also absent when the probe is placed in the affected side (probe effect). The reason for the absence of MMR in the probe ear is that it is not possible to monitor the changes in immittance as a result of the stapedial contraction likely because of the stiffening of the ossicular chain, which prevents stapedial muscle to evoke a measurable change in the immittance.[48]

It should be noted that in early stages of otosclerosis a biphasic reflex response (an on-off effect also known as a diphasic response) has been observed.[49] This effect has been observed even before the commencement of an air-bone gap in the otosclerotic ears.[50] The biphasic middle ear reflex response is characterized by a sudden increase in admittance (a paradoxic response, as stapedial muscle contraction, should result in a decrease in admittance) by switching the stimulus on and off, which surrounds a central plateau at 0.

Wideband Acoustic Immittance

Wideband acoustic immittance (WAI) (**Fig. 2**) is a new middle ear assessment technique that has enabled researchers and clinicians to quantify the reflected, or the absorbed energy in the ear canal across a wide range of frequencies typically between 250 and 8000 Hz.[48] Power absorbance (PA) is a ratio of absorbed power over the incident power and varies between 0 and 1. A value of 0 means all sound energy has been reflected back and a value of 1 means all sound energy has been absorbed by the middle ear system.[48]

WAI has several potential advantages over conventional tympanometry. The technique measures over a large range of frequencies (250–8000 Hz). It is also very fast, taking only a couple of seconds to perform. Additionally, the magnitude of the PA

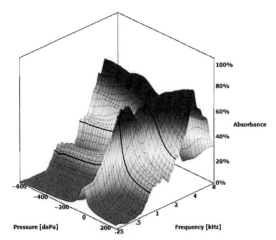

Fig. 2. Wideband acoustic immittance tracings showing three-dimensional multifrequency evaluation and power absorbance of the middle ear. (*Courtesy of* Interacoustics Audiology Solutions, Middelfart, Denmark; with permission.)

does not depend on the distance between the probe tip and the eardrum and so the location of the probe in the ear canal is not as critical as it is in tympanometry in children and adults.[51] Finally, WAI can be run at ambient pressure and does not require pressurization of the ear canal.[52] It is, however, possible to run a pressurized WAI measurement by varying the pressure in a manner identical to tympanometry.[53] At ambient pressures, healthy adults show a pattern of low absorption in the low frequencies, which increases to a maximum between 1000 Hz and 4000 Hz before decreasing again at high frequencies.[54] **Fig. 3** demonstrates this pattern in a normal-hearing individual.

Growing body of the literature suggests that WAI is a good indicator of middle ear pathologies in neonates, children, and adults.[55–63] Compared with conventional 226-Hz tympanometry, WAI may provide for a more sensitive test in evaluating middle ear disorders and conductive hearing loss.[52,64,65] In contrast to conventional 226-Hz tympanometry, WAI is significantly more sensitive to ossicular pathologies.[18] Moreover, the patterns of absorbance vary depending on the status of the middle ear and thus different pathologies result in different patterns of absorbance. Generally, a stiffening pathology results in decreased absorbance over a specific frequency range. For example, otosclerotic ears demonstrate significantly increased reflectance between 400 Hz and 1000 Hz.[18] Researchers found that PA was the most effective way of identifying ears with otosclerosis compared with 226-Hz tympanometry and multifrequency tympanometry.[18] PA was able to identify otosclerosis in 82% of their sample and had a false-positive rate of 17.2%. The research suggests that the use of PA in conjunction with other tools for assessment of middle ear function will improve the identification of otosclerotic ears in a clinical setting.[18] **Fig. 4** demonstrates an example of PA in surgically confirmed otosclerotic ears. The PA was obtained before the surgery and fixation of the stapes was confirmed during the surgery.

AUDIOLOGIC INTERVENTION FOR OTOSCLEROSIS

Auditory complications of otosclerosis include hearing loss and tinnitus. Involved patients rarely complain about sound sensitivity disorders, such as hyperacusis, and the

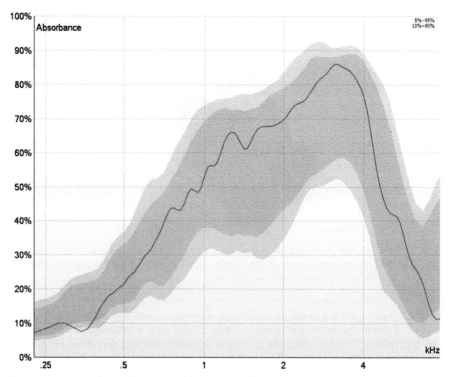

Fig. 3. Power absorbance in a normal-hearing adult. The y-axis is absorbance in % and the x-axis is the frequency in Hz. The shaded areas represent 80% (*dark gray*) and 90% range (*light gray*) of the normative data. (*Courtesy of* Navid Shahnaz, PhD, University of British Columbia, Vancouver, BC, Canada.)

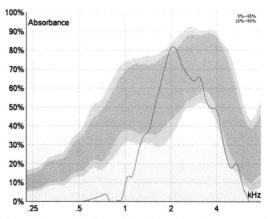

Fig. 4. Power absorbance in a surgically confirmed otosclerotic ear. Note that the absorption less than 1500 Hz is significantly reduced compared with the 90% range for normal individuals (*shaded area*). The y-axis is absorbance in % and the x-axis is the frequency in Hz. (*Courtesy of* Navid Shahnaz, PhD, University of British Columbia, Vancouver, BC, Canada.)

reports of vertigo and balance disorders are not common in presurgical otosclerotic ears. Many patients with otosclerosis are treated with otologic surgery; however, occasionally patients may choose amplification instead of surgery for medical complications, such as stapes gusher or dehiscence of anterior semicircular canals, which may be revealed by high-resolution computed tomography scans.[66] A survey of 184 otologists indicated that hearing aids are advised before surgery.[67]

Hearing Aids and Implantable Auditory Devices

Hearing aid evaluation should always be discussed and offered to have a well-informed consent before to surgery. Occasionally there are patients who do not select surgical management as a solution for their hearing loss and choose amplification. Additionally, because of some unforeseen circumstances, patients' hearing sensitivity does not improve or even worsen after surgical intervention[68] and patients are advised to use hearing aids. Use of hearing aids has been helpful in the management of hearing loss postsurgery.[69–71] Hearing loss caused by otosclerosis can also exacerbate because of sensorineural involvement[72] and this similarly heightens the inclusion of amplification and hearing management protocols in this population.

Modern hearing aids are highly advanced and small.[73] **Fig. 5** demonstrates contemporary hearing aids. Most of today's hearing aids are digital and have the ability of super computation and signal processing. The employment of wireless technology, such as Bluetooth, has enabled users to stream their telephone conversation and music or news to their hearing aids reducing the stigma of hearing aid use. Otologists should encourage their patients to use hearing aids and emphasize the role of neuroplasticity and enhancement of auditory function for the hearing impaired. There is ample evidence in the literature that supports the improvement of auditory function with amplification not only in patients with sensorineural hearing loss but also in those with conductive pathology.[74–77]

Those patients who choose amplification should receive ample amount of time for rehabilitation, orientation, verification, and validation by their audiologists. Successful hearing aid users usually are the ones who communicate effectively with their audiologists about their hearing aids. The advanced clinical standards and practice guidelines emphasize the role of real ear measurements in proper amplification and

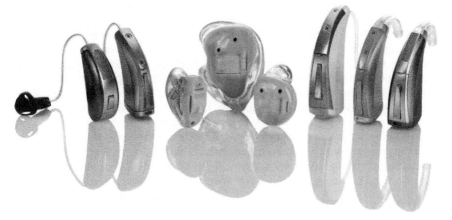

Fig. 5. Modern hearing aids. These hearing aids can stream acoustic signals from electronic devices, such as cell phones and tablets, directly to the hearing aids. (*Courtesy of* Starkey Laboratories, Eden Prairie, MN; with permission.)

verification of hearing devices. Unfortunately, most of the over-the-counter hearing aids lack such standards of care.

The amplification management of hearing loss in otosclerosis can also be accomplished with the use of implantable technology. Auditory prosthesis and implantable devices, such as bone-anchored hearing aids[78] and Bonebridge,[79] have been used as alternatives for conventional hearing aids. These implantable devices provide direct signal transmission through bone conduction (ie, bypassing the middle ear with a conductive pathology, such as otosclerosis), which results in direct stimulation of the cochlea. The bone-anchored hearing aid approach also has been used in pathologies, such as congenital atresia and chronic otitis media.[78] In far advanced otosclerosis, profound or total hearing loss can be detected. These cases of far advanced otosclerotic ears have been managed by cochlear implants with great success.[80,81]

Tinnitus Management in Patients with Otosclerosis

For a large number of patients with otosclerosis, tinnitus can be as annoying as hearing loss. Tinnitus caused by otosclerosis has been associated with reversible modifications in the central auditory pathway because of conductive hearing loss.[82]

In many cases of patients with otosclerosis, tinnitus may improve following surgical intervention.[83] Current research indicated tinnitus improvement of 85% of cases within 6 months following stapedectomy.[83] A recent study has shown improvement of low-frequency tinnitus following stapedectomy; however, the researchers of the same study also reported that high-frequency tinnitus persists following surgical intervention.[84] The improvement of tinnitus also has been reported in patients with stapedotomy.[85]

Tinnitus improvement following stapedectomy is age-related. It has been shown that younger patients with otosclerosis may get relief from tinnitus following surgical intervention when compared with the older subjects.[86] In some cases, tinnitus may persist or even become louder after the surgery. Therefore, tinnitus management and intervention is an important component of the postsurgical management of otosclerosis.

Tinnitus management for patients with otosclerosis falls in the line of tinnitus management protocols that are used for those with sensorineural hearing loss caused by such conditions as noise-induced hearing loss or degenerative changes of the auditory system caused by aging. Tinnitus management includes such approaches as counseling, sound therapy, acoustic enrichment, and use of amplification.[87,88] Many patients report no significant perception of tinnitus with the use of hearing aids. The masking effect of amplification diminishes the patient's awareness of his or her tinnitus. In some cases, particularly in those patients with no significant hearing loss, cognitive behavioral therapy has been used for better coping with tinnitus.[89,90] The cognitive behavioral therapy and potentially sound therapy have been supported as effective methods for tinnitus management by practice guidelines presented by academic and clinical professionals.[91] Many patients habituate to their tinnitus with help and guidance from professionals who are specialized in tinnitus management. Attention to the patients' annoyance from tinnitus is important and clinicians should never dismiss the problem by downplaying tinnitus. Clinicians should avoid such statements as "nothing can be done." Tinnitus is a manageable condition!

Balance Disorders and Otosclerosis

Vertigo is rare in nonoperated otosclerotic ears; however, presence of vertigo may suggest inner ear malformation[92] or vestibular hair cell loss.[93] There is also evidence that otosclerosis is associated with endolymphatic hydrops and use of

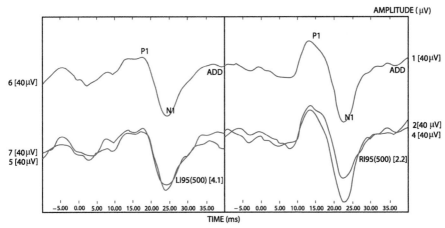

Fig. 6. Cervical vestibular evoked myogenic potential recordings in a confirmed case of superior canal dehiscence. Note the enhanced amplitude on the right side. (*Courtesy of Ali A. Danesh, MS, PhD, Florida Atlantic University, Boca Raton, FL.*)

electrocochleagraphy for better diagnosis has been reported.[94] Occasionally, patients with otosclerosis develop vertigo and dizziness following surgery.[95–97] A recent report has included secondary endolymphatic hydrops following operative interventions for otosclerosis as a pathologic finding.[98] Extensive evaluation and providing vestibular therapy is important for those who suffer from vertigo or other balance disorders. The vestibular evaluation test battery may include such procedures as videonystagmography, caloric tests, video head impulse test, and cervical and ocular vestibular evoked myogenic potential assesments.[99,100] These evaluations, particularly vestibular evoked myogenic potential studies, are helpful in the better diagnosis of such conditions as superior canal dehiscence, which potentially is associated with otosclerosis in some cases.[100–102] In general, low vestibular evoked myogenic potential thresholds and enhanced amplitudes in cases with superior canal dehiscence are expected **(Fig. 6)**.[101–103] For patients with otosclerosis who develop balance disorders, vestibular therapy, balance exercises, and vestibuloadaptive therapy have been shown to be effective in managing their symptoms.[104]

REFERENCES

1. Carhart R. Effects of stapes fixation on bone-conduction responses. In: Schuknecht HF, editor. Otosclerosis. Boston: Little, Brown; 1962. p. 175–97.
2. Hall JW III, Ghorayeb B. Diagnosis of middle ear pathology and evaluation of conductive hearing loss. In: Jacobson J, Northern J, editors. Diagnostic audiology. Austin (TX): Pro-Ed; 1991. p. 161–98.
3. Hall JW III. Introduction to audiology today. Boston: Pearson Educational; 2014.
4. Carhart R. Clinical application of bone conduction audiometry. Arch Otolaryngol 1950;51:798–808.
5. Yasan H. Predictive role of Carhart's notch in pre-operative assessment for middle-ear surgery. J Laryngol Otol 2007;121:219–21.
6. Ahmad I, Pahor AL. Carhart's notch: a finding in otitis media with effusion. Int J Pediatr Otorhinolaryngol 2002;64:165–70.
7. Koshio A, Ito K, Kakigi A, et al. Carhart notch 2-kHz bone conduction threshold dip. Arch Otolaryngol Head Neck Surg 2011;137:236–40.

8. Zhang L, Gao N, Yin Y, et al. Bone conduction hearing in congenital aural atresia. Eur Arch Otorhinolaryngol 2016;273:1697–703.

9. Perez R, de Almeida J, Nedzelski JM, et al. Variations in the "Carhart notch" and overclosure after laser-assisted stapedotomy in otosclerosis. Otol Neurotol 2009;30:1033–6.

10. Shambaugh GE Jr. Surgery of the ear. Philadelphia: WB Saunders; 1959.

11. Hall JW III, Mueller HG III. Audiologists' desk reference. I. Diagnostic audiometry. San Diego (CA): Singular Publishing; 1997.

12. Tillman TW. Clinical applicability of the SAL test. Arch Otolaryngol 1963;78: 20–32.

13. Jerger JF, Anthony L, Jerger S, et al. Studies in impedance audiometry: III. Middle ear disorders. Arch Otolaryngol 1974;99:165–71.

14. Mantzari E, Maragoudakis P, Kandiloros D, et al. The profile of optoacoustic emissions and multifrequency tympanometry in otosclerotic patients undergoing two types of stapes surgery: small fenestra and microtraumatic stapedotomy. Med Sci Monit 2014;20:1613–20.

15. Singh PP, Gupta N, Verma P. Transient evoked and distortion product otoacoustic emission profile in patients of otosclerosis: a preliminary report. Indian J Otolaryngol Head Neck Surg 2012;64:25–30.

16. Jerger J. Clinical experience with impedance audiometry. Arch Otolaryngol 1970;92:311–24.

17. Jerger J. Suggested nomenclature for impedance audiometry. Arch Otolaryngol 1972;96:1–3.

18. Shahnaz N, Bork K, Polka L, et al. Energy reflectance and tympanometry in normal and otosclerotic ears. Ear Hear 2009;30:219–33.

19. Nakajima HH, Pisano DV, Roosli C, et al. Comparison of ear-canal reflectance and umbo velocity in patients with conductive hearing loss: a preliminary study. Ear Hear 2012;33:35–43.

20. Colletti V. Tympanometry from 200 to 2000 Hz probe tone. Audiology 1976;15: 106–19.

21. Colletti V. Multifrequency tympanometry. Audiology 1977;16:278–87.

22. Hunter LL, Margolis RH. Multifrequency tympanometry: current clinical application. Am J Audiol 1992;1:33–43.

23. Lilly D. Multiple frequency, multiple component tympanometry: new approaches to an old diagnostic problem. Ear Hear 1984;5:300–8.

24. Van Camp K, Creten W, Vande Heyning P, et al. A search for the most suitable immittance components and probe tone frequencies in tympanometry. Scand Audiol 1983;12:27–34.

25. Shahnaz N, Polka L. Standard and multifrequency tympanometry in normal and otosclerotic ears. Ear Hear 1997;18:326–41.

26. Shahnaz N, Polka L. Distinguishing healthy from otosclerotic ears: effect of probe-tone frequency on static immittance. J Am Acad Audiol 2002;13:345–55.

27. Alberti PW, Kristansen R. The clinical application of impedance audiometry. A preliminary appraisal of an electro-acoustic impedance bridge. Laryngoscope 1970;80:735–46.

28. Browning GG, Swan IRC, Gatehouse S. The doubtful value of tympanometry with diagnosis of otosclerosis. J Laryngol Otol 1985;99:545–7.

29. Liden G, Peterson JL, Bjorkman G. Tympanometry. Arch Otolaryngol 1970;92: 248–57.

30. Muchnik C, Hildesheimer M, Rubinstein M, et al. Validity of tympanometry in cases of confirmed otosclerosis. J Laryngol Otol 1989;103:36–8.

31. Margolis R, Shanks JE. Tympanometry: principles and procedures. In: Rintelmann WF, editor. Hearing assessment. Austin (TX): Pro-Ed; 1991. p. 179–246.
32. Shanks JE. Tympanometry. Ear Hear 1984;5:268–80.
33. Zhao F, Wada H, Koike T, et al. Middle ear dynamic characteristics in patients with otosclerosis. Ear Hear 2002;23:150–8.
34. Liden G, Harford E, Hallen O. Tympanometry for the diagnosis of ossicular disruption. Arch Otolaryngol 1974;99:23–9.
35. Burke K, Nilges TA. Comparison of three middle ear impedance norms as predictors of otosclerosis. J Aud Res 1970;10:52–8.
36. Margolis R, Osguthorpe J, Popelka G. The effects of experimentally-produced middle ear lesions on tympanometry in cats. Acta Otolaryngol 1978;86:428–36.
37. Zwislocki J. An acoustic method for clinical examination of the ear. J Speech Hear Res 1963;6:303–14.
38. Dieroff H. Differential diagnostic value of tympanometry in adhesive processes and otosclerosis. Audiology 1978;17:77–86.
39. Ivey R. Tympanometric curves and otosclerosis. J Speech Hear Res 1975;18:554–8.
40. Koebsell K, Shanks J, Cone-Wesson BK, et al. Tympanometric width measures in normal and pathologic ears. ASHA 1988;30:99.
41. Lilly D. Measurement of acoustic impedance at the tympanic membrane. In: Jerger J, editor. Modern developments in audiology. New York: Academic Press; 1973. p. 345–406.
42. Shanks JE, Shelton C. Basic principles and clinical applications of tympanometry. Otolaryngol Clin North Am 1991;24:299–328.
43. Colletti V, Fiorino F, Sittoni V, et al. Mechanics of the middle ear in otosclerosis and stapedoplasty. Acta Otolaryngol 1993;113:637–41.
44. Funasaka S, Funai H, Kumakawa K. Sweep frequency tympanometry: its development and diagnostic value. Audiology 1984;23:366–79.
45. Funasaka S, Kumakawa K. Tympanometry using a sweep frequency probe tone and its clinical evaluation. Audiology 1988;27:99–108.
46. Valvik B, Johnsen M, Laukli E. Multifrequency tympanometry. Audiology 1994;33:245–53.
47. Wada H, Koike T, Kobayashi T. Clinical applicability of the sweep frequency measuring apparatus for diagnosis of middle ear diseases. Ear Hear 1988;19:240–9.
48. Hunter LL, Shahnaz N. Acoustic immittance measures: basic and advanced practice. San Diego (CA): Plural Publishing; 2014.
49. Flottorp G, Djupesland G. Diphasic impedance change and its applicability in clinical work. Acta Otolaryngol 1970;263:200–5.
50. Bell J, Causse JR, Michaux P, et al. Mechanical explanation of the on-off effect (diphasic impedance change) in otospongiosis. Audiology 1976;15:128–30.
51. Voss SE, Horton NJ, Woodbury RR, et al. Sources of variability in reflectance measurements on normal cadaver ears. Ear Hear 2008;29:651–65.
52. Shahnaz N, Longridge N, Bell D. Wideband energy reflectance patterns in pre-operative and post-operative otosclerotic ears. Int J Audiol 2009;48:240–7.
53. Keefe DH, Levi E. Maturation of the middle and external ears: acoustic power-based responses and reflectance tympanometry. Ear Hear 1996;17:361–73.
54. Shahnaz N, Bork K. Wideband reflectance norms for caucasian and Chinese young adults. Ear Hear 2006;27:774–88.

55. Hunter LL, Feeney MP, Lapsley Miller JA, et al. Wideband reflectance in new-borns: normative regions and relationship to hearing screening results. Ear Hear 2010;31:599–610.

56. Keefe DH, Abdala C. Theory of forward and reverse middle-ear transmission applied to optoacoustic emissions in infant and adult ears. J Acoust Soc Am 2007;121:978–93.

57. Keefe DH, Folsom R, Gorga MP, et al. Identification of neonatal hearing impairment: ear-canal measurements of acoustic admittance and reflectance in neonates. Ear Hear 2000;21:443–61.

58. Merchant GR, Horton NJ, Voss SE. Normative reflectance and transmittance measurements on healthy newborn and 1-month-old infants. Ear Hear 2010; 31:746–54.

59. Sanford CA, Keefe DH, Liu YW, et al. Sound-conduction effects on distortion-product optoacoustic emission screening outcomes in newborn infants: test performance of wideband acoustic transfer functions and 1-kHz tympanometry. Ear Hear 2009;30:635–52.

60. Hunter LL, Tubaugh L, Jackson JA, et al. Wideband middle ear power measurement in infants and children. J Am Acad Audiol 2008;19:309–24.

61. Keefe DH, Bulen JC, Arehart KH, et al. Ear-canal impedance and reflection coefficient in human infants and adults. J Acoust Soc Am 1993;94:2617–38.

62. Sanford C, Feeney MP. Effects of maturation on tympanometric wideband acoustic transfer functions in human infants. J Acoust Soc Am 2008;124: 2106–22.

63. Van der Werff KR, Prieve BA, Georgantas LM. Test–retest reliability of wideband reflectance measures in infants under screening and diagnostic test conditions. Ear Hear 2007;28:669–81.

64. Beers AN, Shahnaz N, Westerberg BD, et al. Wideband reflectance in normal Caucasian and Chinese school-aged children and in children with otitis media with effusion. Ear Hear 2010;31:221–33.

65. Feeney MP, Grant IL, Marryott LP. Wideband energy reflectance measurements in adults with middle-ear disorders. J Speech Lang Hear Res 2003;46:901–11.

66. Nguyen DQ, Morel N, Dumas G, et al. Dehiscence of the anterior semicircular canal and otosclerosis: a case report. Rev Laryngol Otol Rhinol (Bord) 2006; 127:151–5.

67. Lancer H, Manickavasagam J, Zaman A, et al. Stapes surgery: a National Survey of British Otologists. Eur Arch Otorhinolaryngol 2016;273:371–9.

68. Justicz N, Strickland KF, Motamedi KK, et al. Review of a single surgeon's stapedotomy cases performed with a nickel titanium prosthesis over a 14-year period. Acta Otolaryngol 2017;137:442–6.

69. Johnson EW. Hearing aids and otosclerosis. Otolaryngol Clin North Am 1993;26: 491–502.

70. Redfors YD, Möller C. Otosclerosis: thirty-year follow-up after surgery. Ann Otol Rhinol Laryngol 2011;120:608–14.

71. Redfors YD, Hellgren J, Möller C. Hearing-aid use and benefit: a long-term follow-up in patients undergoing surgery for otosclerosis. Int J Audiol 2013;52: 194–9.

72. Ishai R, Halpin CF, Shin JJ, et al. Long-term incidence and degree of sensorineural hearing loss in otosclerosis. Otol Neurotol 2016;37:1489–96.

73. Saul RS, Danesh AA, Williams DF. The auditory system. In: Williams DF, editor. Communication sciences and disorders: an introduction to the professions. New York: Psychology Press, Taylor & Francis Group; 2012. p. 241–73.

74. Glick H, Sharma A. Cross-modal plasticity in developmental and age-related hearing loss: clinical implications. Hear Res 2017;343:191–201.
75. Lavie L, Banai K, Karni A, et al. Hearing aid-induced plasticity in the auditory system of older adults: evidence from speech perception. J Speech Lang Hear Res 2015;58:1601–10.
76. Leite RA, Magliaro FC, Raimundo JC, et al. Effect of hearing aids use on speech stimulus decoding through speech-evoked ABR. Braz J Otorhinolaryngol 2016 [pii:S1808-8694(16)30236-1].
77. Shiell MM, Champoux F, Zatorre RJ. Reorganization of auditory cortex in early-deaf people: functional connectivity and relationship to hearing aid use. J Cogn Neurosci 2015;27:150–63.
78. Ricci G, Della Volpe A, Faralli M, et al. Results and complications of the BAHA system (bone-anchored hearing aid). Eur Arch Otorhinolaryngol 2010;267:1539–45.
79. Bianchin G, Bonali M, Russo M, et al. Active bone conduction system: outcomes with the Bonebridge transcutaneous device. ORL J Otorhinolaryngol Relat Spec 2015;77:17–26.
80. Berrettini S, Burdo S, Forli F, et al. Far advanced otosclerosis: stapes surgery or cochlear implantation? J Otolaryngol 2004;33:165–71.
81. Calmels MN, Viana C, Wanna G, et al. Very far-advanced otosclerosis: stapedotomy or cochlear implantation. Acta Otolaryngol 2007;127:574–8.
82. Deggouj N, Castelein S, Gerard JM, et al. Tinnitus and otosclerosis. B-ENT 2009;5:241–4.
83. Chang CY, Cheung SW. Tinnitus modulation by stapedectomy. Otol Neurotol 2014;35:1065–9.
84. Ismi O, Erdogan O, Yesilova M, et al. Does stapes surgery improve tinnitus in patients with otosclerosis? Braz J Otorhinolaryngol 2017;83(5):568–73.
85. Bast F, Mazurek B, Schrom T. Effect of stapedotomy on pre-operative tinnitus and its psychosomatic burden. Auris Nasus Larynx 2013;40:530–3.
86. Bagger-Sjöbäck D, Strömbäck K, Hultcrantz M, et al. High-frequency hearing, tinnitus, and patient satisfaction with stapedotomy: a randomized prospective study. Sci Rep 2015;5:13341.
87. Nagashino K, Kinouchi Y, Danesh AA, et al. A computational model for tinnitus generation and its management by sound therapy. Int J Biol Biomed Eng 2014;8:191–6.
88. Sweetow RW, Sabes JH. Effects of acoustical stimuli delivered through hearing aids on tinnitus. J Am Acad Audiol 2010;21:461–73.
89. Cima RF, Andersson G, Schmidt CJ, et al. Cognitive-behavioral treatments for tinnitus: a review of the literature. J Am Acad Audiol 2014;25:29–61.
90. Aazh H, Moore BC, Lammaing K, et al. Tinnitus and hyperacusis therapy in a UK National Health Service audiology department: patients' evaluations of the effectiveness of treatments. Int J Audiol 2016;55:514–22.
91. Tunke DE, Bauer CA, Sun GH, et al. Clinical practice guideline: tinnitus. Otolaryngol Head Neck Surg 2014;151:S1–40.
92. Bertholon P, Karkas A. Otologic disorders causing dizziness, including surgery for vestibular disorders. Handb Clin Neurol 2016;137:279–93.
93. Hızlı Ö, Kaya S, Schachern PA, et al. Quantitative assessment of vestibular otopathology in otosclerosis: a temporal bone study. Laryngoscope 2016;126:E118–22.
94. Shea JJ Jr, Ge X, Orchik DJ. Endolymphatic hydrops associated with otosclerosis. Am J Otol 1994;15:348–57.

95. de Vilhena D, Gambôa I, Duarte D, et al. Vestibular disorders after stapedial surgery in patients with otosclerosis. Int J Otolaryngol 2016;2016:6830648.
96. Grayeli AB, Sterkers O, Toupet M. Audiovestibular function in patients with otosclerosis and balance disorders. Otol Neurotol 2009;30:1085–91.
97. Hirvonen TP, Aalto H. Immediate postoperative nystagmus and vestibular symptoms after stapes surgery. Acta Otolaryngol 2013;133:842–5.
98. Ferster APO, Cureoglu S, Keskin N, et al. Secondary endolymphatic hydrops. Otol Neurotol 2017;38:774–9.
99. Lin KY, Young YH. Role of ocular VEMP test in assessing the occurrence of vertigo in otosclerosis patients. Clin Neurophysiol 2015;126:187–93.
100. Tramontani O, Gkoritsa E, Ferekidis E, et al. Contribution of vestibular-evoked myogenic potential (VEMP) testing in the assessment and the differential diagnosis of otosclerosis. Med Sci Monit 2014;20:205–13.
101. Hope A, Fagan P. Latent superior canal dehiscence syndrome unmasked by stapedotomy for otosclerosis. J Laryngol Otol 2010;124:428–30.
102. Van Rompaey V, Potvin J, van den Hauwe L, et al. Third mobile window associated with suspected otosclerotic foci in two patients with an air-bone gap. J Laryngol Otol 2011;125:89–92.
103. Hunter JB, Patel NS, O'Connell BP, et al. Cervical and ocular VEMP testing in diagnosing superior semicircular canal dehiscence. Otolaryngol Head Neck Surg 2017;156:917–23.
104. Morozova SV, Dobrotin VE, Kulakova LA, et al. Vestibular disorders in patients with otosclerosis: prevalence, diagnostic and therapeutic options. Vestn Otorinolaringol 2009;2:20–2.

Impact of Imaging in Management of Otosclerosis

Amit Wolfovitz, MD[a], Michal Luntz, MD[b],*

KEYWORDS

- Otosclerosis • Computerized tomography • MRI

KEY POINTS

- Imaging is a useful adjunct to the clinical and audiometric information and is often critical to confirm the correct diagnosis and prevent potential complications.
- High-resolution computed tomography (HRCT) without contrast is the modality of choice for the demonstration of fenestral and retro-fenestral (cochlear) spongiotic lesions.
- Both HRCT and MRI are recommended before cochlear implantation surgery in patients with a far-advanced otosclerosis.

INTRODUCTION

Traditionally, imaging was not considered a requirement for the diagnosis of otosclerosis-related hearing loss (ORHL). Histologic changes typical to otosclerosis were described more than 100 years ago,[1–5] although were not found to correlate with the severity of conductive or sensorineural hearing loss[6]; the radiographic findings for otosclerosis were described more than 50 years ago.[7] Nevertheless, controversy exists regarding the correlation between imaging and the degree of hearing loss in otosclerosis.[8–18] Typical otosclerosis-related imaging is useful when evaluating patients with ORHL before primary as well as revision stapes surgery. Imaging is considered the standard of care in far-advanced otosclerosis before cochlear implantation.[8,11,14]

DISEASE OVERVIEW

The pathophysiologic hallmark of the fenestral subtype of otosclerosis is remodeling of the temporal bone that is primarily taking place in the area of the oval window,

Disclosure: The authors have nothing to disclose.
[a] Department of Otolaryngology–Head and Neck Surgery, University of Miami, Miller School of Medicine, 1120 N.W. 14th Street, #5, Miami, FL 33136, USA; [b] Department of Otolaryngology–Head and Neck Surgery, Bnai Zion Medical Center, The Ruth and Bruce Rappaport Faculty of Medicine, Technion, Israeli School of Technology, Golomb 47 Street, Haifa 31048, Israel
* Corresponding author.
E-mail address: michal.luntz@b-zion.org.il

specifically in its anterior part, the fissula ante fenestram, which is a groove between the oval window and the cochleariform process. During the active (otospongiotic) stage of the disease, hypodense foci of bone can be identified in this area.[8] These foci will be replaced later by sclerotic bone in the nonactive (otosclerotic) stage of the disease that can progressively involve the footplate resulting in its thickening and fixation. This stage of the disease is manifested by progressive conductive hearing loss.[9] In 1% to 10% of the cases, a retro-fenestral subtype of the disease occurs with the disease involving the otic capsule, which might become demineralized, leading to far-advanced otosclerosis (defined by House and Sheehy[19] as longstanding hearing loss secondary to otosclerosis with an air conduction [AC] pure tone average of 85 dB or greater and no measurable bone conduction [BC]).[9,19] Diagnosis of the disease is typically based on history, physical examination, and characteristic audiometric findings.[8,9] Occasionally the course of otosclerosis might deviate from the classic presentation, especially in the retro-fenestral subtypes of the disease when mixed or even pure sensorineural hearing loss might occur.[8] The role of imaging in these challenging situations becomes more significant and is further discussed later in this article.

FENESTRAL AND RETRO-FENESTRAL OTOSCLEROSIS: IMAGING DIAGNOSIS

The most common manifestation of fenestral otosclerosis, especially in its spongiotic active stage, is demineralization of the fissula ante fenestram, anterior to the oval window (**Fig. 1**). In the nonactive otosclerosis, this area becomes sclerotic and in advanced stages of the disease this sclerosis can thicken and obliterate the oval window. The former stage of the disease is usually easier to detect, whereas the later becomes detectable only when significant otosclerotic bone causes irregularity and significant thickening of the otic capsule.[10] These lesions can be demonstrated on axial and coronal sections of high-resolution computed tomography (HRCT) without contrast, with a window level at 300 to 400 Hounsfield units (HU) and a width of 2000 to 3000 HU, the modality of choice for otosclerosis, with sensitivity varying from 34% to 91%.[10] A recent study demonstrated sensitivity higher than 90% in

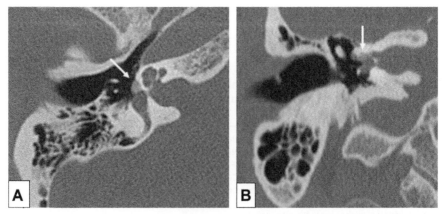

Fig. 1. Fenestral otosclerosis. Axial (*A*) and coronal (*B*) HRCT images of active, spongiotic stage of otosclerosis (*arrow*) with demineralization of the fissula ante fenestram, anterior to the oval window. (*Courtesy of* Simon Angeli, MD, Rita Ghose Bhatia, MD, University of Miami, Miami, FL)

most cases and the ability to describe lesions in the submillimetric scale (using newer computed tomography technology).[9] Another modality based on HRCT is the densitometry measurements of the fissula ante fenestram area, which provides quantitative assessment of the disease and higher sensitivity.[10] Kutlar and colleagues[9] found significantly lower density in active otosclerosis compared with control ears (1131 vs 2091 HU respectively; $P<.05$). The usefulness of densitometry for evaluating outcomes of fluoride treatment is controversial.[10,20] Retro-fenestral (also known as cochlear) otosclerosis is manifested as a lucent area in the normally homogeneously dense, otic capsule. This lucent area might be presenting as focal lucency versus the characteristic double ring/halo sign with lucencies encircling the cochlea (**Fig. 2**).[8,21]

IMAGING-BASED GRADING SYSTEMS FOR OTOSCLEROSIS

Many types of grading systems were developed for otosclerosis based on surgical and histologic findings. Nonetheless, none of these systems are widely accepted. Several radiographic grading systems based on computed tomography were developed in order to describe the location and stage of otosclerosis and often the relationship of the disease radiographic stage and audiometric performance.[9,11–14] Rotteveel and colleagues[14] demonstrated a grading system based on the histologic subdivision of otosclerosis into fenestral and retro-fenestral subtypes (**Table 1**). An additional grading system by Symons and Fanning demonstrated some variation and was found to have excellent interobserver and intraobserver agreement (**Table 2**).[11] Grading systems might seem redundant for most cases with otosclerosis but carry substantial benefits in cases of retro-fenestral (cochlear), far-advanced otosclerosis. In these cases, when patients become potential cochlear implant candidates, the choice of electrode might be influenced based on the extent of the cochlear lesions in order to avoid postoperative facial nerve stimulation with the non-modiolar hugging electrodes.[11]

IMAGING BEFORE REFERRAL FOR STAPES SURGERY

The diagnosis of ORHL and the decision to refer patients for stapes surgery (ie, middle ear exploration with possible stapedectomy/stapedotomy or ossiculoplsty) as part of hearing rehabilitation alternatives have been traditionally defined when patients have a

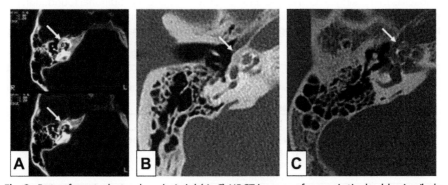

Fig. 2. Retro-fenestral otosclerosis Axial (*A–C*) HRCT images of spongiotic double ring/halo sign with various degrees of lucencies encircling the cochlea in retro-fenestral otosclerosis (*arrow*). (*Courtesy of* Simon Angeli, MD, Rita Ghose Bhatia, MD, University of Miami, Miami, FL.)

Table 1
Rotteveel and colleagues' imaging-based grading systems for otosclerosis[a]

	Otosclerotic Lesions of the Otic Capsule	No. of Ears (%)
Type 1	Solely fenestral involvement (thickened footplate and/or narrowed or enlarged windows)	7 (7)
Type 2	Retro-fenestral with or without fenestral involvement	55 (52)
Type 2a	Double ring effect	26 (25)
Type 2b	Narrowed basal turn	4 (4)
Type 2c	Double ring and narrowed basal turn	25 (23)
Type 3	Severe retro-fenestral (unrecognizable otic capsule), with or without fenestral involvement	27 (25)

Abbreviation: CT, computed tomography.
[a] In 17 (16%) ears, no signs of otosclerosis were detected.
From Rotteveel LJ, Proops DW, Ramsden RT, et al. Cochlear implantation in 53 patients with otosclerosis: demographics, computed tomographic scanning, surgery, and complications. Otol Neurotol 2004;25:946; with permission.

history of conductive or mixed hearing loss (with a significant conductive component) with absent stapedial reflexes (provided pure tone thresholds are still good enough to elicit stapedial reflex), a normal tympanic membrane on otoscopy, a negative Rinne test, and a Weber test that is lateralized toward the ear to be operated.[18,22] Bilateral disease and the presence of a first-degree family member (as exists in 60% of the cases) with similar clinical presentation who underwent a successful stapes surgery are strong confirmatory factors for the presence of otosclerosis.[23] In the absence of the unequivocal clinical presentation, surgeons might need further validation of cause before referral for stapes surgery in order to set realistic expectations as for possible outcomes, to exclude other causes of conductive hearing loss (CHL) in which there is no isolated stapedial fixation; therefore, the chance of achieving complete or near-complete closure of air-bone gap is far lower than in ORHL[8] and, if needed, to direct patients toward a different alternative for hearing restoration.

ALTERNATIVE DIAGNOSIS TO OTOSCLEROSIS DEMONSTRATED WITH IMAGING

Certain clinical situations might lead the clinician to suspect that a nonotosclerosis diagnoses is mimicking an ORHL and should call for imaging as additional foundation for verification of the underlying diagnoses.[8,10] Common examples are summarized in **Box 1** and include mixed hearing loss, significant bilateral conductive or mixed hearing

Table 2
Symons and Fanning's imaging-based grading systems for otosclerosis

CT Grade	Plaques Location
1	Solely fenestral (spongiotic/sclerotic)
2	Patchy localized cochlear disease (± fenestral involvement) • To basal cochlear turn (grade 2A) • To middle/apical turn (grade 2B) • Both (grade 2C)
3	Diffuse confluent cochlear involvement (± fenestral involvement)

Data from Marshall AH, Fanning N, Symons S, et al. Cochlear implantation in cochlear otosclerosis. Laryngoscope 2005;115:1731; with permission.

Box 1
Cases whereby acquiring preoperative imaging is warranted when suspecting otosclerosis

- Mixed hearing loss
- Bilateral significant CHL
- Sensorineural hearing loss
- Children with mixed hearing loss, specifically boys (to rule out X-linked mixed deafness)
- Patients with facial deformity or malformation
- Unstable or fluctuating hearing
- Accompanying vestibular complaint
- History of head trauma
- Revision cases
- History of chronic otitis media

---

loss (in these cases the value of audiometric test might be limited because of the possible masking dilemma); sensorineural hearing loss; children with mixed hearing loss, specifically boys (to rule out X-linked mixed deafness); patients with facial deformity or malformation; unstable or fluctuating hearing; history of head trauma; and patients with vestibular complaints as adjunct to their audiometric complaints.[24] HRCT can identify other middle ear causes of conductive or mixed hearing loss such as ossicular chain discontinuity/fixation (possibly secondary to previous middle ear disease) tympanosclerosis, round window obliteration or cholesteatoma (congenital cholesteatoma still isolated to the attic and hidden medial to an intact scutum) (**Fig. 3**).[8,10] Alternately, imaging can demonstrate different temporal bone pathologies that present with conductive and mixed hearing loss such as superior semicircular canal dehiscence, Osteogenesis imperfecta, Paget disease, fibrous dysplasia, and syphilis, as well as other rare conditions that might cause CHL, such as granulomatous, infectious, neoplastic, and other immunologic pathologies that might affect the temporal bone (**Fig. 4**).[25–27]

Most of these conditions can be at least suspected on HRCT. Therefore, preoperative HRCT is recommended before stapes surgery unless patients underwent a successful contralateral stapedectomy. Adopting this policy improves expectation management as for air-bone gap closure but may also avoid the risk for complications that can be predicted based on HRCT.

THE USE OF PREOPERATIVE IMAGING IN OTOSCLEROSIS TO AVOID INTRAOPERATIVE COMPLICATIONS

Preoperative imaging might also be used to avoid intraoperative complications during procedures for otosclerosis, which is the case with some inner-ear malformations that might jeopardize an outcome like enlarged vestibular aqueduct or X-linked mixed deafness, with accompanying defects in the fundus of the internal auditory canal (**Fig. 5**). These radiographic findings carry with them a significant risk of intraoperative perilymph gusher during stapes surgery and subsequent sensorineural hearing loss.[28] Obliterated round window and fixation of the ossicles might lead to poor results after stapes surgery if not identified before or during the surgery.[21] Evaluating the location of the tympanic segment of the facial nerve is another benefit that can be derived from preoperative HRCT, which can demonstrate an overhanging facial

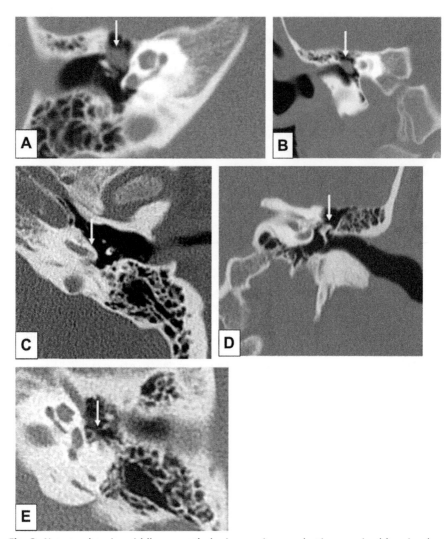

Fig. 3. Nonotosclerosis, middle ear pathologies causing conductive or mixed hearing loss. Axial (*A, C,* and *E*) and coronal (*B, D*) HRCT images demonstrating (*A, B*) congenital cholesteatoma (*arrow*). (*C*) Round window obliteration (*arrow*). (*D*) Incus subluxation (*arrow*). (*E*) Ossicular chain discontinuity with only fibrous connection between the long process of the incus and stapes capitulum (*arrow*). (*Courtesy of* Simon Angeli, MD, Rita Ghose Bhatia, MD, University of Miami, Miami, FL.)

nerve that is obstructing visualization of the oval window, making patients poor surgical candidates (**Fig. 6**).[21,28]

PREOPERATIVE IMAGING ASSESSMENT CHECKLIST

Meticulous and systematic assessment of available preoperative imaging can cover the domains that should be inspected during the diagnostic and surgical planning stage and help avoid the aforementioned misdiagnoses and possible intraoperative complications (**Table 3**).

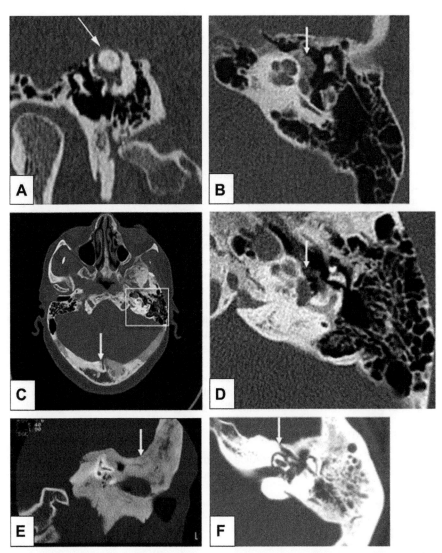

Fig. 4. Temporal bone pathologies that present with conductive and mixed hearing loss. HRCT images demonstrating (*A*) superior semicircular canal dehiscence (*arrow*; Pöschl projection HRCT); (*B*) osteogenesis imperfecta: white arrow points at lucencies anterior to the vestibule; (*C*) Paget disease: diploic widening of the occipital bone (*arrow*) and involving the temporal bone (*square*, see *D*); (*D*) Paget disease involving the temporal bone demonstrating lytic lesions of the inner ear (*arrow*); (*E*) fibrous dysplasia with widened areas of homogeneous ground glass appearance replacing the normal bone (*arrow*); (*F*) syphilitic lesions of the left temporal bone (*arrow*). (*Courtesy of* Simon Angeli, MD, Rita Ghose Bhatia, MD, University of Miami, Miami, FL.)

PREOPERATIVE IMAGING IN RETRO-FENESTRAL (COCHLEAR) OTOSCLEROSIS

When retro-fenestral (cochlear) otosclerosis progresses and cochlear implantation is being considered, imaging (both HRCT and MRI) is of paramount importance. Both imaging modalities might be used to evaluate the patency of the cochlea in cases

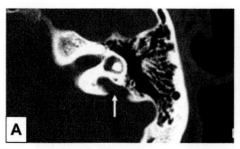
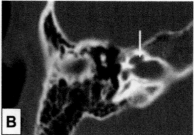

Fig. 5. Inner ear malformation that might jeopardize the outcome. Axial HRCT images demonstrating (A) enlarged vestibular aqueduct (arrow) and (B) X-linked mixed deafness with accompanying defects in the fundus of the internal auditory canal (arrow). (Courtesy of Simon Angeli, MD, Rita Ghose Bhatia, MD, University of Miami, Miami, FL.)

of far-advanced otosclerosis whereby the cochlear lumen may be obstructed (especially when implantation is delayed) and require drill-through or drill-out techniques. It has been demonstrated that these patients have higher numbers of partial electrode insertion or misplacement of the electrode, which might lead to revision surgery.[14,29] Additionally, HRCT might be used to assess the location and extent of hypodense lesions that were found to be correlated with the degree of sensorineural hearing loss.[8–10] Finally, HRCT is useful for patient counseling regarding the chances of facial nerve stimulation following cochlear implantation in patients with retro-fenestral (cochlear) otosclerosis. Marshall and colleagues[11] found a higher risk for facial nerve stimulation after cochlear implantation, with diffuse preoperative confluent involvement of the cochlea. This finding can guide the surgeon in choosing a peri-modiolar electrode rather than using midscala or lateral wall electrodes, as well as for understanding of postoperative possible difficulties during implant programming.[8,14,29]

MRI FOR EVALUATION OF OTOSCLEROSIS

Although HRCT is the modality of choice for most aspects of otosclerosis, additional imaging modalities might be useful for preoperative diagnosis and delineation of

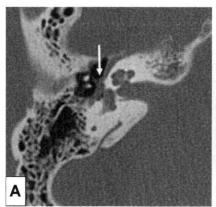
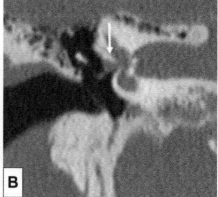

Fig. 6. Overhanging tympanic segment of facial nerve. Axial (A) and coronal (B) HRCT images demonstrating overhanging tympanic segment of the facial nerve (arrow) obstructing visualization of the oval window. Stapes surgery should be avoided in this case. (Courtesy of Simon Angeli, MD, Rita Ghose Bhatia, MD, University of Miami, Miami, FL.)

Table 3
Checklist for preoperative high-resolution computed tomography of the temporal bone in otosclerosis

	Structure	Features Assessed
1	Temporal bone	• Signs of fractures (even if already ossified) • Status of superior semicircular canal (dehiscence?) • Multiple lesions/plaques (other metabolic/infectious/neoplastic bone disease?)
2	Mastoid	• Aerated vs sclerotic/opacified (suspected of chronic otitis media) • Intact air cells vs bony erosion (cholesteatoma)
3	Middle ear	• Aerated vs sclerotic/opacified (suspected of chronic otitis media) • Abnormal vascular structures (high-riding jugular bulb)
4	Ossicular chain	• Continuity • Abnormal morphology • Fixation, dislocation • Fractures • Erosion (cholesteatoma)
5	Stapes	• Position (dislocated) • Morphology • Adjacent structures (position of facial nerve) • Floating footplate (in children) • Erosion (cholesteatoma)
6	Oval window	Thickness and level of obliteration (drilling needed?)
7	Round window	Obliteration? (avoid stapes surgery)
8	Facial nerve	• Tympanic segment: overhanging (avoid stapes surgery) • Mastoid segment: abnormal position (might influence on choice of approach)
9	Inner ear	• Malformation • Enlarged vestibular aqueduct (consider avoiding stapes surgery) • Enlarged cochlear duct and pattern of X-linked mixed hearing loss (avoid stapes surgery) • Obliterated cochlea (especially before cochlear implant)
10	Otosclerotic lesions	Size and location: correlation with grading system and hearing outcome (especially before cochlear implant)
11	Opposite ear	Disease is bilateral in 80%–85% cases, even in absence of symptoms

anatomy in otosclerosis. MRI will often be the first modality to assess patients with sensorineural or mixed hearing loss; hence, knowing to identify otosclerosis in this modality is important.[30] Although MRI is less useful for the demonstration of bony pathology and anatomy, it is very useful for the evaluation of the patency of cochlear lumen before cochlear implantation in patients with far-advanced otosclerosis (**Fig. 7**).[10] Cochlear otosclerosis might be appreciated as a ring of isointense signal in the peri-cochlear and peri-labyrinthine regions on T1-weighted images with mild to moderate enhancement with gadolinium related to hypervascularity and inflammatory response in cases of large otospongiotic peri-cochlear foci. T2-weighted images might demonstrate hyperintensity as well.[10,27] Three-dimensional fluid attenuation inversion recovery sequence with and without gadolinium using 3T MRI was found by Lombardo and colleagues[30] to be advantageous for the demonstration of the altered composition of the endocochlear fluid due to inflammation and blood-labyrinth barrier breakdown, which was demonstrated in 81.8% of their patients. Several studies even considered MRI to be superior to HRCT in demonstrating lesions in the lateral wall of the labyrinth, where partial-volume effects could be troublesome

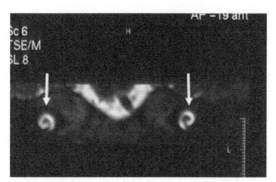

Fig. 7. Patent cochlear lumen in far-advance otosclerosis (*arrow*). Coronal MRI, T2-weighted images demonstrating hyperintensity and normal potency of cochlear lumen bilaterally. (*Courtesy of* Simon Angeli, MD, Rita Ghose Bhatia, MD, University of Miami, Miami, FL.)

using HRCT.[31] MRI might also be considered preoperatively in cases of suspected otosclerosis and symptoms associated with endolymphatic hydrops. In these circumstances, a delayed MRI 4 hours after intravenous injection of gadolinium can demonstrate endolymphatic hydrops. Stapes surgery should be avoided in these patients because of the increased risk of postoperative sensorineural hearing loss.[32] De Oliveira Vicente and colleagues,[33] in a pilot study, demonstrated that MRI analysis using specific software is an objective method that has higher sensitivity than the audiometric test for follow-up on the activity of otospongiotic treatment with fluorides and is the most accurate method available.

SINGLE-PHOTON EMISSION COMPUTED TOMOGRAPHY FOR EVALUATION OF OTOSCLEROSIS

Single-photon emission computed tomography (SPECT) using 99 technetium-diphosphonates (because diphosphonates are highly adsorbed by the immature hydroxyapatite of active otospongiotic foci).[10] Scintigraphic examination using similar agents were tried but suffered from poor spatial orientation.[10] Berrettini and colleagues[10] suggested this option for diagnostic purposes in difficult cases and for medical treatment follow-up. In this study, SPECT exhibited high sensitivity and specificity (95.2% and 96.7%, respectively) in identifying otospongiotic foci in the otic capsule. A higher uptake index on SPECT was also correlated with significantly poorer BC and with retro-fenestral compared with fenestral lesions.[10]

POSTOPERATIVE IMAGING IN OTOSCLEROSIS: COMPLICATIONS AND RESULTS ASSESSMENT

Stapes surgery is a relatively safe procedure with a high rate of air-bone gap closure, and greater than 90% of patients report better hearing 1 year after the surgery.[34] Profound sensorineural hearing loss occurs in less than 1% of the cases, and worsening of the BC thresholds greater than 5 dB occur in about 5% of the cases.[34–36] Incomplete closure of air-bone gap and a remaining conductive or mixed hearing loss occur in 6.5% to 27.0% of the cases.[34,37] Both sensorineural hearing loss and vertigo might occur following deep insertion of the prosthesis, labyrinthitis, perilymphatic fistula, and intralabyrinthine hemorrhage and can be demonstrated in postoperative HRCT.[21,35,36] Yehudai and colleagues[38] demonstrated in their study that the prosthesis depth can be well demonstrated using postoperative HRCT. In this study, it

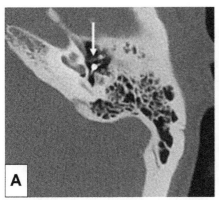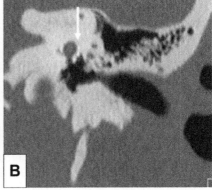

Fig. 8. Stapes prosthesis dislocation. Axial (*A*) and coronal (*B*) HRCT images of the left tempo-ral bone demonstrating dislocated stapes prosthesis (*arrow*) posterior to the oval window. (*Courtesy of* Simon Angeli, MD, Rita Ghose Bhatia, MD, University of Miami, Miami, FL.)

was further demonstrated that deeper protrusion of the prosthesis into the vestibule correlated with better hearing results at several frequencies. HRCT demonstrates pneumo-labyrinth, which might signify possible perilymphatic fistula (especially after the first postoperative week) and is considered as one of the most common causes of postoperative sensorineural hearing loss.[35,36] Hearing deterioration following suc-cessful surgery might be explained by prosthesis dislocation. This complication can occur at any time postoperatively and can be easily demonstrated using HRCT (**Fig. 8**).[21,37] Moreover, erosion of the long process of the incus occurring long after the surgery might present as conductive or mixed hearing loss after successful sur-gery. Another explanation might be an overlooked obliteration of the round window or ossicular fixation or other temporal bone entity as was previously described (see **Figs. 3** and **4**). The common denominator for all of these complications is their excel-lent demonstration using HRCT. Reparative granuloma is an unusual complication, characterized by hearing loss, occurring 1 to 2 weeks after the surgery, related to a severe inflammatory response near the vestibule; it might be well demonstrated us-ing MRI with gadolinium demonstrating enhancement of the otic capsule and middle ear, whereas HRCT demonstrating bony erosion in the middle ear.[39] As a general rule, the authors recommend obtaining HRCT before revision stapes surgery in order to rule out the aforementioned pathologies and avoid additional complication and pa-tient frustration.

SUMMARY

The use of imaging in otosclerosis for diagnosis, preoperative assessment, and follow-up gives the clinician an additional tier of validation and evaluation of pa-tients' diagnoses. This evaluation might help in offering the correct solution for hearing-impaired individuals whose type of hearing loss is likely to be ORHL. The use of imaging in otosclerosis is expected to reduce complication rates, failures, and disappointment. Imaging might be also used following an unsuccessful stapes procedure or hearing deterioration following a primarily successful procedure in or-der to get better insight about the probable cause. HRCT is the modality of choice in otosclerosis. Before cochlear implantation, both MRI and HRCT should be considered.

REFERENCES

1. Politzer A. Uber primare erkrankung der knockernen labyrinthkapsel. Zeitschrift Fur Ohrenheilkunde 1893;25:309–27.
2. Siebenman F. Totaler knocherner verschluss beider labyrinthfester und labyrinthitis serosa infolge progessiver spongiosierung. Verhanlungen Deutschen Otologischenn Gesellschaft 1912;6:267–83.
3. Manasse P. Die osteitis chronica metaplastica der labyrinthkapsel. Wiesbaden (Germany): JF Bergmann; 1912.
4. Jenkins GJ. Serial microscopic sections of the labyrinth and middle ear, showing ankylosis of the stapes; Otosclerosis. Proc R Soc Med 1914;7:40–1.
5. Fraser JS. The pathology of otosclerosis, congenital syphilitic deafness, and paralabyrinthitis. Proc R Soc Med 1916;9:43–61.
6. Schuknecht HF, Barber W. Histologic variants in otosclerosis. Laryngoscope 1985;95:1307–17.
7. Mundnich K. Die Radiologie der Otosklerose. Fortschr Hals Nasen Ohrenheilkd 1961;8:328.
8. Lee TC, Aviv RI, Chen JM, et al. CT grading of otosclerosis. AJNR Am J Neuroradiol 2009;30:1435–9.
9. Kutlar G, Koyuncu M, Almeli M, et al. Are computed tomography and densitometric measurements useful in otosclerosis with mixed hearing loss? A retrospective clinical study. Eur Arch Otorhinolaryngol 2014;271:2421–5.
10. Berrettini S, Ravecca F, Volterrani D, et al. Imaging evaluation in otosclerosis: single photon emission computed tomography and computed tomography. Ann Otol Rhinol Laryngol 2010;119:215–24.
11. Marshall AH, Fanning N, Symons S, et al. Cochlear implantation in cochlear otosclerosis. Laryngoscope 2005;115:1728–33.
12. Shin YJ, Fraysse B, Deguine O, et al. Sensorineural hearing loss and otosclerosis: a clinical and radiological survey of 437 cases. Acta Otolaryngol 2001;121:200–4.
13. Kiyomizu K, Tono T, Yang D, et al. Correlation of CT analysis and audiometry in Japanese otosclerosis. Auris Nasus Larynx 2004;31:125–9.
14. Rotteveel LJ, Proops DW, Ramsden RT, et al. Cochlear implantation in 53 patients with otosclerosis: demographics, computed tomographic scanning, surgery, and complications. Otol Neurotol 2004;25:943–52.
15. Naumann IC, Porcellini B, Fisch U. Otosclerosis: incidence of positive findings on high-resolution computed tomography and their correlation to audiological test data. Ann Otol Rhinol Laryngol 2005;114:709–16.
16. Marx M, Lagleyre S, Escudé B, et al. Correlations between CT scan findings and hearing thresholds in otosclerosis. Acta Otolaryngol 2011;131:351–7.
17. Wycherly BJ, Berkowitz F, Noone AM, et al. Computed tomography and otosclerosis: a practical method to correlate the sites affected to hearing loss. Ann Otol Rhinol Laryngol 2010;119:789–94.
18. Karosi T, Csomor P, Sziklai I. The value of HRCT in stapes fixations corresponding to hearing thresholds and histologic findings. Otol Neurotol 2012;33:1300–7.
19. House HP, Sheehy JL. Stapes surgery: selection of the patient. Ann Otol Rhinol Laryngol 1962;70:1062–8.
20. Derks W, De Groot JAM, Raymakers JA, et al. Fluoride therapy for cochlear otosclerosis? An audiometric and computerized tomography evaluation. Acta Otolaryngol 2001;121:174–7.
21. Purohit B, Hermans R, Op de beeck K. Imaging in otosclerosis: a pictorial review. Insights Imaging 2014;5:245–52.

22. Luntz M, Yehudai N, Most T. Hearing rehabilitation counseling for patients with otosclerosis-related hearing loss. Otol Neurotol 2009;30:1037–43.
23. Rudic M, Keogh I, Wagner R, et al. The pathophysiology of otosclerosis: review of current research. Hear Res 2015;330:51–6.
24. De la Cruz A, Angeli S, Slattery WH. Stapedectomy in children. Otolaryngol Head Neck Surg 1999;120:487–92.
25. Merchant SN, Nadol JB Jr. Otologic manifestations of systemic disease. In: Flint PW, Haughey BH, Lund V, et al, editors. Cummings otolaryngology–head & neck surgery. Philadelphia: Elsevier Saunders; 2015. p. 2301–18.
26. Mafee MF, Valvassori GE, Deitch RL, et al. Use of CT in the evaluation of cochlear otosclerosis. Radiology 1985;156:703–8.
27. Goh JP, Chan LL, Tan TY. MRI of cochlear otosclerosis. Br J Radiol 2002;75: 502–5.
28. House JW, SN, Cunningham CD III. Otosclerosis. In: Flint PW, Haughey BH, Lund V, et al, editors. Cummings otolaryngology–head & neck surgery. Philadelphia: Elsevier Saunders; 2015. p. 2211–9.
29. Ruckenstein MJ, Rafter KO, Montes M, et al. Management of far advanced otosclerosis in the era of cochlear implantation. Otol Neurotol 2001;22:471–4.
30. Lombardo F, De Cori1 S, Aghakhanyan G, et al. 3D-Flair sequence at 3T in cochlear otosclerosis. Eur Radiol 2016;26:3744–51.
31. Ziyeh S, Berlis A, Ross UH. MRI of active otosclerosis. Neuroradiology 1997;39: 453–7.
32. Sone M, Yoshida T, Sugimoto S, et al. Magnetic resonance imaging evaluation of endolymphatic hydrops and post-operative findings in cases with otosclerosis. Acta Otolaryngol 2017;137:242–5.
33. De Oliveira Vicente A, Chandrasekhar SS, Yamashita HK, et al. Magnetic resonance imaging in the evaluation of clinical treatment of otospongiosis: a pilot study. Otolaryngol Head Neck Surg 2015;152:1119–26.
34. Strömbäck K, Lundman L, Bjorsne A, et al. Stapes surgery in Sweden: evaluation of a national-based register. Eur Arch Otorhinolaryngol 2017;274:2421–7.
35. Vandevoorde A, Williams MT, Ukkola-Pons E, et al. Early postoperative imaging of the labyrinth by cone beam CT after stapes surgery for otosclerosis with correlation to audiovestibular outcome. Otol Neurotol 2017;38:168–72.
36. Bain MD, Mocan BO, Sarac S, et al. Early computed tomography findings of the inner ear after stapes surgery and its clinical correlations. Otol Neurotol 2013;34: 639–43.
37. Vincent R, Sperling NM, Oates J, et al. Surgical findings and long-term hearing results in 3,050 stapedotomies for primary otosclerosis: a prospective study with the otology-neurotology database. Otol Neurotol 2006;27:S25–47.
38. Yehudai N, Masoud S, Most T, et al. Depth of stapes prosthesis in the vestibule: baseline values and correlation with stapedectomy outcome. Acta Otolaryngol 2010;130:904–8.
39. Watts E, Powell HRF, Saeed SR, et al. Post-stapedectomy granuloma: a devastating complication. J Laryngol Otol 2017;20:1–4.

Special Anatomic Considerations in Otosclerosis Surgery

Helge Rask-Andersen, MD, PhD[a],*, Nadine Schart-Morén, MD[b],
Karin Strömbäck, MD, PhD[b], Fred Linthicum, MD[c], Hao Li, PhD[b]

KEYWORDS

- Micro-CT • Human • Temporal bone • Otosclerosis • Otolith organ

KEY POINTS

- Micro–computed tomography and 3-dimensional rendering revealed the relationship between the otolith organs and the oval window.
- Besides saccule, awareness of the position of the utricle macula near the superior margin of the footplate is essential to avoid damage during stapes surgery.
- A step-by-step consideration of the anatomy in otosclerosis surgery is important.
- Calcification of the anterior malleolar ligament seems to be a normal finding. Fixation should therefore be substantiated by palpation at surgery.

INTRODUCTION

After primary stapes surgery, sensorineural hearing loss associated with vertigo is a rare complication today, with rates ranging from 0.2% to 3%.[1] The underlying causes of this complication include intravestibular protrusion of the prosthesis, damage to the membrane labyrinth, surgical manipulation of the floating footplate, perilymph fistula, immune system, or unexpected conditions such as a perilymph gusher. A gusher is often caused by modiolar defects and can likely be prevented by the use of preoperative computed tomography (CT). Damage to the saccule is a concern in stapes surgery, particularly in stapedectomy procedures.[2] A displaced, incorrectly sized, or

Disclosure: This article was supported by ALF grants from Uppsala University Hospital and Uppsala University and by the Foundation of "Tysta Skolan," Sellanders Foundation, and the Swedish Deafness Foundation (Drs. H.R. Andersen and H. Li).

[a] Department of Surgical Sciences, Head and Neck Surgery, Section of Otolaryngology, Uppsala University Hospital, SE-75185 Uppsala, Sweden; [b] Department of Otolaryngology, Uppsala University Hospital, Uppsala SE-751 85, Sweden; [c] Department of Head and Neck Surgery, David Gefin School of Medicine, University of California, Los Angeles, 1000 Veteran Avenue, Room 32-28, Los Angeles, CA 90024, USA

* Corresponding author.

E-mail address: helge.rask-andersen@surgsci.uu.se

unnecessarily long prosthesis can induce irritation or even disrupt the membrane labyrinth and cause hearing loss, and a reduced distance between the stapes and the membrane labyrinth may ensue. The prevalence of such anatomic variations is not well understood. Trauma to the utricle at the upper rim of the oval window (OW) is less often described. A surgical checklist presented by Linder and Fisch[3] highlighted the importance of visualizing the anterior malleolar process and ligament, the incudo-malleolar joint, the exposure of the entire stapes, and the pyramidal process as well as identifying sclerosis of the round window (RW). With this checklist, the surgeon can identify those at risk of middle ear structure impairment (**Table 1**).

The anatomy of the ear varies markedly. The size and shape of the inner ear, including those of the cochlea, OW, and RWs, can vary. Consequently, a hole drilled in the footplate could appear at different positions inside the vestibule. In "small" cochleae, the windows are smaller and are positioned closer to each other.[4,5] In addition, the distance from the OW to the sensory areas should be smaller in those with small cochleae. These areas include the base of the cochlea (high-frequency region), the saccule, the utricle, and the 2 ampullas of the superior and lateral semicircular canals. Therefore, surgery in a small ear is more challenging, and the surgeon needs to be acquainted with the anatomy behind the stapes footplate. However, it is difficult to conceptualize in 3 dimensions the projection of these inner ear structures in different planes. The membrane labyrinth is mostly studied in 2-dimensional (2D) temporal bone sections that provide limited information on spatial relationships. The present study was performed to provide more information on the 3-dimensional (3D) relationship between the vestibule and OW. For this purpose, the authors used micro-CT with a 3D rendering technique to study human temporal bones. 3D reconstructions and orthogonal sectioning, or a "cropping technique," provided additional information on the projections of the vestibular organs on the medial wall of the middle ear.

Techniques Used in the Study

Temporal bone microdissections

A total of 113 archival specimens of macerated human temporal bones were analyzed. Fifty were from nonselected autopsy specimens (mean age of 56 years; 9 bilateral cases). The specimens were kindly provided by the Uppsala Medical Museum. The collection of temporal bones was established by the late Dr Herman Wilbrand and one of the present authors (H.R.-A.) during the 1970s and 1980s at the Department of Diagnostic Radiology and Otolaryngology at the Uppsala University Hospital. The

Table 1	
Step-by-step considerations of the anatomy in otosclerosis surgery	
Malleus	Head fixation, anterior spine, anterior ligament
Incus	Head fixation, ligament
Incudostapedial joint	Erosion, fixation
Facial nerve	Bone dehiscence, herniation
Stapes tendon	Stapes fixed against the pyramidal process
Stapes	Crural anatomy, fixation, thick crura, otosclerotic lesion
Fissula ante fenestram, otic capsule	Otosclerotic lesions
Round window	Otosclerotic obliteration
Utricle	Superior rim of the OW ("no-go")
Saccule	Anterior rim of the OW ("no-go")

Preoperative CT if an SSCD is suspected.

results obtained from this collection were previously published.[6,7] Seventy-eight bones were dissected using a dental drill. The microdissected temporal bones were evaluated using a Zeiss V20 microscope (Germany). Sixty bones were not dissected and were observed using micro-CT without prior drilling. In addition, 3 cadaver temporal bones were investigated by soft tissue analyses. These bones were also obtained from the collection. Moreover, the authors analyzed 300 middle ear ossicles (triplets) for varying morphology (**Fig. 1**).

Micro–computed tomography

A total of 113 macerated temporal bones underwent micro-CT and 3D reconstruction. The bones were scanned with micro-CT (SkyScan 1176; Bruker, Belgium) using the following parameters: 65-kV source voltage, 385-μA current, 9-μm pixel size, 1-mm Al filter, 1-second exposure time, 2-frame averaging, and a 0.30° rotation step. The projection images were acquired over an angular range of 360°, with an angular step of 0.3°. In the resultant images, the image size was 4000 × 2672 pixels, and the pixel size was 9 μm. Projections were reconstructed using the software NRECON ver. 1.7.0.4 (Bruker) based on the Feldkamp algorithm. A volume-rendering technique was used to present the 2D projection of a 3D discretely sampled data set produced by the micro-CT scanner and visualized using the CTvox application (version 3.0; Bruker). Opacity and grayscale values were adjusted to create a realistic 3D view that was as similar to the real bones as possible. Geometric measurements were performed and images were obtained with the 3D Slicer program (Slicer 4.6; www.slicer. org). 3D Slicer is an open software platform for medical image informatics, image processing, and 3D visualization.[8] The visualization of the surface anatomy of the temporal bone was performed from the micro-CT. The images were resized at a 4:1 ratio before 3D reconstruction, owing to hardware and software limitations. Opacity and grayscale values were adjusted during the volume rendering. The application displays reconstructed slices as a 3D object and provides a realistic 3D visualization of scanned objects. Virtual sectioning of the petrous bone revealed internal areas of the bone. The 3D modeling software was equipped with tools that allowed geometric measurements in 3D. For the cadaver bones, the authors also used a soft tissue paradigm with micro-CT to visualize the inner ear soft tissue as well as the middle ear ossicles and their ligaments.

Anatomy of the Malleus and Incus and Incus-Malleolar Fixation

During surgery, alternative reasons for conductive hearing loss should be excluded. For this purpose, inspection of the anatomy of the middle ear from the lateral to the medial may be necessary (**Fig. 2**). Guilford[9] described fixation of the malleus head to be associated with stapedial otosclerosis. Guilford and others[10] thought that otosclerosis was responsible for, and resulted from, long fixation. Tos[11] described 4 types of bony fixation in the epitympanum: isolated fixation of the incus, isolated fixation of the malleus, fixation of both the incus and malleus, and ossification of the ligaments. Malleus ankylosis in the epitympanic space may be caused by a bony spur in the lateral epitympanic wall or tegmen.[12,13] Such bone spurs may be congenital or caused by fibrosis (the formation of new bone as a result of chronic infection or trauma). According to Subotic and colleagues,[14] bony fixation of the malleus head was found in only 14 of 1108 bones (1.2%), and it varied from a bony lamella to a solid bony bridge. In the authors' collection of more than 300 unselected middle ear ossicular triplets, only one malleus showed a bony spur (see **Fig. 1**).

There are 3 human ossicular ligaments: namely, *the superior malleolar ligament*, *anterior malleolar ligament*, and *posterior incudal ligament*. Fibrosis may lead to

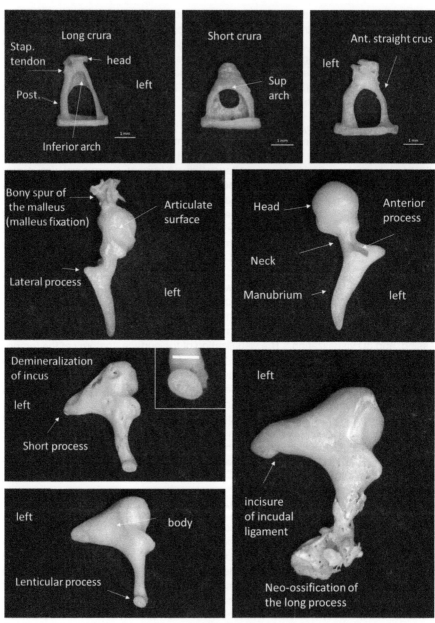

Fig. 1. Anatomy of human middle ear ossicles (from the Uppsala collection; the scale bar is 1 mm). One malleus head shows a bony spur. Ant.straight crus, anterior straight crus; Post, posterior; Stap.tendon, stapedial tendon; Sup arch, superior arch. One incus displays neomineralization of the long process. The lenticular disc is surrounded by a cartilage ring.

reduced ossicular mobility. According to Nandapalan and colleagues,[15] Huber and colleagues,[16] and Nakajima and colleagues,[17] experiences from revision surgery show that partial or complete fixation of the anterior malleolar ligament is more common than previously thought. Fixation of the malleus toward the anterior tympanic

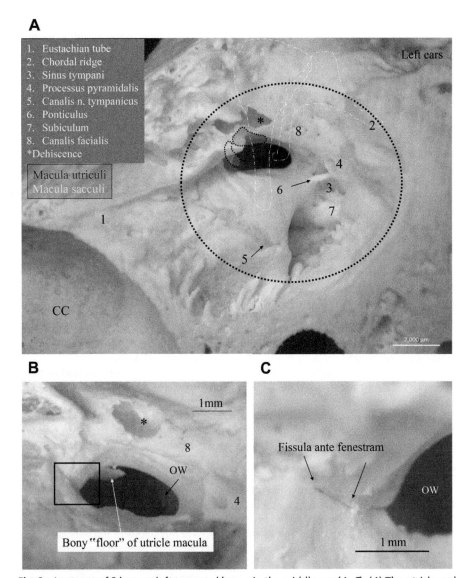

Fig. 2. Anatomy of 2 human left temporal bones in the middle ear (A–C). (A) The utricle and saccule maculae are projected onto the medial wall. (B) The inferior view through the OW shows the bony floor of the utricle macula near its superior rim. (C) A slit-form impression can be seen at the anterior rim of the OW. Otosclerotic lesions were previously thought to originate from this location. CC, common crus.

spine was present in up to 30% of primary stapes surgeries. Severe hyalinization of the anterior malleolar ligament was found in otosclerotic bones, in contrast to minimal hyalinization of this ligament in nonotosclerotic bones. Superior ligament hyalinization was associated with anterior ligament hyalinization. The severity of otosclerosis was not related to the severity of hyalinization. A difficulty faced by surgeons is distinguishing partial fixation of the ligament from complete rigidity. According to Fisch and colleagues,[18] partial fixation was present in 38% of 80 patients undergoing revision surgery. The investigators recommend visualization and palpation, which often necessitate a canaloplasty. If there is reduced mobility, separation of the incudostapedial joint should be followed by reevaluation of mobility.

According to Victor Goodhill,[19] the complex supportive system in the middle ear "makes it clear that there are a number of anatomic factors predisposing to malleus fixation." Anterior fixation may be caused by persistent bone of the anterior spine that is anchored anteriorly to a calcification of the anterior ligament or anterior fold. The anterior ligament in children is described as a long elastic strip of bone (Meckel's cartilage arising from the first pharyngeal arch), and this is contracted in adults. It runs within the anterior malleolar ligament. The ligament courses close to the chorda tympani and inserts at the petrotympanic fissure and sphenoid bone[20] near and lateral to the exit canal of the chorda tympani, called the anterior canaliculus.[21] In Goodhill's description,[19] the *anterior ligament* runs somewhat parallel to the course of the *anterior process*, is attached to the neck of the malleus just above the anterior process, and extends to the anterior tympanic wall, close to the petrotympanic fissure. Some of its fibers extend through this fissure to reach the angular spine of the sphenoid. Micro-CT performed in the authors' laboratory shows frequent calcification of the anterior malleolar ligament (**Fig. 3**). The matching clinical data for these specimens indicate no previous history of ear disease, and there were no signs of malleus fixation, which may suggest that the radiographic calcification of the ligament has insignificant diagnostic value and still permits normal malleus motions. Furthermore, there is a complex interface between the ligament and its insertion on the neck and anterior spine of the malleus. Soft tissue connects and spreads to the malleolar neck, which explains the preserved mobility that is often observed (see **Fig. 3**B).

Incus ankylosis to the epitympanic wall may arise from bony spurs[22] as well as from ligament fixation in the incudal fossa.[23] Isolated otosclerosis may affect the stapes, whereas this effect occurs less frequently in the incus and malleus. In the authors' collection, one incus demonstrated neo-ossification of the long process of the incus (see **Fig. 1**). Proctor's[24] descriptions of the tympanum helped to better understand the complex anatomy of the mucosal folds and suspensory apparatus of the lateral ossicular chain.

Pyramidal Process and Chordal Ridge

The size and length of the bony tube surrounding the stapedius tendon vary greatly. Stapes fixation can be due to an unusual long pyramidal process causing fixation of the capitulum.[25] Laterally, the chorda tympani enters the middle ear under the bony chordal ridge or eminence. The bony opening lies near the sulcus of the annulus fibrosus. It sometimes lies inside the groove, where it can easily be damaged when loosening the tympanic ring. The chordal ridge often obstructs the surgeon's view of the OW and needs to be removed by curettage or a chisel. The nerve overlies the long process of the incus and courses through the posterior malleolar fold (chordal fold). It passes between the incus and malleus neck, near its anterior process, and courses parallel to the anterior ligament, leaving through the petrotympanic fissure (see **Fig. 3**). Its postganglionic fibers innervate the submandibular and sublingual glands as well as the minor glands in the oral cavity. If damaged, impairment of the sense of taste varies. Bilateral transection of the nerve may result in dry mouth, and there seems to be little reinnervation of the taste buds.

Persistent Stapedial Artery

A persistent stapedial artery was reported by Moreano and colleagues.[26] The artery can have different sizes, and it often runs in a small bony channel along the anterior segment of the facial nerve through the stapes from the carotid to the facial canal

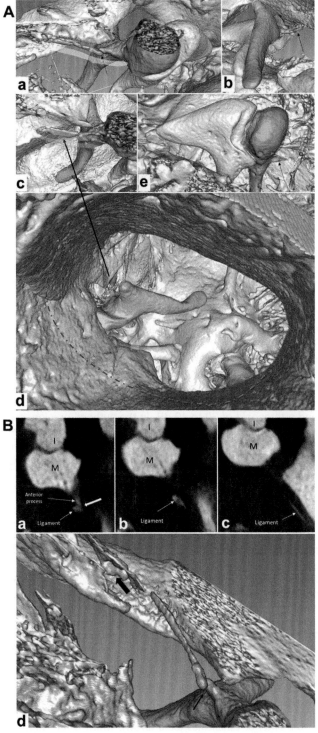

Fig. 3. (*A*) Micro-CT image with 3D rendering of 3 human cadaver temporal bones. (*a*, specimen 1) The supero-medial projection and (*b*) inferolateral projection. The ligament is completely

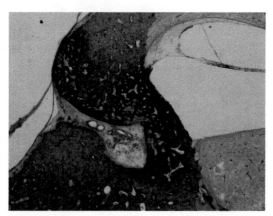

Fig. 4. Otosclerotic obliteration of the RW. The organ of Corti is degenerated.

and the geniculate ganglion to the middle cranial fossa. It may cause conductive hearing loss due to stapes ankylosis,[27,28] and it may be associated with carotid artery aberrations.[29] Depending on its size, surgery may involve risks for facial palsy.

The Round Window

The RW is a site that is often afflicted by otosclerotic lesions.[30] In the literature, it is stated that RW engagement may be a cause of unsuccessful hearing restoration after stapes surgery[2] (**Fig. 4**). Surgery should allow for visualization of the RW niche and exclude obliterative otosclerosis or congenital RW atresia. Congenital obliteration seems to lead to both conductive and sensorineural hearing loss, but this is somewhat debatable.[31] Usually, individuals with such obliteration present with a mixed hearing impairment and a threshold of 30 to 40 dB. In the authors' opinion, opening the RW with a diamond drill should be avoided. Assuming that there is no additional pressure outlet, it seems that the cochlea can be sensitive to alternative, as yet unknown, stimuli. A partial stenosis of the RW may not affect hearing because its size is normally wide ranging with little effect on hearing.[4,5]

The Facial Nerve

Dehiscence of the Fallopian canal was observed in 55% of 535 bones by Baxter.[32] The most frequent site of dehiscence was the posterior half of the inferior or inferolateral aspects of the canal. Dehiscence of the horizontal segment of the facial canal in otosclerosis was found in 14 of 427 patients (3.27%),[33] and similar findings were made by Nomiya and colleagues.[34] A facial canal dehiscence and nerve herniation of the second portion or a narrow niche may limit surgical access to the OW and

---

ossified, but the malleus is not fixed. (c, d, specimen 2) These images show a partly ossified ligament. (e, specimen 3) There is no ossification of the ligament, and the anterior process is short. (d) Proposed skin incision line for visualization of middle ear structures, according to Linder and Fisch.[3] (B) (a–c) Horizontal micro-CT sections at the level of the anterior malleolar ligament in specimen 1. Note the presence of a jointlike structure (*bold arrow*) in the transmission zone between the anterior process of the malleus and the ligament. (d) Corresponding 3D renderings show the anterior ligament, its insertion on the sphenoid, and its relationship to the anterior canaliculus (*bold arrow*), which is the chorda tympani nerve exit medial to the petrotympanic fissure. The thin arrow shows the relationship between the anterior ligament and the spine of the malleus. I, incus; M, malleus.

challenge the optimal placement of the prosthesis (**Fig. 5**). Partial nerve prolapse into the OW niche may occur with or without dehiscence.[35] In 32 cases of partial nerve prolapse, a small piston (0.4 mm) was placed in the lower part of the OW, which was sometimes enlarged toward the promontory. There was a total prolapse of the OW in 0.3% of cases. Projection of the saccule and utricle maculae in an ear with simulated facial nerve herniation is presented in **Fig. 5**. In the authors' collection of human temporal bones, the anterior niche of the OW is sometimes narrowed through a bone apposition from the facial canal wall, without nerve herniation. This bone can be safely drilled away to expose the OW.

Anatomy of the Stapes – Surgical Challenges

The anatomy of the stapes is highly variable (see **Fig. 1**). The plate is often slightly skewed and shaped like a "child's sole" with its heel directed posteriorly. The stapediovestibular joint consists of a fibrous annular ligament. Congenital stapes fixation may develop as a result of the inadequate differentiation of the annular ligament.[36] In 11.2% of ears in patients undergoing surgery for congenital stapes fixation, an anomalous facial nerve was found.[37] There is an anterior and posterior crus, with the anterior crus generally appearing more slender. The head or capitulum surface contains cartilage and forms the incudostapedial joint together with the cartilage-surfaced lenticular disc of the long process of the incus. It is associated with a ring of softer tissue (see **Fig. 1**). The stapedial tendon attaches to the head of the stapes, the upper part of the posterior surface of the posterior crus, or even the incudostapedial joint.

The crura can be long or short. Removal of the crura is a critical step in stapes surgery. It may be more difficult when the anterior crus is robust and the crura are short (see **Fig. 1**), and it can lead to fracture and a "floating plate." An anterior fragment is particularly demanding because it can be difficult to remove without jeopardizing the saccule. Plate fragments may also enter the vestibule superiorly

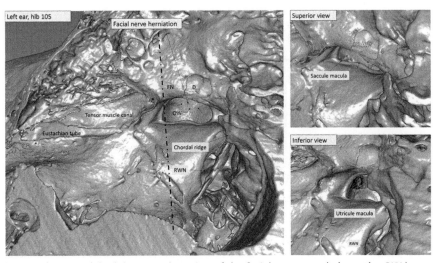

Fig. 5. Dehiscence (*D*) of the second portion of the facial nerve canal above the OW is common. Its mean size is approximately 0.9 mm. The interrupted line represents a cross-section that is demonstrated in **Fig. 7**. FN, facial nerve canal; OW, oval window; RWN, round window niche.

(**Fig. 6**). These fragments should be left behind because the distance between the utricle macula and upper rim of the window is sometimes only 0.5 mm (**Fig. 7**). The opening of the vestibule with a perilymph drain carries a risk for sensorineural deafness. The extraction of an intact stapes plate should always be avoided owing to a "corkscrew or vacuum effect" that may break the thin-membraned labyrinth and cause hearing loss and tinnitus (see **Fig. 6**). It is not absolutely clear that a rupture of the saccule leads to deafness.[2] The stapes footplate can sometimes be the only focus of otosclerosis, without involvement of the OW rim, but with fixation to the otic capsule bone.[38] Likewise, otosclerotic capsule lesions may fix the footplate but with no extension of otosclerosis into the footplate itself. No isolated otosclerotic lesions were found among the authors' stapes specimens. Hearing loss in osteogenesis imperfecta type I is indistinguishable from otosclerosis, and it typically occurs from atrophic crura with a thick, fixed, and pathologically changed stapes plate.[39]

Fissula Ante Fenestram

In the literature, it is often stated that a predilection for otosclerosis occurs between the OW and the cochleariform process, where the tensor tympani tendon turns toward

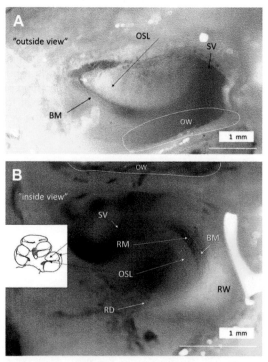

Fig. 6. A fresh human cochlea opened at the level of the OW. The osseous spiral lamina (OSL) and the basilar membrane (BM) are exposed. (*A*) The "outside" superolateral view. (*B*) The "inside" or medial view. The pressure pulse into the scala vestibule (SV) is assimilated by the basilar membrane, which is narrow and slightly tense in this region. Direct surgical damage to the scala media is unlikely, but the gracile membranes could theoretically be damaged during the elimination of the stapes footplate ("corkscrew" effect). RD, reunion duct; RM, Reissner membrane.

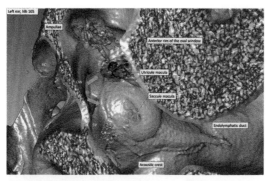

Fig. 7. A lateral view of the medial wall of the vestibule (*blue arrows*) near the anterior rim of the OW. The positions of the maculae were artificially reconstructed. The distance between the anterior rim of the OW and the saccular membrane is approximately 1 mm. The utricle macula lies above the upper rim of the OW and, due to perspective, looks smaller than its actual size. FC, facial canal; SV, scala vestibuli.

the malleus. This small cleft is known as the fissula ante fenestram (see **Fig. 2**C), which is a slitlike fold of soft tissue extending across the endochondral layer. It was considered a persistent synchondrosis between the primordial cochlear and vestibular parts of the cartilaginous otic capsule, and the surrounding bone may contain immature cartilage.[40] The area should be surveilled because there are other causes of stapes ankylosis. There seems no evidence that nonotosclerotic stapes fixation represents a significant distinct pathologic diagnosis.[38]

Utricle and Saccule

The utricle (pars superior) lies in the upper space of the vestibule, whereas the saccule (pars inferior) occupies the lower anterior space of the vestibule. Utricle and saccule are parts of the membrane labyrinth and contain the otolith organs (statoconial). The membrane consists of an inner layer of polygonal flat cells and an outer fibrous layer separated by a basal lamina. The fibrous layer has some contact points with the surrounding bone. The utricle and saccule maculae are approximately 1.5 to 2 × 2- to 3-mm large patches that are situated medially in the vestibule.[41] The surfaces of the maculae are perpendicular to each other. The macula of the utricle contains approximately 30,000 hair cells, whereas the macula of the saccule contains 16,000 hair cells.[42] Each macula is a paired organ with sensory cells polarized toward a dividing line (striola) in the utricle macula and away from the dividing line in the saccule macula. The hair bundles extend into a gelatinous sheet called the *statoconial membrane*. According to Lindeman,[42] the sensory cells of the macula utriculi are morphologically polarized in all directions. This means that any horizontal displacement of the statoconial membrane tangential to the surface of the epithelium will result in both the excitation and the inhibition of particular cells. The polarization vectors in the saccule are mainly in the posterosuperior and anteroinferior directions (**Fig. 8**). Millions of 0.5- to 10-μm-long calcium carbonate crystals (and an organic matrix) give the macula a chalky appearance during surgery. The saccule macula can be observed through the OW when viewed posterosuperiorly (surgical view). The shape of the maculae was described by Retzius,[41] Lorente de No,[43] Hardy,[44] and Lindeman.[42]

Utricle and Oval Window

The utricle is an oblong cylindrical tube (larger than the saccule) that forms a shallow elliptical recess, the recessus ellipticus, in the vestibular bone surface (**Fig. 9**, *inset*).

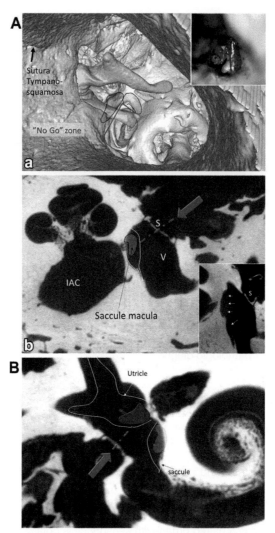

Fig. 8. (*A*) (*a*) A micro-CT image with 3D rendering of a human right temporal bone from a surgeon's view. The maculae are projected onto the medial wall. Red lines mark surgical "no-go" zones. (*b*) A micro-CT section at the level of the stapes. The saccule and its macula are delineated. The anterior angulation of the prosthesis should be avoided to protect the saccule macula. The lower inset shows the saccule membrane derived from different algorithms. The upper inset shows the corresponding surgical field in a right ear. (*B*) Micro-CT section shows the relationship between the stapes footplate and the utricle macula in the vertical projection.

The macula is somewhat rhomboid and lies mostly horizontal. It rests on a thin bony ledge (the "trampoline") projecting into the upper vestibule at the floor of the utricle. It is susceptible to external perilymph uproars and vertical impacts. It is located at the superior rim of the OW, with a distance to the OW as small as 0.5 to 1 mm (**Fig. 10,** *insets*). The utricle macula is difficult to observe during surgery, but the bony ledge can be visualized through the OW in temporal bone specimens using an inferior view (see **Fig. 5**).

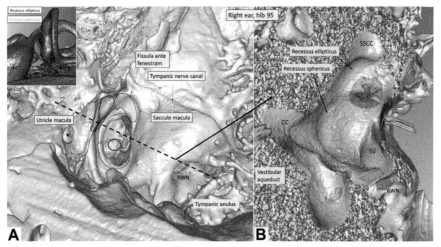

Fig. 9. A micro-CT image enhanced using a 3D rendering algorithm of a right temporal bone. (*A*) A surgeon's view of the middle ear showing the OW and stapes. The utricle and saccular maculae are plotted and shown in violet and blue, respectively. The interrupted line represents a cross-section through the bone viewed in (*B*). (*B*) The lateral view of the medial wall of the vestibule and the anterior part of the stapes. The utricle macula appears smaller because it lies in the same optical plane. Red circle shows authors' recommended site for stapedotomy drilling. Inset shows inner ear cast with recessus ellipticus and sphericus outlined in red. Asterisk points to artefact drilling; CC, common crus; IAC, internal auditory canal; RWN, round window niche; SSCC, superior semicircular canal; SV, scala vestibuli.

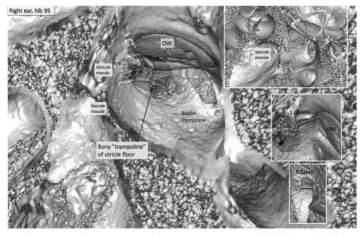

Fig. 10. A higher magnification of a slightly more superiorly sectioned temporal bone than that in **Fig. 11**, showing the location of the utricle and macula relative to the stapes footplate (*red circle*). The utricle macula lies horizontally on a thin bony "trampoline" that can be seen as bony spiculae situated at the level of the superior rim of the OW. The distance between the lateral rim of the utricle macula and superior rim of the OW in this bone was 1.08 mm (*red line*). The lower inset shows another bone in which the distance was 0.5 mm.

Saccule and Oval Window

The saccule is a flat sac located in a fovea in the bone of the medial wall of the vestibule. The macula lies at the level of or inferior to a horizontal line drawn through the stapes crura. It is orientated almost vertically in a convex surface (recessus sphericus) of the medial wall, directed posteromedially. It is shaped like a hook with the anterior part of the epithelium bulging outward in a superior direction.[42] In macerated bones, the cribriform area of the saccule nerve is well defined. The risk of perforating the saccule is greatest at the anterior rim of the OW, where the distance to the footplate is 1 to 1.5 mm, but this can vary (see **Figs. 7** and **9**; **Fig. 11**). The saccule communicates with the cochlea through the reunion duct and with the endolymphatic duct and sac through the sinus of the endolymphatic duct. There is also communication with the utricle through the utriculosaccular duct. Interestingly, the saccule seems to be innervated by 3 nerve trunks, one of which is derived from the cochlea[44].

During revision surgery, the RW niche should be inspected in detail to rule out a window obliteration. The anatomy of the RW and its niche is highly variable. The entire RW is seldom visible during surgery without drilling down the overhang. A fold usually conceals the membrane. Superior semicircular canal dehiscence (SSCD) should be excluded when clinically indicated. These patients usually, but not always, have vestibular symptoms.[45]

A thorough audiologic examination, including acoustic stapedius reflex testing, should be performed. Elicited reflexes rule out stapes fixation, except for the rare case of a softened stapes crura in osteogenesis imperfecta. A CT before revision surgery may confirm SSCD. Atypical audiometry with combined sensorineural and conductive hearing loss may warrant suspicion of disturbed inner ear fluid homeostasis. Modiolar malformation or an enlarged cochlear aqueduct can prevail, and CT may prevent an unexpected perilymph gusher.

The maculae are located near the anterior and superior rims of the OW. They are easily injured by a slanted, protruding intravestibular prosthesis. This "no-go" zone should be avoided, as should the surgical manipulation of plate fragments and the possibility of a floating plate reaching the vestibule. Small fenestra prostheses should

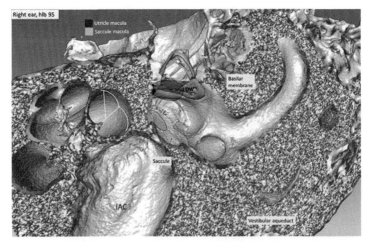

Fig. 11. A horizontal section through the same bone shown in **Fig. 9**. The stapes is viewed from the vestibule. The position of the basilar membrane can be seen at a distance far from the lower rim of the OW. IAC, internal acoustic canal.

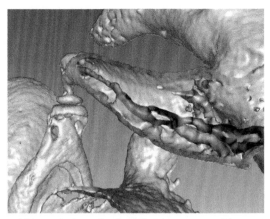

Fig. 12. Micro-CT and 3D rendering of a fresh human temporal bone. A surface paradigm was used to visualize the interior vessel (*red*) in the long process of the incus running to the lenticular process. Feeders are invariably seen on the ventromedial surface of the long process.

be introduced perpendicular to the plane of the footplate, at a maximum of 0.25 mm into the vestibule in routine cases, posterior to its midportion (**Fig. 9**A). The saccule is thought to be more at risk than the utricle, which was found from the horizontal temporal bone sections. Owing to the supraplate position of the utricle, there is generally less awareness of its location near the superior margin of the footplate. This part of the labyrinth is probably more often damaged or concussed during stapes surgery.

Calcification of the anterior malleolar ligament seems to be a normal finding. Fixation should therefore be substantiated by palpation at surgery. The surgeon also has to keep in mind that the long process of the incus is always susceptible for necrosis (**Fig. 12**).

Necrosis of the long process of the incus, at the site of the attachment of the prosthesis may cause a "loose wire syndrome".[46] It can be related to the pressure induced by the prosthesis.[47] Critical may be the variable shape of the shaft[48,49] or vascular supply to the lenticular and long process[50,51] or vessels running in the joint mucosal network. There are different opinions as to its development. Nutritive foramen invariably exist at the ventromedial side at the middle–inferior third of the long process. These contain feeding arteries that together with superficial arteries may be compressed by excessive crimping (see **Fig. 12**).

ACKNOWLEDGMENTS

The authors acknowledge the kind donations of private funds by Börje Runögård and David Giertz of Sweden.

REFERENCES

1. Vincent R, Sperling NM, Oates J, et al. Surgical findings and long-term hearing results in 3,050 stapedotomies for primary otosclerosis: a prospective study with the otology-neurotology database. Otol Neurotol 2006;27(8 Suppl 2):S25–47.

2. Merchant S, Nadol J. Schuknecht's pathology of the ear. China: People's Medical Publishing House-USA; 2010.

3. Linder TE, Fisch U. A checklist for surgical exposure in stapes surgery: how to avoid misapprehension. Adv Otorhinolaryngol 2007;65:158–63.

4. Atturo F, Barbara M, Rask-Andersen H. Is the human round window really round? An anatomic study with surgical implications. Otol Neurotol 2014;35:1354–60.

5. Atturo F, Barbara M, Rask-Andersen H. On the anatomy of the 'hook' region of the human cochlea and how it relates to cochlear implantation. Audiol Neurootol 2014;19:378–85.

6. Wilbrand HF. Multidirectional tomography of the facial canal. Acta Radiol Diagn (Stockh) 1975;16:654–72.

7. Rask-Andersen H, Stahle J, Wilbrand H. Human cochlear aqueduct and its accessory canals. Ann Otol Rhinol Laryngol Suppl 1977;86:1–16.

8. Fedorov A, Beichel R, Kalpathy-Cramer J, et al. 3D Slicer as an image computing platform for the Quantitative Imaging Network. Magn Reson Imaging 2012;30: 1323–41.

9. Guilford FR. Personal experiences with the Shea oval window-vein graft technique. Laryngoscope 1961;71:484–503.

10. Goodhill V. The fixed malleus syndrome. Trans Am Acad Ophthalmol Otolaryngol 1966;70:370–80.

11. Tos M. Bony fixation of the malleus and incus. Acta Otolaryngol 1970;70(2): 95–104.

12. Guilford FR, Anson BJ. Osseous fixation of the malleus. Trans Am Acad Ophthalmol Otolaryngol 1967;71:398–407.

13. Vincent R, Lopez A, Sperling NM. Malleus ankylosis: a clinical, audiometric, histologic, and surgical study of 123 cases. Am J Otol 1999;20:717–25.

14. Subotic R, Mladina R, Risavi R. Congenital bony fixation of the malleus. Acta Otolaryngol 1998;118:833–6.

15. Nandapalan V, Pollak A, Langner A, et al. The anterior and superior malleal ligaments in otosclerosis: a histopathologic observation. Otol Neurotol 2002;23: 854–61.

16. Huber A, Koike T, Wada H, et al. Fixation of the anterior mallear ligament: diagnosis and consequences for hearing results in stapes surgery. Ann Otol Rhinol Laryngol 2003;112:348–55.

17. Nakajima HH, Ravicz ME, Rosowski JJ, et al. Experimental and clinical studies of malleus fixation. Laryngoscope 2005;115:147–54.

18. Fisch U, Acar GO, Huber AM. Malleostapedotomy in revision surgery for otosclerosis. Otol Neurotol 2001;22:776–85.

19. Goodhill V. In anatomical aspects. Acta Otolaryngol 1966;62(sup 217):7–8.

20. Schuknecht H, Gulya A. Anatomy of the temporal bone with surgical implications, vol. 45. Philadelphia: Lea & Febiger; 1986.

21. Mudry A. Glaser fissure, Huguier canal, and Civinini canal: a confused eponymical imbroglio. Otol Neurotol 2015;36:1115–20.

22. Staecker H, Merchant SN. Temporal bone pathology case of the month. Congenital fixation of the incus. Am J Otol 2000;21:137–8.

23. House HP. Diagnostic aspects of congenital ossicular fixation. Trans Am Acad Ophthalmol Otolaryngol 1956;60:787–90.

24. Proctor B. Surgical anatomy and embryology of the middle ear. Trans Am Acad Ophthalmol Otolaryngol 1963;67:801–14.

25. Schuknecht HF, Trupiano S. Some interesting middle ear problems. Laryngoscope 1957;67:395–409.

26. Moreano EH, Paparella MM, Zelterman D, et al. Prevalence of facial canal dehiscence and of persistent stapedial artery in the human middle ear: a report of 1000 temporal bones. Laryngoscope 1994;104:309–20.

27. Breheret R, Bizon A, Tanguy JY, et al. Persistent stapedial artery with otosclerosis. Ann Otolaryngol Chir Cervicofac 2009;126:259–63 [in French].

28. Sugimoto H, Ito M, Hatano M, et al. Persistent stapedial artery with stapes ankylosis. Auris Nasus Larynx 2014;41:582–5.

29. Roll JD, Urban MA, Larson TC 3rd, et al. Bilateral aberrant internal carotid arteries with bilateral persistent stapedial arteries and bilateral duplicated internal carotid arteries. AJNR Am J Neuroradiol 2003;24:762–5.

30. Stewart TJ, Belal A. Surgical anatomy and pathology of the round window. Clin Otolaryngol Allied Sci 1981;6:45–62.

31. Linder TE, Ma F, Huber A. Round window atresia and its effect on sound transmission. Otol Neurotol 2003;24:259–63.

32. Baxter A. Dehiscence of the Fallopian canal. An anatomical study. J Laryngol Otol 1971;85:587–94.

33. Tange RA, de Bruijn AJ. Dehiscences of the horizontal segment of the facial canal in otosclerosis. ORL J Otorhinolaryngol Relat Spec 1997;59:277–9.

34. Nomiya S, Cureoglu S, Kariya S, et al. Histopathological incidence of facial canal dehiscence in otosclerosis. Eur Arch Otorhinolaryngol 2011;268:1267–71.

35. Ballester M, Blaser B, Hausler R. Stapedotomy and anatomical variations of the facial nerve. Rev Laryngol Otol Rhinol (Bord) 2000;121:181–6 [in French].

36. Harada T, Black FO, Sando I, et al. Temporal bone histopathologic findings in congenital anomalies of the oval window. Otolaryngol Head Neck Surg 1980; 88:275–87.

37. An YS, Lee JH, Lee KS. Anomalous facial nerve in congenital stapes fixation. Otol Neurotol 2014;35:662–6.

38. Quesnel AM, Ishai R, Cureoglu S, et al. Lack of evidence for nonotosclerotic stapes fixation in human temporal bone histopathology. Otol Neurotol 2016;37: 316–20.

39. Vincent R, Gratacap B, Oates J, et al. Stapedotomy in osteogenesis imperfecta: a prospective study of 23 consecutive cases. Otol Neurotol 2005;26:859–65.

40. Anson BJ, Wilson G. The fissula ante fenestram in an adult human far. Anat Rec 1933;56:383–93.

41. Retzius G. Das Gehörorgan der Wirbelthiere: morphologisch-histologische Studien, vol. II. Stockholm (Sweden): Samson and Wallin; 1884.

42. Lindeman HH. Studies on the morphology of the sensory regions of the vestibular apparatus with 45 figures. Ergeb Anat Entwicklungsgesch 1969;42:1–113.

43. Lorente de N6 R. Etudes sur l'anatomie et la physiologie du labyrinthe de l'oreille et du VIIIe nerf. Deuxieme partie. Quelques donn6es au sujet de l'anatomie des organes sensoriels du labyrinthe. Trav Lab Rech Biol Univ Madrid 1926;24:53.

44. Hardy M. Observations on the innervation of the macula sacculi in man. Anat Rec 1934;59:403–18.

45. Palma Diaz M, Cisneros Lesser JC, Vega Alarcon A. Superior semicircular canal dehiscence syndrome - diagnosis and surgical management. Int Arch Otorhinolaryngol 2017;21:195–8.

46. McGee TM. The loose wire syndrome. Laryngoscope 1981;91:1478–83.

47. Morgenstein KM, Manace ED. Incus necrosis following stapedectomy. Laryngoscope 1968;78:600–19.

48. Kwok P, Fisch U, Strutz J, et al. Comparative electron microscopic study of the surface structure of gold, Teflon, and titanium stapes prostheses. Otol Neurotol 2001;22:608–13.

49. Toth M, Moser G, Rösch S, et al. Anatomic parameters of the long process of incus for stapes surgery. Otol Neurotol 2013;34:1564–70.

50. Alberti PW. The blood supply of the incudostapedial joint and the lenticular process. Laryngoscope 1963;73:605–28.

51. Lisonek P. The intraosseous canals and vessels of the incus and head of the stapes [in German]. Acta Univ Palacki Olomuc Fac Med 1985;111:89–100.

Stapedectomy Versus Stapedotomy

Horace C.S. Cheng, MD, MASc, Sumit K. Agrawal, MD, FRCSC,
Lorne S. Parnes, MD, FRCSC*

KEYWORDS

• Stapes surgery • Stapedectomy • Stapedotomy • Otosclerosis

KEY POINTS

• Stapedectomy and stapedotomy represent the standard surgical procedures to address conductive hearing loss in otosclerosis.
• Stapedotomy provides better high frequency hearing improvement compared with stapedectomy.
• Both stapedectomy and stapedotomy have proven long-term stability in conductive hearing improvements.
• Stapedotomy has lower rates of complication compared with stapedectomy.
• Minimally invasive approaches may represent the next major development in stapes surgery in a selected patient population.

 Video content accompanies this article at http://www.oto.theclinics.com.

INTRODUCTION

Some of the most illustrious physicians and otologists from the 18th and 19th centuries, including Valsalva, Toynbee, Troltsch, and Politzer, all played key roles in furthering the understanding of otosclerosis.[1,2] Despite some early promise, the morbidity and even mortality of stapes surgery made it too dangerous, and further attempts were subsequently abandoned. As the understanding of otologic physiology and medical technology improved, attempts to correct the cause of the conductive hearing loss were renewed in the 20th century. These efforts were supported by the introduction of precision surgical tools, better visualization with operating loupes, advances in the field of anesthesia, and the advent of antibiotics.

Disclosure: The authors have nothing to disclose.
Department of Otolaryngology–Head and Neck Surgery, Schulich School of Medicine and Dentistry, Western University, London, Ontario, Canada
* Corresponding author. London Health Sciences Centre, University Hospital, B1-333, 339 Windermere Road, London, Ontario N6A 5A5, Canada.
E-mail address: parnes@uwo.ca

Otolaryngol Clin N Am 51 (2018) 375–392
https://doi.org/10.1016/j.otc.2017.11.008
0030-6665/18/© 2017 Elsevier Inc. All rights reserved.

The fenestration operation was the operation of choice in the mid 20th century. This procedure restored hearing by creating a new route for acoustic energy to propagate into the inner ear, bypassing the fixed stapes footplate. However, Rosen's discovery of hearing improvement from an accidental mobilization of the stapes in 1952[3] led to renewed interests in the mobilization procedures. Various new techniques and tools were introduced to improve the outcomes. However, they failed to address the recurrent ankylosis of the stapes footplate, the Achilles heel in the mobilization procedure. This factor ultimately led to the deterioration of hearing improvement in a significant proportion of patients.

It was Shea who performed the first stapedectomy in 1956,[4] heralding the modern era of stapes surgery. His first attempts were made with a Teflon replica of the stapes made by Harry Treace. His subsequent vein graft and polyethylene tube prostheses have since been modified with other graft materials and more standardized prefashioned prostheses (**Fig. 1**). Further modifications using micro hand drills, electric micro drills, and various lasers paved the way for the next innovation in stapes surgery whereby small openings just large enough to allow the insertion of piston like prostheses were made in the stapes footplate. Thus stapedotomy, or small fenestra stapedectomy as it was known at the time, was born. Marquet was generally considered to be the pioneer of this technique with his initial attempts in 1963.[5] This technique is illustrated in **Fig. 2**. Subsequent innovations including different prostheses materials and designs have further improved surgical outcomes and reduced complications.

The aim of this article is to provide an informed discussion about the differences between stapedectomy and stapedotomy. Short- and long-term surgical outcomes, and complications are the key areas for review. Furthermore, interesting aspects of stapes surgery such as the size of the prosthesis and the anesthetic choice are also discussed. We provide a brief overview of the modified stapes mobilization procedures and conclude the article with a "How I Do It" description of our own technique accompanied by an edited video of an operation.

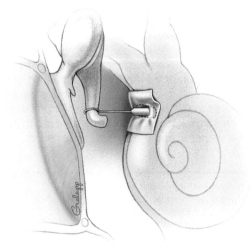

Fig. 1. Schematic diagram of total stapedectomy. Note the prosthesis inserted between the long process of the incus and the tissue graft over the oval window. (©Christine Gralapp.)

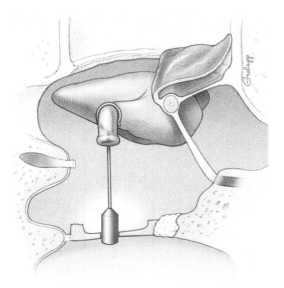

Fig. 2. Schematic diagram of stapedotomy. The prosthesis is inserted through a small opening in the stapes footplate to recreate the mobile ossicular chain movement into the labyrinth. (©Christine Gralapp.)

INDICATIONS AND CONTRAINDICATIONS
Indications

- Confirmed diagnosis of otosclerosis.
- A 25 dB or greater conductive hearing loss in frequencies 250 Hz to 1 kHz with negative Rinne at 512 Hz.[6,7]
- Mixed hearing loss not serviceable by hearing aid unless conductive hearing loss is reduced[8] (far advanced otosclerosis).

Contraindications

- Only hearing ear.
- Active infection of external and/or middle ear.
- Concomitant Meniere's disease with hearing loss of 45 dB or greater at 500 Hz and with high-tone loss.[9]
- Poor overall medical condition.
- Occupational requirement for intact vestibular function.

OUTCOME COMPARISON

Numerous studies have been conducted to assess the outcome of stapedectomy and stapedotomy procedures. Among them are studies that directly compared the 2 approaches. The focus of this section is to summarize the short- and long-term outcome data from such comparison studies. In addition, complications reported from these studies are also discussed.

Short-Term Results

A summary of key studies that compared short-term outcomes of stapedectomy and stapedotomy is provided in **Table 1**.

Table 1
Short-term outcome differences for STE and STO

	Number STE/STO	Pure Tone Audio (Technique with Better Outcome at Listed Frequencies)	Air–Bone Gap (Technique with Better Outcome at Listed Frequencies)	Speech Discrimination Results	Incidence of SNHL STE/STO (%)
House et al,[10] 2002	134/75	NS	STO: 4 kHz	NS	9.8/5.9[b] (NS)
Fisch,[11] 1982	170/170	—	STO; 4 kHz	—	0.6/0 (NS)
Colletti & Fiorino,[12] 1994	428/1030	STO: 8 kHz	NS	STO	—
Somers et al,[13] 1994	165/1429	STO; 4 and 8 kHz	—	—	Total STE: 2.56 Partial STE: 0.71 STO: 0.68
Bailey et al,[14] 1981	50/50	STO: 2, 4, and 8 kHz	STO: 4 kHz	STE: 81% STO: 96%	6/2
McGee,[15] 1981	141/139	—	STO; 0.5–2 kHz	STE: 83.7% STO: 92.8%	—
Moon & Hahn,[16] 1984	106/264	STO: 2, 4, and 8 kHz	STO; 1–4 kHz and 4 kHz	STE: 83% STO: 95%	0/0.3
Persson et al,[17] 1997	275/162	STE: 0.25, 0.5, 1, 2, and 4 kHz	STE; 0.25, 0.5, 1, and 2 kHz	—	Total STE: 6.2[a] Partial STE: 3.8[a] STO: 5.4[a]
Kos et al,[18] 2001	51/553	—	NS	—	5.9/3.1
Sedwick et al,[19] 1997	227/323	NS	STE; 250 and 500 Hz	NS	11.9/6.9[b]
Cremers et al,[20] 1991	150/161	NS	—	—	2.1/0.6
Quaranta et al,[21] 2005	72/79	NS	STO; 4 kHz	—	1.4/1.3
Spandow et al,[22] 2000	60/55	—	—	—	5/0
Levy et al,[23] 1990	50/50	—	STO	STO	5/0
Vasama et al,[24] 2006	47/47	NS	NS	NS	0/0
Pedersen & Elbrønd,[25] 1983	30/30	STO; 4 and 8 kHz	NS	—	0/0

Abbreviations: NS, no statistical difference; SNHL, sensorineural hearing loss; STE, stapedectomy; STO, stapedotomy.
[a] A ≥15 dB BC decrease.
[b] A ≥10 dB BC decrease.

House and colleagues[10] performed an in-depth study of the surgical outcomes of their patients who had undergone stapedectomy and stapedotomy procedures. Stapedectomy was defined as removal of 25% or more of the footplate. One hundred thirty-four stapedectomy cases were compared against 75 stapedotomy cases. At early follow-up between 3 and 12 months, the improvement in pure tone average (PTA) of the air–bone gap was 16.9 dB for stapedectomy and 16.4 dB for stapedotomy. No differences were found in PTA and speech discrimination score between the groups. The percentage of patients with an air–bone gap closure to within 10 dB per frequency showed no significant difference except at 4 kHz, where the stapedotomy group demonstrated a higher closure rate. A unique aspect of this study was the subgroup comparison of 42 patients who had both procedures performed, stapedectomy in 1 ear and stapedotomy in the other, for bilateral otosclerosis. Thus, each patient acted as self-control, although stapedectomy was performed as the first surgery in all cases, so there may have been learning bias favoring the stapedotomy. Similar findings with no significant difference in PTA were found for all paired cases. Improvement of air–bone gap at 4 kHz was once again noted for stapedotomy group reaching statistical significance.

Fisch[11] conducted a similar study with 340 cases equally divided among 2 groups. Both total and partial stapedectomy were included under the stapedectomy group. Stapedotomy was performed using the 0.6-mm diameter prosthesis. Air–bone gap measurements at 0.5 to 2 kHz and 4 kHz were calculated. The percentage of patients achieving air–bone gap closure to within 10 dB at 1 year was 54% for stapedectomy and 58% for stapedotomy. There was no significant difference for the 0.5 to 2 kHz range at 3 weeks to 3 years. However, the stapedotomy group performed significantly better at 4 kHz at 1 year follow-up. This study also included further discussion and analysis of stapedotomy using a 0.4-mm diameter prosthesis. The impact of prosthesis diameter on hearing outcome is discussed elsewhere in this article.

Colletti and Fiorino[12] published a large surgical series comparing stapedectomy and stapedotomy, with additional analysis performed on stapedius tendon preservation within the stapedotomy group. They reviewed 1459 cases consisting of 428 stapedectomies, 561 stapedotomies with stapedius tendon section, and 470 stapedotomies in which they preserved the incudostapedial joint and stapes head and neck, keeping the tendon attached. Audiometric results at 0.5 to 2 kHz, 4 kHz, and 8 kHz were analyzed 6 months after surgery. The result showed stapedectomy achieving a slightly higher rate of air–bone gap closure at 0.5 to 2 kHz, although this difference did not attain statistical significance. The converse is true with a stapedotomy air–bone gap closure performing better at 4 kHz, although this difference was not statistically significant. Air conduction at 8 kHz was found to be significantly better for the stapedotomy group. Thirty subjects in each group were chosen randomly to undergo speech audiometry 1 to 2 years after surgery. With ipsilateral masking, there was a statistically significant decrease in speech discrimination scores in the stapedectomy group compared with the stapedotomy group. A subgroup analysis of the stapedotomy cohort showed that those with stapedius tendon preservation performed better still.

Somers and colleagues[13] published an in-depth statistical analysis of otosclerosis surgery performed by Jean Marquet, who pioneered the stapedotomy procedure. A total of 1681 surgical procedures were included in the analysis. Total stapedectomy, partial stapedectomy, and stapedotomy accounted for 4.1%, 5.8%, and 85% of the cases, respectively. At the follow-up period of 6 to 12 months, the stapedotomy group demonstrated better postoperative air conduction with statistical significance compared with both the partial and total stapedectomy groups at 4 kHz, and over the total stapedectomy group at 8 kHz. Clearly, however, with the vast majority being stapedotomy cases, practice bias must be considered in the results.

Bailey and colleagues[14] compared the results of stapedectomy and stapedotomy in 100 patients randomized into the 2 surgical arms. The short-term results from 1 to 12 months demonstrated significant improvement in the stapedotomy group in terms of postoperative air conduction at 2, 4, and 8 kHz. The percentage of air–bone gap closure was also superior in the stapedotomy group at 4 kHz. The mean speech discrimination score was increased by 11.8% in the stapedotomy group, whereas a slight decrease of 0.4% was observed in the stapedectomy group.

McGee[15] reviewed his surgical series consisting of 280 total cases of stapedectomy and stapedotomy. At 6 months of follow-up, the percentages of air–bone gap closures to within 10 dB over the 0.5 to 2.0 kHz frequency range were 85.8% for the stapedectomy group and 96.4% for the stapedotomy group. Additionally, only 83.7% of stapedectomy patients achieved a speech discrimination score within 10% or better of preoperative score, compared with 92.8% of patients in stapedotomy patients. The differences in the air–bone gap and speech audiometry were statistically significant.

Moon and Hahn[16] performed a similar study with 106 cases of stapedectomy and 264 cases of stapedotomy. In this study, stapedectomy was defined as greater than 50% of footplate removal. At the 6-month follow-up, the gain in air conduction in the stapedotomy group demonstrated significant improvement over its counterpart at 2, 4, and 8 kHz. The percentage of air–bone gap closure in the stapedotomy group was also significantly higher than the stapedectomy group at 1 to 4 kHz range, and at 4 kHz. The percentage of patients with better or same speech discrimination scores was 83% for stapedectomy, compared with 95% for stapedotomy.

Persson and colleagues[17] published a detailed analysis comparing total stapedectomy (n = 205), partial stapedectomy (n = 70), and stapedotomy (n = 162). A stainless steel wire prosthesis (House wire) and fascia to cover the oval window was used for stapedectomy, whereas a 0.4-mm Teflon-platinum piston (Fisch piston) without a graft was used for stapedotomy. At the 1-year follow-up, the gain in PTA was greater in both the total and partial stapedectomy cohorts compared with the stapedotomy procedure. The air–bone gap showed better performance of stapedectomy, except at 4 kHz. The overall rates of air–bone gap closure to within 10 dB were 94.0% with total stapedectomy, 83.9% with partial stapedectomy, and 82.8% with stapedotomy. The authors also observed a statistically significant improvement of postoperative bone conduction in favor of the stapedectomy groups at frequencies lower than 4 kHz.

Kos and colleagues[18] analyzed a series of 51 cases of stapedectomy with 553 cases of stapedotomy. The surgical series included operations by 19 surgeons including residents. At 6 weeks of follow-up, the percentages of patients achieving air–bone gap closure within 10 dB was comparable between the groups.

Sedwick and colleagues[19] compared a series of 227 stapedectomy and 323 stapedotomy procedures from the House ear clinic. At 4 months of follow-up, the percentages of air–bone gap closure over 0.5 to 2.0 kHz were similar with 78.7% for stapedectomy and 77.8% for stapedotomy. However, the rate of air–bone gap closure was statistically higher at 250 and 500 Hz for the stapedectomy group.

Cremers and colleagues[20] analyzed a series of 311 primary operations for otosclerosis consisting of 48 total stapedectomy, 102 partial stapedectomy, and 161 stapedotomy procedures. In addition, a subgroup of 114 cases, 38 from each of the operative techniques, were carefully matched for patient characteristics, clinical type of otosclerosis, and prosthesis design and selected for further analysis. No significant difference was noted in the overall patient groups in terms of PTA at the 6- to 12-month follow-up. However, the matched subgroup analysis showed the total stapedectomy group was outperformed by both of the 2 other groups with a statistically significant difference of 7.4 dB in mean hearing gain. No significant difference in hearing gain was observed between the stapedotomy and partial stapedectomy groups.

The following are the key findings from several smaller studies. Quaranta and colleagues[21] compared the results of 72 partial stapedectomy with 79 stapedotomy procedures. At the 6-week follow-up, the percentage of air–bone gap closure did not reveal any statistical difference. However, the proportion of air–bone gap closure achieved statistical significance at 4 kHz with superior result for the stapedotomy group. The change in air–bone gap was also compared, and it showed statistically significant superior results in the stapedotomy group at 2, 3, and 4 kHz. In addition, the mean postoperative change in bone conduction over 1, 2, and 4 kHz was significant, showing an improvement of bone conduction for the stapedotomy group. Spandow and colleagues[22] compared 60 stapedectomy with 55 stapedotomy procedures. The results of air conduction and residual air–bone gap pointed to superior performance of the stapedotomy group, especially in the high-frequency range. Levy and colleagues[23] reported the results from 100 procedures with 50 cases from each procedure randomly selected from their case archive. At the 8-week follow-up, the percentage of patients with air–bone gap closure to within 10 dB was 92% for stapedotomy and 68% for stapedectomy. This difference was statistically significant. No statistical difference was noted in speech discrimination. Vasama and colleagues[24] conducted a study with 47 stapedectomies and 47 stapedotomies. There were no statistically significant differences in terms of PTA for air conduction, PTA for bone conduction, or percentage of patients with an air–bone gap closure between groups. Pedersen and Elbrønd[25] compared the outcome of 60 procedures, 30 of which were done using a stapedectomy technique with the House prosthesis and 30 using a stapedotomy using the Fisch prosthesis. By analyzing the data at 3 weeks and 3 months, a statistically significant improvement of postoperative hearing was noted at 4 and 8 kHz in the stapedotomy group compared with the stapedectomy cohort. Moreover, improvement in the air–bone gap was noted to be superior in the stapedotomy group at 4 kHz, although the P value was not reported. Esquivel and colleagues[26] analyzed a series of 17 stapedectomy and 18 stapedotomy procedures. At the initial 6- to 12-month follow-up of this long-term study, the PTA of air conduction was compared between groups and no statistical significance was detected.

The body of literature suggests that both stapedectomy and stapedotomy provide excellent outcomes in addressing conductive hearing loss owing to otosclerosis. In most studies, stapedotomy using a 0.6-mm diameter prosthesis provides superior audiometric responses and air–bone gap closures in the higher frequencies. The restoration of high-frequency hearing is thought to have a direct impact on improved speech discrimination.[14,15] However, these findings are all based on case series analyses. There are currently no studies with a high level of evidence to support these observations in an unequivocal manner.

Long-Term Results

Shea,[27] the pioneer of the stapedectomy procedure, published his long-term results comparing stapedectomy versus stapedotomy in 200 patients, 100 from each cohort. Patients, were randomly selected for long-term audiometric analysis. The percentages of air–bone gap closure and further cochlear loss were found to be stable over the period of 5 to 15 years in stapedectomy, and from 5 to 20 years in stapedotomy.

Key findings about the stability of both stapedectomy and stapedotomy from other relevant long-term studies are summarized in **Table 2**. There remain disagreements in terms of which of the 2 procedures provides better long-term outcome. However, the

Table 2
Long-term outcome differences for STE and STO

	Number STE/STO	Follow-up Period STE/STO (y)	Pure Tone Audio (Technique with Better Outcome at Listed Frequencies)	Air–Bone Gap (Technique with Better Outcome at Listed Frequencies)	Speech Discrimination Results
Colletti & Fiorino,[12] 1984	188/191	10/10	—	STO; 4 kHz	—
McGee,[15] 1981	22/18 at 4 y 22/20 at 5 y 26/24 at 6 y 5/11 at 7 y	7/7	—	STO (years 4–6) NS (year 7)	STO (years 4–7)
Spandow et al,[22] 2000	60/55	5/5	STO; 4 and 6 kHz	STO; 0.5–3 kHz	—
Kürsten et al,[28] 1994	22/35	9.3/6.2	STO; 4 kHz	—	—
House et al,[10] 2002	134/75	11.5/6.0	NS; 0.5–2 kHz STO; 4 kHz	NS	NS
House et al,[10] 2002	42/42[a]	10.4/6.8	NS	NS	—
Esquivel et al,[26] 2002	17/18	7.6/7	NS	NS	—
Kos et al,[18] 2001	41/400	7/7	—	NS	—

Abbreviations: NS, no statistical difference; STE, stapedectomy; STO, stapedotomy.
a Patients with stapedectomy in 1 ear and stapedotomy in the other ear.

long-term stability of the 2 approaches has been unambiguously demonstrated in the studies included in **Table 2**.

Stapedotomy Long-Term Superiority

Colletti and Fiorino[12] reviewed their surgical series with a follow-up period of 10 years. The percentage of patients with air–bone gap closure to within 10 dB remains equivalent between the groups in the 0.5 to 2.0 kHz range. However, a statistically significant difference at 4 kHz was noted with a better air–bone gap closure rate in the stapedotomy group. The difference was approximately 20%. This result is consistent with the series by the same group at a 5-year follow-up interval,[29] demonstrating a stable trajectory over the long term.

McGee[15] reported his series of 280 patients with long-term data of 7 years. Comparing the percentage of patients with air–bone gap closure to within 10 dB, the group of patients undergoing stapedotomy performed better (P<.05) compared with the group that had undergone stapedectomy at years 4 to 6. The stapedotomy group also performed better in speech discrimination between years 4 and 7. Similar results showing the improvement of air conduction in stapedotomy over stapedectomy was demonstrated by Spandow and colleagues.[22] In their series of 115 patients over a period of 5 to 10 years of long-term follow-up, improved audiometric outcomes in the stapedotomy group was noted in the high frequencies. Kürsten and colleagues[28] drew similar conclusions with their study of 57 patients. The mean follow-up duration was 6.2 years for stapedotomy and 9.3 years for stapedectomy. The 2 surgical groups had similar long-term results in 0.5 to 2.0 kHz, but an improved outcome at 4 kHz in the stapedotomy group. Consistent in all the studies mentioned was the stability of the long-term outcomes for both stapedectomy and stapedotomy.

No Difference Between Stapedectomy and Stapedotomy

House and colleagues[10] noted no statistical differences in PTA at the 0.5 to 2 kHz, air–bone gap, and speech discrimination in their long-term surgical series of 209 patients. The only result with statistically significant difference was for air conduction at 4 kHz, with a superior performance of the stapedotomy group. However, this observation might be influenced by the difference in late follow-up period of 11.5 years in the stapedectomy compared with only 6 years in the stapedotomy group. A further subgroup analysis of 42 patients who had received stapedectomy in one ear and stapedotomy in the other ear again failed to demonstrate any significant difference in PTA, air–bone gap, and speech discrimination in the long term. Esquivel and colleagues[26] conducted a long-term study with 34 patients. The mean follow-up duration was 7.6 years for stapedectomy and 7 years for stapedotomy. The stability of the hearing results from both groups was maintained over the study duration, and no statistical difference in hearing deterioration rate between the 2 groups was found. Kos and colleagues[18] analyzed the long-term results from their series consisting of 41 stapedectomy and 400 stapedotomy procedures. The follow-up duration ranged between 1 and 21 years with a mean of 7 years. They found no difference between groups in terms of percentage air–bone gap closure at 0.5 to 2.0 kHz.

In summary, all the studies reviewed consistently demonstrate stable long-term hearing results for both stapedectomy and stapedotomy, although overall stapedotomy provided better long-term audiometric results, especially in the high-frequency range. It should always be kept in mind that, over the long term, bone conduction thresholds, and in turn air conduction thresholds will deteriorate in most otosclerotic ears with or without stapes surgery compared with normal ears because of the disease's effect on the cochlea.

SENSORINEURAL HEARING LOSS

Although the majority of patients with otosclerosis achieve a good outcome after stapedectomy and stapedotomy, some unfortunately suffer early and/or late complications. A detailed account on the complications of otosclerosis surgery is beyond the scope of this article; a limited review of sensorineural hearing loss based on the studies included is provided instead. Most authors defined sensorineural hearing loss as a more than 20-dB decrease in postoperative bone conduction, although other definitions have also been used. The rates of sensorineural hearing loss for the studies reviewed are summarized in **Table 1**. Sensorineural hearing loss of 20 dB or more occurred in approximately 6% of the stapedectomy procedures in the series by Bailey and coworkers[14] and Kos and associates.[18] The rate of sensorineural hearing loss was lower for stapedotomy at 2.0% and 3.1%, respectively. Results by Fisch,[11] Somers and associates,[13] Cremers and colleagues,[20] and Spandow and coworkers[22] also demonstrated the higher rate of sensorineural hearing loss with stapedectomy. Results from House and colleagues[10] and Sedwick and associates[19] provided additional information about the rate of sensorineural hearing loss with 10 dB or more. Based on these 2 studies, the rate of sensorineural hearing loss with a 10-dB or greater decrease occurred in 9.8% to 11.9% for stapedectomy, and 5.9% to 6.9% for stapedotomy. Overall, higher rates of sensorineural hearing loss are observed in stapedectomy compared with stapedotomy. One potential explanation of this phenomenon is the greater mechanical trauma on the inner ear structures during footplate manipulation and removal.

Mann and colleagues[30] performed a careful review of their surgical series involving 1229 cases, including 691 stapedectomies, 234 stapedotomies, and 304 revision procedures. Twenty cases of moderate to severe sensorineural hearing loss with a greater than 40-dB decrease in bone conduction were identified and underwent to careful analysis. Some of the factors identified as potential causes of hearing deterioration including revision status, increased intraoperative bleeding, and obliterative otosclerosis requiring significant drilling were deemed unmodifiable. However, postoperative acute otitis media was identified as a potentially modifiable cause of sensorineural hearing loss. The authors have, therefore, advocated for routine perioperative antibiotic prophylaxis in stapes surgery.

ASPECTS OF STAPES SURGERY
Prosthesis Size

A key consideration in stapedotomy is the size of prosthesis. The diameter of the prosthesis is thought to have an integral role in the outcome. The overall size could also influence surgical approach. For instance, Fisch[11] proposed a technique consisting of reversal of the classic steps of stapedectomy made possible by the smaller 0.4-mm piston. Throughout the evolution of stapes surgery, different surgeons had proposed different-sized prosthesis as being the optimal design. Those who favored the larger diameter piston pointed to larger surface area of contact and theoretic benefit in the transmission of mechanical energy. However, those who advocate for a smaller diameter claimed that a smaller prosthesis induces less trauma to the inner ear,[31] and that the smaller size may allow modification of surgical approach to improve stability and improved safety.[11] Numerous experimental studies have been performed to model the biomechanics of stapes surgery. An excellent summary of this body of literature was captured in a review article by Hüttenbrink.[32]

Despite all the elegant models proposed by the scientists, the restoration of hearing remains the gold standard for surgical success. Using this as the metric, Laske and colleagues[33] conducted a metaanalysis on the outcome of stapedotomy procedures based on prosthesis diameter. Five controlled studies[11,34–37] consisting of 590 cases were selected for the metaanalysis comparing the surgical outcomes between 0.4-mm and 0.6-mm diameter prosthesis. In these studies, success was defined as closure of air–bone gap to less than 10 dB. The success rate was 67% for a 0.6-mm diameter prosthesis versus 58% for a 0.4-mm diameter prosthesis, achieving statistical significance of $P = .05$. Further analysis of the odds ratio was performed with events defined as surgical success and exposure defined as a 0.4-mm diameter prosthesis usage. The overall odds ratio of the metaanalysis was 0.68 (95% confidence interval, 0.46–1.00), indicating that exposure to a 0.4-mm diameter prosthesis is associated with lower odds of surgical success. The results show that a 0.6-mm diameter prostheses are associated with a higher success rate.

Laske and colleagues[33] also performed a pooled data analysis consisting of 62 studies with 9536 cases. The analysis revealed that a 0.6-mm prosthesis was used in 58.8% and a 0.4-mm prosthesis in 34.4% of cases. In contrast, the combined number of 0.3-mm, 0.5-mm, and 0.8-mm prostheses accounted for only 6.9% of the total cases. The small number of 0.3-mm, 0.5-mm, and 0.8-mm diameter prosthesis groups were too small to reach statistical significance in subsequent analyses. The 0.6-mm diameter prosthesis group once again demonstrated significantly higher success rate of 81.1% compared with 75.1% in the 0.4-mm diameter prosthesis group. Further analysis of air–bone gap per frequencies shows statistical significance at 0.5, 1, and 2 kHz between groups. No statistical difference was observed at 0.25 and 4 kHz. A potential selection bias within studies could influence study outcomes. For instance, a 0.4-mm diameter prosthesis might have been selected preferentially in cases with difficult anatomy.

Based on the results from this metaanalysis and the pooled data analysis, the use of a 0.6-mm diameter prosthesis was associated with a higher rate of surgical success. However, this conclusion must be interpreted with the view that no randomized controlled trial on this topic has been conducted to date.

General Versus Local Anesthesia

The anesthetic used for stapes surgery is another factor to be considered. Both modalities offer unique benefits and drawbacks.[38] Stapes surgery is suitable for conditions provided by local anesthetic mainly owing to the limited surgical field. The most commonly used agent is 1% to 2% lidocaine with 1:100,000 epinephrine injection. Most patients are able to tolerate the procedure with local anesthesia alone, but some surgeons prefer additional intravenous sedation to achieve greater patient comfort. The main advantage of performing the surgery under local anesthesia is the immediacy of feedback from patients during prosthesis placement. Improvements in hearing can be with from patient feedback. Tuning fork examination can also be done to confirm improvement of conductive hearing loss. Patient report of vestibular symptoms can also alert surgeons during the footplate manipulation[39] or prosthesis insertion. Corrective maneuvers such as reducing further footplate manipulation or reducing the length of the prosthesis can be attempted to minimize the risks. In addition, local anesthetic also reduces the theoretic risk of prosthesis displacement during emergence from general anesthesia.

One major drawback of performing local anesthetic is the limited duration of action by the anesthetic agent. Lidocaine with epinephrine mixture has a duration of 2 to 6 hours depending on the volume and concentration infused, the location of administration, and tissue pH.[40] This finding was further characterized in a study by Collins and colleagues,[41] whereby the onset and duration of local anesthetic agents were tested intradermally. The duration of 1% lidocaine with 1:100,000 epinephrine was found to have a range of 3.22 to 10.32 hours with a mean of 6.63 hours. The surgeon must be able to finish the entire surgery within this time frame, which could be stressful in difficult cases. Patients under local anesthesia need to cooperate throughout the entire case by laying still. They might become physically or emotionally distressed from the experience despite the surgeon's and anesthesiologist's best efforts.

General anesthesia is superior in terms of control over the depth and duration of anesthesia. Stillness of the surgical field can be achieved with use of paralytic agents. The senior author had a case under local anesthesia in which the patient sat up during the crucial footplate drilling. The drill entered the inner ear leading to a profound sensorineural hearing loss. Postoperative amnesia and patient comfort are also key considerations. However, the surgeon loses direct feedback from patient under general anesthesia. There are also increased overall risks of general anesthesia, although these risks are very low compared with the early years of stapes surgery because of safer anesthetic agents and techniques for securing airways.

In a systematic review by Wegner and colleagues,[42] 3 studies with a total of 417 procedures were selected to compare the effect of anesthesia on surgical outcomes. The pooled analysis did not demonstrate any statistically significant differences in postoperative air–bone gap, rate of sensorineural hearing loss, or vertigo between the 2 anesthetic approaches. One of the 3 studies found a statistically significant difference in the incidence of postoperative dead ear with 1.87% in the general anesthesia group compared with 0% in the local anesthesia group.[39]

Overall, it seems that there is no significant surgical outcome difference attributable to the anesthetic administered. From a practical logistic perspective, it seems self-evident that cases done under local anesthesia will be faster, with quicker turnovers between cases. However, cases done under local anesthesia may be more stressful not just for the patient, but also the surgeon, depending on the degree and type of associated conscious sedation. In many institutions, anesthesiologists administer the sedation, and their protocols can vary widely. Surgeons should work together with the anesthesiologists in determining the optimal approach specific to their experiences and skill sets to achieve the best possible surgical outcomes.

MODIFIED STAPES MOBILIZATION PROCEDURES

Since the original discovery of hearing restoration from stapes mobilization by Rosen,[3] attempts at mobilization of the stapes have been made with varying degrees of success. The theoretic advantage of restoring the body's native ossicular chain and avoiding the use of prostheses is intrinsically appealing. However, the long-term preservation of hearing gain in the era of stapes mobilization was limited by recurrent ankylosis of the stapes footplate. It was discovered that patients with otosclerotic foci limited to the anterior aspects of the footplate along with a fracture of the footplate outside of the foci had longer lasting hearing improvement.[43] Several novel procedures were devised to achieve this result. These procedures all involved resection of the anterior crus and isolation of the otosclerotic focus. The isolation was achieved by intentional fracturing of the footplate by some, and partial stapedectomy by others. Although some investigators simply mobilized the posterior segment, others elected to remove the entire footplate and interposed a piece of tragal perichondrium between the posterior crus and the oval window. These procedures were technically challenging owing to the limited exposure with poor optics at the time and challenges discerning the diseased structures from those that were to be intentionally left intact. After the invention of stapedectomy by Shea, its simplicity, superior results, and long-term stability soon made stapes mobilization obsolete.

In the last 2 decades, some surgeons have returned to the concept of stapes mobilization. Key technological breakthroughs that enabled these attempts include use of the laser in stapes surgery, fiberoptic delivery of laser energy, and the high-resolution otoendoscope. Using these technologies, stapes mobilization can be performed as a minimally invasive procedure. Silverstein and coworkers[36] described the laser stapedotomy minus prosthesis (laser STAMP) operation and its preliminary outcomes in 1998. Poe[43] published the result of his investigative work and prospective study of laser stapedioplasty in 2000. The basic concept and goals of the 2 surgical approaches were similar: to mobilize and isolate the posterior crus and posterior segment of the footplate using precise surgical techniques and instrumentations. Patient selection was paramount in ensuring surgical success. The otosclerotic foci must be limited to the anterior footplate. A thin blue footplate with proper visualization must be present for separation of the posterior footplate from its anterior otosclerotic foci. In laser STAMP, an Argon laser was used to vaporize the anterior crus via an endoprobe. Visualization was provided by either microscopy or otoendoscopy. The laser was also used to divide the anterior and posterior segments of the footplate, leaving a 0.5-mm gap. In laser stapedioplasty, a prototype Argon laser endoscope was used to provide visualization as well as instrumentation in the small surgical field. Because the suitability for a minimally invasive procedure was determined intraoperatively, all patients were counseled for possible stapedotomy. In the prospective study by Poe, 11 of the 34 patients were deemed suitable for laser stapedioplasty, whereas the remaining 68% of patients underwent conventional stapedotomy.

The initial results from these 2 procedures were promising. In the laser stapedioplasty study, the postoperative results of laser stapedioplasty and stapedotomy in the control arms showed no statistically significant differences. Both groups achieved a mean air–bone gap closure to less than 10 dB at 6 weeks after surgery.[43] From the first 12 patients who had undergone the laser STAMP procedure, the postoperative mean air–bone gap improved significantly by 17.4 dB.[44] None of the patients who had undergone the laser STAMP procedure developed hyperacusis. This was thought to be due to the preservation of the stapedius tendon and hence the acoustic reflex. Additionally, the laser STAMP procedure demonstrated statistically significant improvement in the 6 to 8 kHz range compared with laser stapedotomy.[45]

The rate of refixation was also investigated by Silverstein and colleagues.[46] Over a follow-up interval of 5 to 53 months (mean, 25.6 months), only 1 of the 46 patients who had undergone the laser STAMP procedure developed worsening of conductive hearing consistent with refixation.[46] A subsequent long-term study[47] of 43 patients showed that only 3 patients developed refixation over a 12- to 140-month follow-up (median, 33 months). All 3 patients were successfully revised with stapedotomy with 1 revision performed 12 years after the laser STAMP procedure.

The development of modified mobilization prosthesis-free procedures may represent yet another breakthrough in the surgical management of otosclerosis. These novel approaches have been shown to provide good hearing outcome in a selected group of patients. It was estimated that these approaches could be used in 45% to 50% of all cases of otosclerosis cases requiring surgery.[44] Further studies to address preoperative patient selection as well as to confirm the long-term stability would further advance this exciting area of innovation.

"HOW I DO IT"

Stapes surgery is a technically challenging operation with little margin for error. It has undergone a fascinating evolution since its inception by Dr John Shea in 1956. Major advancements have included the development of micro drills, the use of various lasers, variations in prostheses materials and styles, and, perhaps most important, much improved visualization with brighter, clearer microscopes and most recently with rigid endoscopes.

Back in its heyday in the 1960s through the 1980s there was such a huge backlog of patients, the surgery went under the purview of most community otolaryngologists. Now that the procedure is much less commonly performed, for the younger generation of surgeons it has almost become an otologic subspecialty procedure. Our informal survey of fellowship-trained otologists in Canada suggests that an annual of volume of at least 10 cases is required to maintain skills, maximize results, and minimize complications.

There are many variations of the technique, instruments, and prostheses. Each can be very effective in different hands depending on the experience of the surgeon. The following is a synopsis of how this author (LSP) performs a stapedotomy with prosthesis. Patients must meet audiological criteria and have no general or regional anesthetic contraindications. I perform primary stapes surgery under general anesthesia. For most revision cases, and in some special circumstances, I operate using local anesthesia with conscious sedation.

Almost all my cases are done as day surgery. I work in a teaching hospital and have residents partake in my cases. Each case is scheduled for 1.5 hours, including turnaround time. Patients are typically discharged home 2 to 3 hours after the procedure. I do not routinely use perioperative antibiotics or corticosteroids. Patients are positioned supine on the operating table with the head turned away from the operative ear. The head is placed in a ring headrest in a laterally flexed position to angle the ear canal away from the shoulder.

The description of the surgery that follows is accompanied by a video (Video 1). I use povidone-iodine 7.5% to prep the pinna and periauricular skin, but do not take any extra measures to prep the deeper ear canal or tympanic membrane. I inject the ear canal skin inferiorly, posteriorly, and anteriorly with 1% lidocaine in 1:40,000 adrenaline with a 26-G 1.5-inch needle on a 1-mL tuberculin syringe. Injections require no more than a total of 1.0 to 1.5 mL of local anesthesia. Slow, gentle injections are crucial to prevent blebs in the canal skin and to ensure medial diffusion for hemostasis along the entire incisions.

I always work through a speculum. I freehand the speculum for the first part of the case, but then secure it in a speculum holder once I have maximized the exposure. It is always best to fit in the largest diameter speculum to maintain its stability and maximize exposure. The minimum working diameter speculum is 5 mm, but 8 mm is ideal.

I make the superior and inferior canal incisions with a sagittal roller knife and join them horizontally with a triangle knife, making the flap about 6 mm in length. I elevate the meatal flap evenly throughout its width with a McCabe flap knife elevator so that the flap falls forward onto the tympanic membrane before I enter the middle ear. Before elevating the annulus, I enter the middle ear superiorly near the notch of Rivinus to identify the chorda tympani. I divide the mucosa and find the top of the annulus, and then bluntly elevate it inferiorly out of its sulcus with the flap knife down to the bottom end of the incision.

Not uncommonly, ear canal tortuosity can obscure the inferior exposure so that some of the flap elevation has to be done blindly. This highlights the importance of elevating in the proper plane under the annulus so as to not tear the flap or tympanic membrane. After its elevation, the tympanomeatal flap is folded forward at the malleus attachment to expose the entire posterior one-half of the middle ear. The incus and stapes are identified and palpated with a Rosen needle or equivalent before curetting the bone. A fixed stapes with a mobile lateral chain confirms the diagnosis, as does the observation of white otosclerotic bone anterior to the footplate at the fissula ante fenestrum.

In most cases, posterior/superior ear canal bone needs to be excavated to improve exposure. Although some use a drill for this part, I always use a small sharp bone curette. The curetting action should be away from the chorda tympani and ossicles. All attempts should be made to preserve the chorda and not stretch it, which means working around the chorda without retracting it. Required exposure includes the pyramidal process and stapedius tendon posteriorly, the facial nerve canal superiorly, and the anterior footplate anteriorly.

After maximizing the exposure, I secure the speculum in the speculum holder. I separate the incudostapedial joint using a 45° pick with great care to not rock the stapes so as to not mobilize the footplate. I cut the stapedius tendon with small Bellucci scissors. I do not use a laser in my practice and I do not create a control hole in the footplate. Thus, my next step is to down fracture the superstructure toward the promontory with a 45° pick. So as to not avulse the chorda, the pick is inserted inferior to the chorda and then up under the stapes neck. The suprastructure is flicked off the footplate, as opposed to pushed off the footplate, to minimize the chances of footplate mobilization.

I use a prosthesis with a 0.6-mm piston diameter. Thus, I create a stapedotomy with a 0.8-mm diameter stapedotomy with a diamond drill bit on the Skeeter drill. The wider opening accommodates a piston angle that is not orthogonal to the footplate. Ideally, the opening is centered in the footplate, although sometimes its location must be altered by limitations in the overall exposure or local factors like a facial nerve canal overhang. For a typical thin footplate, very little drilling is required to create the fenestra. Visual and tactile feedback determines the right amount of pressure. Once the vestibule is open, great care must be taken to not aspirate perilymph. This occurrence is best prevented by using a 24-G suction with thumb off the thumb plate hole when removing the fluid from around or over the stapedotomy.

I do not routinely measure the distance from footplate to incus. In the majority of cases I use a 4.5-mm long piston prosthesis. I use a De La Cruz style piston because it has the shortest piston segment at 1.27 mm, making it easy to determine how much of the piston is lateral and medial to the footplate. I prefer the Eclipse prosthesis (Grace Medical, Memphis, TN) made with a Teflon piston and nitinol wire that can be hand or heat crimped. The crimped wire should be secure enough to not fall off the incus but not be constrictively tight. After crimping, the incus should be gently balloted to ensure free movement of the piston in the stapedotomy. I do not routinely place tissue under or around the prosthesis unless the stapedotomy is inadvertently made too large. In these latter instances, I typically use a blood patch acquired by venopuncture by the anesthesiologist, which I instill with a 26-G needle on the tuberculin syringe.

I carefully reposition the tympanomeatal flap and pack the canal by injecting a paste made from Gelfoam powder, saline, and antibiotic ointment through a 16-G blunt needle loaded onto a 3-mL syringe. Patients are seen about 9 or 10 days postoperatively for follow-up to remove the packing and then about 2 to 3 months later for follow-up audiometric testing.

SUMMARY

Stapedectomy and stapedotomy represent the state-of-the-art surgical procedures in addressing the conductive hearing loss caused by otosclerosis. Their high rates of success and long-term stability have been demonstrated repeatedly in many studies. In comparing the short- and long-term results of the 2 procedures, it is evident that stapedotomy confers better hearing gain at the high frequencies as well as lower complication rates. Over time, many innovations by otologists have further improved the surgical outcomes and led to dramatic improvements in patent's quality of life. Modified stapes mobilization approaches may represent the next major development in stapes surgery in a select patient population.

SUPPLEMENTARY DATA

Supplementary data related to this article can be found online at https://doi.org/10.1016/j.otc.2017.11.008.

REFERENCES

1. Shea JJ. A personal history of stapedectomy. Am J Otol 1998;19(5 Suppl):S2–12.
2. Glasscock ME, Storper IS, Haynes DS, et al. Twenty-five years of experience with stapedectomy. Laryngoscope 1995;105(9 Pt 1):899–904.
3. Rosen S. Mobilization of the stapes to restore hearing in otosclerosis. N Y State J Med 1953;53:2650–3.
4. Shea JJ. Fenestration of the oval window. Ann Otol Rhinol Laryngol 1958;67:932–51.
5. Marquet J. "Stapedotomy" technique and results. Am J Otol 1985;6:63–7.
6. Gulya AJ, Minor LB, Poe DS. Glasscock-Shambaugh surgery of the ear. PMPH-USA; 2010.
7. Nadol JB, McKenna MJ. Surgery of the ear and temporal bone. Lippincott Williams & Wilkins; 2004.
8. Sziklai I. Surgery of stapes fixations. Springer; 2016.
9. Issa TK, Bahgat MA, Linthicum FH Jr, et al. The effect of stapedectomy on hearing of patients with otosclerosis and Meniere's disease. Am J Otol 1983;4(4):323–6.
10. House HP, Hansen MR, Al Dakhail AA, et al. Stapedectomy versus stapedotomy: comparison of results with long-term follow-up. Laryngoscope 2002;112(11):2046–50.
11. Fisch U. Stapedotomy versus stapedectomy. Am J Otol 1982;4(2):112–7.
12. Colletti V, Fiorino FG. Stapedotomy with stapedius tendon preservation: technique and long-term results. Otolaryngol Head Neck Surg 1994;111(3 Pt 1):181–8.
13. Somers T, Govaerts P, Marquet T, et al. Statistical analysis of otosclerosis surgery performed by Jean Marquet. Ann Otol Rhinol Laryngol 1994;103):945–51.
14. Bailey HA, Pappas JJ, Graham SS. Small fenestra stapedectomy. A preliminary report. Laryngoscope 1981;91:1308–21.
15. McGee TM. Comparison of small fenestra and total stapedectomy. Ann Otol Rhinol Laryngol 1981;90(6 Pt 1):633–6.
16. Moon CN, Hahn MJ. Partial vs. total footplate removal in stapedectomy: a comparative study. Laryngoscope 1984;94:912–5.
17. Persson P, Harder H, Magnuson B. Hearing results in otosclerosis surgery after partial stapedectomy, total stapedectomy and stapedotomy. Acta Otolaryngol 1997;117:94–9.
18. Kos MI, Montandon PB, Guyot JP. Short- and long-term results of stapedotomy and stapedectomy with a Teflon-wire piston prosthesis. Ann Otol Rhinol Laryngol 2001;110:907–11.

19. Sedwick JD, Louden CL, Shelton C. Stapedectomy vs stapedotomy. Do you really need a laser? Arch Otolaryngol Head Neck Surg 1997;123:177–80.

20. Cremers CW, Beusen JM, Huygen PL. Hearing gain after stapedotomy, partial platinectomy, or total stapedectomy for otosclerosis. Ann Otol Rhinol Laryngol 1991;100:959–61.

21. Quaranta N, Besozzi G, Fallacara RA, et al. Air and bone conduction change after stapedotomy and partial stapedectomy for otosclerosis. Otolaryngol Head Neck Surg 2005;133:116–20.

22. Spandow O, Söderberg O, Bohlin L. Long-term results in otosclerotic patients operated by stapedectomy or stapedotomy. Scand Audiol 2000;29:186–90.

23. Levy R, Shvero J, Hadar T. Stapedotomy technique and results: ten years' experience and comparative study with stapedectomy. Laryngoscope 1990;100(10 Pt 1):1097–9.

24. Vasama JP, Kujala J, Hirvonen TP. Is small-fenestra stapedotomy a safer outpatient procedure than total stapedectomy? ORL J Otorhinolaryngol Relat Spec 2006;68:99–102.

25. Pedersen CB, Elbrønd O. Large versus small fenestration technique in stapedectomy. A comparative investigation of House and Fisch prostheses in stapedectomy. Clin Otolaryngol Allied Sci 1983;8:21–4.

26. Esquivel CR, Mamikoglu B, Wiet RJ. Long-term results of small fenestra stapedectomy compared with large fenestra technique. Laryngoscope 2002;112(8 Pt 1):1338–41.

27. Shea JJ. Stapedectomy - long-term report. Ann Otol Rhinol Laryngol 1982;91(5 Pt 1):516–20.

28. Kürsten R, Schneider B, Zrunek M. Long-term results after stapedectomy versus stapedotomy. Am J Otol 1994;15:804–6.

29. Colletti V, Sittoni V, Fiorino FG. Stapedotomy with and without stapedius tendon preservation versus stapedectomy: long-term results. Am J Otol 1988;9:136–41.

30. Mann WJ, Amedee RG, Fuerst G, et al. Hearing loss as a complication of stapes surgery. Otolaryngol Head Neck Surg 1996;115:324–8.

31. Smyth GD, Hassard TH. Eighteen years experience in stapedectomy. The case for the small fenestra operation. Ann Otol Rhinol Laryngol Suppl 1978;87(3 Pt 2 Suppl 49):3–36.

32. Hüttenbrink KB. Biomechanics of stapesplasty: a review. Otol Neurotol 2003;24:548–57 [discussion: 557–9].

33. Laske RD, Röösli C, Chatzimichalis MV, et al. The influence of prosthesis diameter in stapes surgery: a meta-analysis and systematic review of the literature. Otol Neurotol 2011;32:520–8.

34. Mangham CA. Reducing footplate complications in small fenestra microdrill stapedotomy. Am J Otol 1993;14:118–21.

35. Casale M, De Franco A, Salvinelli F, et al. Hearing results in stapes surgery using two different prosthesis. Rev Laryngol Otol Rhinol (Bord) 2003;124:255–8.

36. Silverstein H, Hester TO, Rosenberg SI, et al. Preservation of the stapedius tendon in laser stapes surgery. Laryngoscope 1998;108:1453–8.

37. Shabana YK, Ghonim MR, Pedersen CB. Stapedotomy: does prosthesis diameter affect outcome? Clin Otolaryngol Allied Sci 1999;24:91–4.

38. Mathews SB, Rasgon BM, Byl FM. Stapes surgery in a residency training program. Laryngoscope 1999;109:52–3.

39. Vital V, Konstantinidis I, Vital I, et al. Minimizing the dead ear in otosclerosis surgery. Auris Nasus Larynx 2008;35:475–9.

40. Cousins MJ, Bridenbaugh PO. Neural blockade in clinical anesthesia and management of pain, vol. 494. Lippincott Williams & Wilkins; 1998.
41. Collins JB, Song J, Mahabir RC. Onset and duration of intradermal mixtures of bupivacaine and lidocaine with epinephrine. Can J Plast Surg 2013;21:51–3.
42. Wegner I, Bittermann AJ, Zinsmeester MM, et al. Local versus general anesthesia in stapes surgery for otosclerosis: a systematic review of the evidence. Otolaryngol Head Neck Surg 2013;149:360–5.
43. Poe DS. Laser-assisted endoscopic stapedectomy: a prospective study. Laryngoscope 2000;110(5 Pt 2 Suppl 95):1–37.
44. Silverstein H. Laser stapedotomy minus prosthesis (laser STAMP): a minimally invasive procedure. Am J Otol 1998;19:277–82.
45. Silverstein H, Hoffmann KK, Thompson JH, et al. Hearing outcome of laser stapedotomy minus prosthesis (STAMP) versus conventional laser stapedotomy. Otol Neurotol 2004;25:106–11.
46. Silverstein H, Jackson LE, Conlon WS, et al. Laser stapedotomy minus prosthesis (laser STAMP): absence of refixation. Otol Neurotol 2002;23:152–7.
47. Silverstein H, Van Ess MJ, Alameda YA. Laser stapedotomy minus prosthesis: long-term follow-up. Otolaryngol Head Neck Surg 2011;144:753–7.

The Stapes Prosthesis
Past, Present, and Future

Alexander Sevy, MD[a,b,*], Moises Arriaga, MD, MBA[a,b]

KEYWORDS

- Stapes • Prosthesis • Stapedectomy • Stapedotomy • Otosclerosis

KEY POINTS

- In 1956, Shea and Treace made a stapes prosthesis using a Teflon piston and vein graft over the oval window after stapedectomy for otosclerosis, as an alternative to fenestration.
- Further iterations of stapes prostheses followed, by Shea, House, Robinson, McGee, Schuknecht, and many others.
- A wide array of biomaterial availability influenced stapes surgery techniques, especially methods for incus attachment.
- Stapes prosthesis has many shapes and sizes; titanium, nitinol, and Teflon are popular materials. There are also powered implant options.
- Excellent results can be achieved with prostheses designed to rest on tissue grafts in stapedectomy techniques or pass through the footplate in stapedotomy techniques.

NASCENCE OF STAPES SURGERY

Although Valsava first described stapes ankylosis leading to hearing loss in 1703 and Meniere described mobilization of the stapes with a gold rod in 1842, stapes surgery is regarded to have begun in 1876 when Kessel developed the removal of the stapes after mobilization to address hearing loss. Hearing improvement with mobilization alone was fleeting; however, with stapedectomy, results were more durable and the practice spread through Europe and even to the United States. Unfortunately, without antibiotics, hearing loss and lethal intracranial complications led to the condemnation of stapes surgery in 1899 by Politzer, Siebenmann, and Moure at the International Otology Congress in London.[1,2] There was a shift to fenestration techniques from 1900s until the 1950s. Rosen rediscovered stapes mobilization in 1952, and notably in 1956 Shea revisited stapes surgery using a carved Teflon (DuPont, Wilmington,

Disclosure Statement: The authors have nothing to disclose.
[a] Department of Otolaryngology–Head and Neck Surgery, Louisiana State University School of Medicine, 533 Bolivar Street, New Orleans, LA 70112, USA; [b] Our Lady of the Lake Hearing and Balance Center, 7777 Hennessy Boulevard, Suite 709, Baton Rouge, LA 70808, USA
* Corresponding author. Our Lady of the Lake Hearing and Balance Center, 7777 Hennessy Boulevard, Suite 709, Baton Rouge, LA 70808.
E-mail address: asevy@lsuhsc.edu

Otolaryngol Clin N Am 51 (2018) 393–404
https://doi.org/10.1016/j.otc.2017.11.010
0030-6665/18/© 2017 Elsevier Inc. All rights reserved.

oto.theclinics.com

Delaware) stapes prosthesis (**Fig. 1**B) made by Treace with a vein graft over the oval window after stapedectomy to restore hearing in the setting of otosclerosis.

NATURAL OR NO MATERIALS

Although utilization of a prosthesis to replace the stapes is the most common technique, some surgeons developed stapes surgeries that did not require the implantation of foreign material. Partial footplate removal developed by Plester and then fenestration of the footplate was advanced by Shea, Marquet, and Martin. In the late 1950s. Portman, Hough, Juers, and others advanced a posterior crus interposition stapedioplasty with anterior curotomy and partial stapedectomy.[3] In those techniques, the anterior crurotomy freed the stapes superstructure from the anterior otosclerosis fixation and the remaining posterior crus provided ossicular connection to the partial footplate removal, which had been sealed with a vein graft. More recently, Silverstein described laser stapedotomy minus prosthesis (STAMP) in cases of minimal otosclerosis with transection of the blue footplate and anterior crurectomy to mobilize the stapes with preservation of the stapedial tendon.[4,5]

EARLY PROSTHESES

The basic physical requirement of a stapes prosthesis is to achieve a secure connection between the mobile incus and the sealed perilymph in the oval window. More than 100 other stapes prostheses have been developed since Shea and Treace's original carved Teflon stapes replica (see **Fig. 1**B). The evolution of Shea's personal stapedectomy technique over time provides a window to the confluence of changing concepts of the physical requirements of stapes prostheses as well as the changes in biomaterial availability and surgical equipment capabilities. Shea himself started to use a pointed polyethylene tube strut in 1958 (**Fig. 1**C) and then a Teflon piston prosthesis in 1962, followed by a Teflon cup prosthesis in 1964; then he added microsurgical laser techniques in 1993.

House popularized a stainless steel wire-loop prosthesis (**Fig. 1**D) that could be crimped onto the long process of the incus in 1960. This crimp-on prosthesis type used in a total stapedectomy technique has provided excellent long-term results, including paired comparisons in patients undergoing total stapedectomy on one

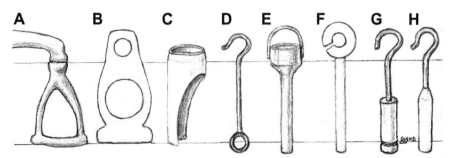

Fig. 1. Early and representative stapes prostheses. (*A*) Human stapes and incus long process; (*B*) first stapes prosthesis, Shea and Treace, carved Teflon fluoroplastic; (*C*) Shea strut, polyethylene; (*D*) House wire loop, stainless steel; (*E*) Robinson bucket handle, titanium; (*F*) fluoroplastic loop; (*G*) platinum wire hook, stainless steel piston; and (*H*) nitinol wire hook and fluoroplastic piston. (*Courtesy of* Alexander Sevy, MD, Louisiana State University School of Medicine, New Orleans, LA.)

side and stapedotomy on the other.[6] Attempts to improve the procedure by adhering Gelfoam resulted in increased complications.[7] In 1962, Schuknecht developed a steel wire prosthesis and template, which allowed surgeons to custom-make their steel wire prostheses and affix fat or Gelfoam to expedite sealing the oval window without a separate tissue graft.[2,8–10]

FURTHER ITERATIONS

The large backlog of otosclerosis patients in the 1960s created a push for innovation to improve the techniques and outcomes of stapedectomy. Although the success rate was in the 90% range, challenges included necrosis of the incus (particularly with the polyethylene strut), postoperative dizziness, loosening of the wire loop, fistula, and granuloma formation with Gelfoam prostheses. In 1960, McGee (Olympus, Bartlett, TN) developed a stainless steel piston with a wire hook and then, in 1963, Schuknecht developed the Tef-wire with a Teflon piston attached to a wire hook (**Fig. 1**H). The McGee prosthesis was modified to include a burnishing to the distal tip of the prosthesis to indicate the appropriate depth of penetration of the vestibule (**Fig. 1**G). De La Cruz also developed a piston prosthesis with a short piston to alert the surgeon to excessive depth in the vestibule. Fisch modified the wire hook from a round cross-section to a flattened metal ribbon attached to a piston. In 1961, Robinson developed a bucket handle prosthesis (**Fig. 1**E) which was subsequently modified by Lippy with a notch to better accommodate the incus, especially in revisions with distal incus necrosis (**Fig. 2**). Aspects from different prostheses (**Fig. 3**) were often combined, such as with the previously discussed Shea Teflon piston with a bucket-like cup to accommodate the incus. Causse championed the all-Teflon prosthesis with a piston and a C-shaped hook

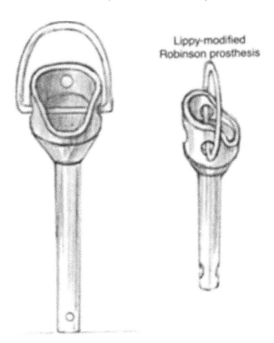

Lippy-modified
Robinson prosthesis

Fig. 2. Lippy-modified Robinson prosthesis. (*Courtesy of* Grace Medical, Memphis, TN; with permission.)

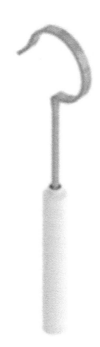

Fig. 3. Grace Tef-ribbon. (*Courtesy of* Grace Medical, Memphis, TN; with permission.)

for the incus developed originally by Shea in 1962 (**Fig. 1**F).[11] The self-crimping feature of this prosthesis provided technical consistency to the fixation of the prosthesis onto the incus. Later, Causse[8] refined the design to include a Polycel stapedius tendon attachment on the shaft to maintain stapedius function and the acoustic reflex. A unique stapedectomy challenge occurs when the incus is absent. Fenestration included incus removal; thus, previous fenestration patients required a mechanism to attach the stapes prosthesis to the mobile malleus. The initial incus replacement prosthesis was a modified wire loop, which was placed on the malleus under a periosteal pocket and bent to contact an oval window vein graft. This has since followed the same pattern as stapedectomy prosthesis with pistons that can fit through a stapedotomy and alternative crimping techniques with heat-activated biomaterials (**Fig. 4**).

MATERIAL CONCERNS

In 1987 there was the accidental manufacture of several lots of McGee pistons with a magnetic alloy stainless steel. There are 2 variants of stainless steel commonly used in medicine, the 300 and 400 series. In the 300 series, microdipoles are arranged more randomly reducing its magnetism but the 400 series has greater microdipole alignment and greater magnetism. The 400 series is typically used for instruments and the 300 series for implants; however, 28 lots of McGee pistons in 1987 were accidentally made with 400 series stainless steel and there was a worldwide recall. This becomes a safety concern for MRI with any ferromagnetic implant. In magnetic exposure experiments, 400 series stainless steel moved the most with a small amount of movement with 300 series steel, and no movement from titanium platinum or tantalum. Although the 300 series stainless steel seems safe in MRI movement

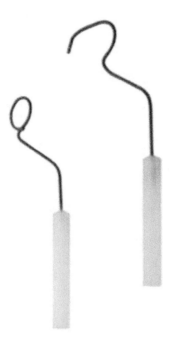

Fig. 4. Malleus to footplate piston. Open (*right*) and closed (*left*) nitinol images. (*Courtesy of* Grace Medical, Memphis, TN; with permission.)

studies, titanium has become one of the primary metal materials used in ossicular chain reconstruction due in large part to its nonferromagnetic properties, in addition to its strength and weight.[12]

Nitinol is an alloy metal (titanium and nickel) that returns to its original shape when heated. Thus, a stapedectomy prosthesis wire can be manufactured to the size of the incus diameter, then stretched to the size necessary for placement during surgery, and then heated with a laser during surgery to return to its original shape and size (see **Fig. 4**; **Fig. 5**).[13] Nitinol allows for circumferential crimping of a wire hook around the incus without overly squeezing the incus during manual crimping. Stapes crimpers often have jaws that do not meet to prevent the application of too much force but sometimes the wire hook can be loose and still require additional crimping with an alligator forceps. Changing the material of the hook from stainless steel to platinum (**Fig. 6**) is one strategy to facilitate an appropriate crimp onto the incus. In cases of partial erosion of the incus, the long process may prove too short or thin for the designed method of incus fixation. Materials, such as hydroxyapatite and ionomeric cements, have been used in primary and revision surgeries to aid prosthesis attachment to the incus (ionomeric cement should be used judiciously because fatal neurotoxicity from the high aluminum content has been reported with use of large amounts during cranioplasty). Prostheses, such as the Kraus K-Helix piston, have been designed to work in conjunction with cements in situations with a shortened incus (**Fig. 7**).

PROSTHESIS-SPECIFIC TECHNIQUE HIGHLIGHTS

Stapedectomy prostheses are associated with specific technical maneuvers (see **Table 1** for highlights of different surgeons and stapes prostheses). The common

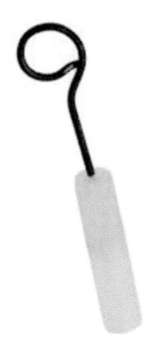

Fig. 5. Closed nitinol piston (closed image of nitinol Eclipse piston). (*Courtesy of* Grace Medical, Memphis, TN; with permission.)

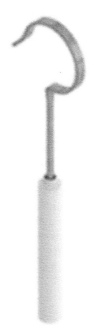

Fig. 6. Platinum ribbon piston prosthesis. (*Courtesy of* Grace Medical, Memphis, TN; with permission.)

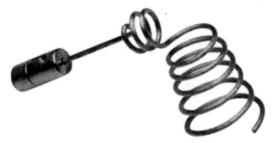

Fig. 7. Stapes prosthesis designed for shortened incus and cement adhesion. (*Courtesy of Grace Medical, Memphis, TN; with permission.*)

Table 1				
Stapes surgery technique highlights				
Surgeon/ Inventor, Year	**Prosthesis**	**Stapes**	**Graft/Material at Round Window**	**Attachment to Incus**
Shea, 1956	Carved Teflon piston	Stapedectomy	Vein graft	Placed long process through hole
House, 1960	Wire loop, stainless steel	Stapedectomy	Vein graft	Crimp wire onto long process
McGee, 1960	Shepherd's crook + piston, stainless steel	Stapedectomy	Vein graft	Crimp wire (shepherd's crook) onto long process
Robinson, 1961	Bucket handle, stainless steel (now titanium)	Stapedectomy	Vein graft	Lift incus vs push prosthesis down, slide lenticular process into cup and bucket handle over long process
Schuknecht, 1962	Wire loop stainless steel, Gelfoam	Stapedectomy	Vein graft, Gelfoam at end of wire loop	Crimp wire onto long process
Shea, 1962 (popularized and later modified by Causse)	Teflon loop + piston	Stapedectomy	Vein graft	C-shaped hook onto long process, no crimping. Option to attach stapedial tendon to prosthesis
Silverstein, 1989	STAMP	Laser stapedotomy/ anterior crurectomy	Fat graft	I-S joint not divided, stapedial tendon preserved
Wengen, 1997	aWengen clip, titanium	Stapedotomy		Spring allows clipping onto LP without crimping
Knox, 1999	Nitinol heat-activated wire, Teflon piston	Stapedotomy		Place hook over long process, then heat-activated crimping; can use laser

Abbreviations: I-S, incudostapedial; LP, long process.
Data from Refs.[2,4,7,8,10,11,13]

features of the surgical techniques are exposure of the incudo-stapedial joint, footplate, facial nerve, and stapedius tendon. Once stapes fixation and lateral ossicular mobility are confirmed, the incudo-stapedial joint is separated and the stapedius muscle is sectioned. The stapes superstructure can be down fractured with or without dividing the posterior crus. At this point, depending on the selected prosthesis and surgeon preference, a total stapedectomy, footplate drill out, partial stapedectomy, or stapedotomy can be performed using picks, hooks, hand drills, drills, or a laser. It is paramount to minimize instrumentation or suction around and especially beyond the footplate to minimize risk of perilymph removal and sensorineural hearing loss. If a vein graft or other material has been obtained, it can be placed over the oval window prior to prosthesis placement and thus quickly seal the vestibule, whereas in stapedotomy technique, the oval window is open until the prosthesis is placed requiring care to avoid suctioning the fenestra until the prosthesis is placed. With total stapedectomy techniques with a bucket handle–type prosthesis, some surgeons focus first near the footplate and push the prosthesis on the tissue graft medially until the depth relative to the incus is correct; others lift the incus first and place the prosthesis and release the incus to have the lenticular process rest in the bucket handle.

Crimping

Regarding attachment to the incus, since House's description there has been an option of a malleable hook that can be crimped over the incus long process. Alligator forceps have been used to crimp these prostheses; however, this step is not trivial, with technical articles, instructional courses, and instrument design devoted to the topic of crimping techniques to avoid excessive force, inadequate crimping, and incorrect shape of the crimp. Complications of incus necrosis and loose wire syndrome often are attributed to the crimping technique. Numerous specialized crimpers have been designed to optimize crimping, such as the birdbeak McGee and off-axis Juers crimpers, with limits on closure and groves to aid in control without overcrimping and improved visualization during crimping. Several options avoid mechanical crimping altogether, such as Shea-Causse Teflon piston, bucket handle prostheses, and heat activated crimping, with materials such as nitinol. With heat-activated prostheses, a laser (or other heat source) in lieu of a mechanical crimper to close the hook end of the prosthesis around the long process as developed by Knox and Reitan.[13] A newer variation of the heat-activated prosthesis design has the hook slightly off axis to accommodate a wider array of incus diameters so that the hook is not limited in closure by the wire overriding itself (Eclipse piston) (see **Fig. 5**). Another option is the àWengen clip (**Fig. 8**) that uses a spring mechanism clip onto the incus without

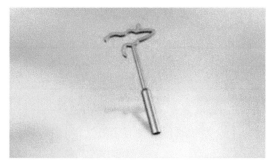

Fig. 8. àWengen clip-on prosthesis. (*Courtesy of* Kurz Medical Inc., Tucker, GA; with permission.)

crimping or a nitinol version, which has a looser clip tightened by sequential laser applications.

Sealing the Oval Window

The original stapedectomy prostheses were designed for total footplate removal with vein or other tissue grafts on which the prostheses were placed. With stapedotomy, it is possible to use autologous blood, presized sized tissue graft, which adheres to the piston, or small pieces of tissue around the entry point of the prosthesis into the fenestra.

PROSTHESIS DIMENSIONS
Diameter

Stapes prostheses are manufactured with a range of piston diameters from 0.3 mm to 0.8 mm. Some surgeons have advocated smaller diameters to reduce the size of stapedotomy fenestration and potentially also the risk to hearing loss. In tissue-seal prostheses, Fucci and colleagues[14] noted no statistical difference in air bone gap closure between Robinson prostheses with 0.4-mm versus 0.6-mm shaft diameters. Wegner and colleagues[15] performed a cadaveric study comparing 0.4-mm, 0.6-mm, and 0.8-mm pistons with varying fenestration sizes. A larger-diameter piston can displace a larger volume for a given stroke distance and the investigators noted improved sound transmission with the large diameters. All prostheses fared at least as well as a mobile stapes below 700 Hz but had a relative drop-off for higher frequencies approaching the noise floor above 6000 Hz. Regardless of the piston diameter, there is phase delay for all sizes of pistons relative to a mobile native stapes, particularly from 500 Hz to 4000 Hz. Although some investigators have argued that smaller piston diameter provides enhanced, high-frequency results, a recent meta-analysis of surgical results with stapedotomy demonstrated an advantage for 0.6-mm versus 0.4-mm diameter pistons in overall hearing results, air-bone gap (ABG) closure, and even high-frequency results.[16]

Length

Length of the prosthesis also plays a role and manufacturers provide a variety of methods to allow surgeons to tailor the length. The prosthesis must be long enough to stay in the fenestra but short enough not to intrude excessively within the vestibule and risk injury to the saccule. McGee and De La Cruz addressed this issue by markers on their prosthesis or a designed shorter length piston to avoid overinsertion. Whether there are different length prostheses produced, or the material allows cutting with a knife or is engineered to be trimmed with clippers, manufacturers allow surgeons to select different sizes at the time of surgery. The shaft can also be designed to allow for adjustment of length.[17] Measurements can be taken in surgery from stapes footplate to the lateral or medial side of the incus to determine the length needed. Shape can also be a factor particularly to avoid contact with the facial nerve, and the shaft can be bent or offset as in the Robinson-Moon prosthesis (Medtronic Xomed, Jacksonville, FL). Surgeons must understand the prosthesis design with respect to measurement of the incus to the footplate because this relationship is not standard. A recent example was an initial higher-than-expected failure rate with Gyrus Smart Piston Nitinol prostheses (Olympus, Bartlett, TN) attributable to prosthesis shortening with heat activation; thus, the usual measurement technique yields a 0.25-mm shorter length, which made lateral displacement more likely.[18]

PROSTHESES COMPARED

With many implant options available and few well-designed head-to-head studies of prostheses, a true comparison of outcomes cannot be achieved, especially because surgical technique and operator experience heavily influence hearing results and risk profiles. Forton and colleagues[19] achieved an 87% rate postoperative closure of ABGs to within 10 dB when using a laser for stapedotomy compared with another group's rate at 56.5% ABG closure using the same prosthesis but a micropick for the stapedotomy. In a longer-term study using nitinol prostheses, their patients achieved 94% ABG less than or equal to 10 dB at 1 year and maintained that level at 5 years.[20]

Results from surgeons using different prostheses, however, can be difficult to compare for many reasons. Rothbaum and colleagues[21] found that senior surgeons demonstrated significantly less displacement when targeting of fenestra (0.10 mm vs 0.24 mm,) decreased movement of the prosthesis during crimping (0.27 mm vs 0.40 mm), and a decreased rate of dislodgement of the prosthesis (6.7% vs 46.7%) compared with junior surgeons.

An opportunity to see the relative efficacy of specific prostheses is to consider studies comparing their experience with different stapes prostheses placed by the same group of surgeons. Lippy found no significant difference between the Gyrus titanium versus Robinson stainless steel implants (Medtronic Xomed, Jacksonville, FL) with mean 4-tone improvements of 27.7 dB versus 27.8 dB and postoperative ABG of 2.56 dB versus 2.60 dB.[22] There can also be conflicting findings between groups. One study comparing Teflon to nitinol detected no significant difference in ABG closure at 1 month, 2 month, 3 months, and 6 months.[23] Another group showed ABG closure less than 10 for only 36% of fluoroplastic implants but achieved 84% success with NiTiBOND (Kurz Medizintechnik, Dusslingen, Germany) and also included early and late groups of titanium pistons with 44% success initially that improved up to 92% with their more recent group. This study reveals evidence of a learning curve with their surgeons and the titanium implants.[24] In another study, nitinol prostheses performed better versus platinum ribbon manual crimp with better results short term (ABG 7.127 vs 11.692, respectively) and long term (ABG of 6.094 vs 8.936, respectively).[25] Rajan and colleagues[26] achieved ABG less than 10 dB 89% with nitinol and 74% titanium.

Failure Rates

One group found failure rates at 10 years were 11.2% for stainless steel McGee with platinum ribbon, with an average time to fail of 2.5 years (these tended to displace laterally and the malleable crimped platinum ribbon loosened over time), whereas they were 9.5% for stainless steel Robinson bucket handle, with a longer average time to fail of 8.6 years.[27] Ying and colleagues[18] found 11% revision rates with their noncrimp nitinol pistons and 4% with their crimped platinum wire prostheses, which may be attributable to learning curve issues of length selection and laser energy selection, as discussed previously.

POWERED IMPLANTS

To further tailor the frequency response curve and provide higher energy, particularly in the middle and higher frequencies, powered middle ear implants have been applied to stapes surgery. The direct acoustic cochlear stimulator with an implantable electromagnetic transducer was designed to be placed on the oval window after stapedectomy, actuated using an external behind-the-ear processor.[28] Alternatively, a floating mass transducer that was applied to round window vibratory stimulation can be attached to an ossicular prosthesis, such as a partial ossicular replacement prosthesis or total ossicular replacement prosthesis, with improved results over round window placement.[29]

FUTURE DIRECTIONS

In addition to inevitable mixing and matching of various design elements and the development of new materials, the future of stapes implants may incorporate pharmaceutical or growth factor delivery with drug-eluting prostheses or pumps that could be incorporated with implants. Additionally, powered implants could be combined with cochlear implants for acoustic and electric stimulation in hybrid implant candidates.

SUMMARY

Excellent stapedectomy results can be obtained with a wide range of prostheses and techniques. The data have not identified an inherently superior prosthesis. Stapes surgeons can remain confident in the old adage that if they are obtaining excellent results with their current technique and prosthesis, there is no reason to change. Furthermore, prior to changing which prosthesis is used, surgeons must consider overall implications in terms of length measurement, long-term stability, and tissue-material interactions.

REFERENCES

1. Arnold W, Häusler R. Otosclerosis and stapes surgery. Basel (Switzerland): Karger; 2007.
2. Shea JJ Jr. A personal history of stapedectomy. Am J Otol 1998;19:S2–12.
3. Juers AL. Stapedioplasty. A new concept for stapes surgery. Laryngoscope 1959;69:1180–93.
4. Silverstein H. Laser stapedotomy minus prosthesis (laser STAMP): a minimally invasive procedure. Am J Otol 1998;19:277–82.
5. Silverstein H, Van Ess MJ, Alameda YA. Laser stapedotomy minus prosthesis: long-term follow-up. Otolaryngol Head Neck Surg 2011;144:753–7.
6. House HP, Hansen MR, Al Dakhail AA, et al. Stapedectomy versus stapedotomy: comparison of results with long-term follow-up. Laryngoscope 2002;112: 2046–50.
7. Sheehy JL, Nelson RA, House HP. Stapes surgery at the otologic medical group. Am J Otol 1979;1:22–6.
8. Fritsch MH, Naumann IC. Phylogeny of the stapes prosthesis. Otol Neurotol 2008; 29:407–15.
9. Shea JJ. Thirty years of stapes surgery. J Laryngol Otol 1988;102:14–9.
10. Shea JJ Jr. Forty years of stapes surgery. Am J Otol 1998;19:52–5.
11. Causse J. Present problems in the surgery of otosclerosis. J Laryngol Otol 1965; 79:265–99.
12. Fritsch MH. MRI scanners and the stapes prosthesis. Otol Neurotol 2007;28: 733–8.
13. Knox GW, Reitan H. Shape-memory stapes prosthesis for otosclerosis surgery. Laryngoscope 2005;115:1340–6.
14. Fucci MJ, Lippy WH, Schuring AG, et al. Prosthesis size in stapedectomy. Otolaryngol Head Neck Surg 1998;118:1–5.
15. Wegner I, Eldaebes MM, Landry TG, et al. The effect of piston diameter in stapedotomy for otosclerosis: a temporal bone model. Otol Neurotol 2016;37: 1497–502.
16. Laske RD, Roosli C, Chatzimichalis MV, et al. The influence of prosthesis diameter in stapes surgery: a meta-analysis and systematic review of the literature. Otol Neurotol 2011;32:520–8.

17. Gottlieb PK, Li X, Monfared A, et al. First results of a novel adjustable-length ossicular reconstruction prosthesis in temporal bones. Laryngoscope 2016;126: 2559–64.
18. Ying YL, Hillman TA, Chen DA. Patterns of failure in heat-activated crimping prosthesis in stapedotomy. Otol Neurotol 2011;32:21–8.
19. Forton GE, Wuyts FL, Delsupehe KG, et al. CO2 laser-assisted stapedotomy combined with aWengen titanium clip stapes prosthesis: superior short-term results. Otol Neurotol 2009;30:1071–8.
20. Lavy J, Khalil S. Five-year hearing results with the shape memory nitinol stapes prosthesis. Laryngoscope 2014;124:2591–3.
21. Rothbaum DL, Roy J, Hager GD, et al. Task performance in stapedotomy: comparison between surgeons of different experience levels. Otolaryngol Head Neck Surg 2003;128:71–7.
22. Lippy WH, Burkey JM, Schuring AG, et al. Comparison of titanium and Robinson stainless steel stapes piston prostheses. Otol Neurotol 2005;26:874–7.
23. Brar T, Passey JC, Agarwal AK. Comparison of hearing outcome using a Nitinol versus Teflon prosthesis in stapedotomy. Acta Otolaryngol 2012;132:1151–4.
24. Canu G, Lauretani F, Russo FY, et al. Early functional results using the nitibond prosthesis in stapes surgery. Acta Otolaryngol 2017;137:259–64.
25. Tenney J, Arriaga MA, Chen DA, et al. Enhanced hearing in heat-activated-crimping prosthesis stapedectomy. Otolaryngol Head Neck Surg 2008;138: 513–7.
26. Rajan GP, Diaz J, Blackham R, et al. Eliminating the limitations of manual crimping in stapes surgery: mid-term results of 90 patients in the Nitinol stapes piston multicenter trial. Laryngoscope 2007;117:1236–9.
27. Raske M, Welling JD, Gillum T, et al. Long-term stapedectomy results with the McGee stapes prosthesis. Laryngoscope 2001;111:2060–3.
28. Hausler R, Stieger C, Bernhard H, et al. A novel implantable hearing system with direct acoustic cochlear stimulation. Audiol Neurootol 2008;13:247–56.
29. Shimizu Y, Puria S, Goode RL. The floating machss transducer on the round window versus attachment to an ossicular replacement prosthesis. Otol Neurotol 2011;32:98–103.

Use of Lasers in Otosclerosis Surgery

Kestutis Paul Boyev, MD

KEYWORDS

- Laser • Stapedotomy • Otosclerosis • Hearing loss

KEY POINTS

- Lasers were initially used for otosclerosis surgery starting in the late 1970s and quickly became popular as a no-touch alternative to conventional instrumentation.
- Technological advances in laser types and delivery systems have proliferated, and a preference for handheld delivery systems seems to have emerged.
- Currently, it is not possible to demonstrate a clear advantage among the various available laser systems; however, there is some evidence that suggests using a laser could lead to better surgical outcomes.

 Video content accompanies this article at http://www.oto.theclinics.com.

INTRODUCTION

The introduction of an operating microscope and a powered drill by William House clearly revolutionized otology and neurotology, empowering and inspiring surgeons to perfect techniques that had previously been impossible or simply too dangerous. Arguably, the invention and application of the laser (light amplification by stimulated emission of radiation) was the third major revolution of twentieth century otology.

THE INVENTION OF THE LASER

In 1958, Arthur Schawlow and Charles Townes applied for a patent for the laser[1] as a modification of an earlier technology, the maser, which used stimulated emissions of microwave radiation. By adapting the principles of the maser to instead use light, of shorter wavelength than microwave radiation, their device acquired properties that were extremely useful for industry and medicine alike.

Disclosure Statement: The author has nothing to disclose.
Division of Otology/Neurotology, Department of Otolaryngology–Head and Neck Surgery, The Morsani College of Medicine, University of South Florida, 12901 Bruce B. Downs Boulevard, MDC 73, Tampa, FL 33612, USA
E-mail address: pboyev@health.usf.edu

Otolaryngol Clin N Am 51 (2018) 405–413
https://doi.org/10.1016/j.otc.2017.11.009
0030-6665/18/© 2017 Elsevier Inc. All rights reserved.

The first working laser was built by Theodore Maiman at Hughes Research Laboratories. On May 16, 1960, he was able to demonstrate the linear transmission of a beam of light that had a severely restricted spectrum of wavelength. Maiman built on the invention of Schawlow and Townes, introducing a method to pump energy into a ruby rod with mirrored ends to excite the medium into higher energy states. The energy emitted by the transitions between these states was the source of delivery of extremely high-power densities. Investigators had to wait until later that year before they could enjoy the sight of a thin beam of red light, the first manufactured light to display the characteristics that define laser radiation: monochromaticity, directionality, coherence, and brightness.[2]

HISTORICAL ASPECTS OF STAPES SURGERY

Occurring nearly contemporaneously with the invention of laser technology, the advent of the era of otologic microsurgery was underway. John J. Shea had applied microsurgical techniques to the otosclerotic human stapes and, in 1956, he demonstrated it could be safely removed and replaced with a Teflon prosthetic stapes, thus providing an effective alternative to the fenestration operations promoted by Julius Lempert and others.[3] Although both the invention of laser and the development of modern stapes surgery can be dated to within 2 years, it took 2 decades of refinements before these innovations were combined.

Rodney C. Perkins[4] performed the first laser stapedotomy operation on August 8, 1978. In 1980, he published a report of the first 11 subjects whom he treated with what he called an argon laser microscope, which was built in collaboration with Jack Urban, among others. During the years when stapedectomy was the dominant approach to otosclerosis surgery, there had been no real impetus to investigate instruments other than picks and/or drills. In the 1960s, Plester[5] advocated partial stapedectomy (small fenestra), the removal of the posterior one-third of the footplate, and Shea and colleagues[6] developed a Teflon piston to replace Shea's original replacement prosthesis, which looked very much like an actual stapes. In the 1970s, Fisch,[7] among others, favored minimalist approaches based on histopathologic studies that noted adhesions between the otosclerotic foci and the underlying saccular membrane near the anterior footplate. It was suspected that removal of the entire footplate could fistulize the endolymphatic space and lead to deafening as potassium-rich endolymph poured into the perilymphatic space. These developments enhanced the popularity of piston prostheses over fat-wire because the former were more easily accommodated by the increasingly smaller openings. As small-fenestra approaches gained currency and as the adverse effects of mechanical trauma associated with removal or drilling of the footplate were recognized, the obvious advantages of laser became manifest: it is an instrument that can precisely apply energy to vaporize the posterior crus, transect the stapedius tendon, and create a stapedotomy. These properties further inspired or enabled innovative refinements of work around the footplate, such as the technique of stapedotomy minus prosthesis (STAMP).[8]

LASER TECHNICAL CONSIDERATIONS

Lasers made an attractive alternative or supplement to the existing mechanical technology of drills and microperforation because of the potential to avoid trauma to the inner ear and thus to reduce the incidence of postoperative hearing loss or dizziness. Risk of complications, such as floating footplate, could also be minimized if a no-touch modality could be substituted. It was acknowledged, however, that the nature of laser energy could have undesirable thermal and acoustic effects. The effects of temperature changes on cochlear function had been investigated thoroughly in animal models before the advent of laser ear microsurgery; however, the specific changes in temperature imparted by laser followed somewhat later and remain an active subject of investigation.

When a beam of laser light strikes tissue, it is transmitted, reflected, or absorbed. It is the latter 2 interactions that influence suitability of a given laser for otologic surgery; it is the property of transmission that can put deeper structures at risk. Ossicular bone and perilymph are the 2 main substances of concern because they are routinely encountered; the interactions of laser with mucosa and blood (in hemostasis) are subsidiary factors. As laser energy strikes tissue and is absorbed, the predominant effect is that heat is generated. Depending on factors, such as average power, this heat can coagulate proteins at lower power levels but can vaporize or even melt bone at higher levels. Furthermore, heat will dissipate after the exposure but the dynamics of dissipation of this heat are mediated by pulse duration, pulse timing, and spot size.[9]

The use of carbon dioxide (CO_2) lasers in otolaryngology dates back to use in endolaryngeal surgery in the early 1970s by Strong and Jako,[10] who first studied the effects of the laser in cadaveric specimens and then canine larynges before using them in the operating theater. Although the CO_2 laser was invented in 1965, a key development was Bredemeier's invention of the micromanipulator.[11] Because CO_2 laser energy is invisible to the human eye, it needed to be paired to a coaxial helium-neon aiming beam (632.8 nm), which is visible as a red beam. The difference in wavelength (and therefore in the respective properties of diffraction) between these 2 beams led to technical challenges in maintaining parfocality. They were subject to chromatic aberration as they traveled through a path of lenses and mirrors incorporated in the aiming mechanism of the micromanipulator. This made calibration of the beams a critical task and confirmation of the integrity of this calibration was necessary. This was done by aiming a few pulses at a wooden tongue depressor before its use in a patient. Once spot size could be reduced to the tolerances of stapes surgery, an instrument already familiar to otolaryngologists could find a new indication. Because of its properties of tissue interaction and its absorption by water, the CO_2 laser was thought by some surgeons to possess advantages over the potassium-titanyl-phosphorus (KTP) and argon lasers. However, to some surgeons, these advantages were mitigated by the inability of the CO_2 laser to be incorporated into a handheld instrument until relatively recently.

LASER–TISSUE INTERACTIONS IN THE EAR

Lesinski[12] characterized the ideal stapedotomy laser as one whose energy should (1) be completely absorbable by the footplate; (2) would not impart heat to the perilymph; and (3) would not damage facial nerve, inner ear sensory epithelium, or saccular membranes. In addition, he identified 5 variables that the surgeon controls: (1) pulse timing, (2) pulse duration, (3) mode (continuous, chopped, or pulsed), (4) average power, and (5) spot size. (**Fig. 1**). Light of a given wavelength is most readily absorbed by its complementary color and thus the blue-green argon laser was for many years the instrument of choice; for example, vitreoretinal surgeons operating on a target that was mostly red. The off-white of otic capsule bone was found to reflect this wavelength, thus requiring greater energy to penetrate the bone. This led to great concern regarding thermal damage to surrounding structures and prompted several studies that measured the increase in temperature after a sequence of laser applications, such as would typically be necessary during surgery. Vollrath and Schreiner[13] studied these temperature effects in guinea pigs and were able to make several observations that were subsequently corroborated. Perhaps the most alarming was that laser

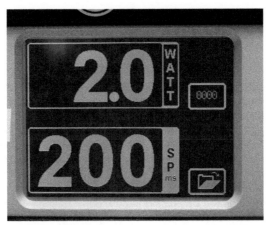

Fig. 1. Control panel of CO_2 fiber-guided laser system in pulse (SP) mode, showing user-defined parameters of 2 W and 200 millisecond pulses.

energy directly applied to perilymph without any interposed tissue could boil the perilymph; however, more typical exposures showed safer, tolerable temperature increases. In subsequent studies, they investigated the physiologic effects of these temperature increases by looking at the cochlear microphonic (CM) and the compound action potential (CAP).[14] They found that both CM and CAP immediately became depressed with the application of the laser impulse, with the CM recovering very rapidly after the impulse ceased. In contrast, the CAP remained reduced for a longer time, with a time constant roughly 7 times as long as that of the CM (15.2 seconds for CAP vs 2.2 seconds for CM). Additionally, they observed cumulative effects, such as increases in temperature for short duration impulses if the intervals between impulses were short.

Lesinski and Palmer[15] used a thermocouple in a cochlear model to investigate the temperature increase imparted by the argon and KTP lasers. Whereas the KTP laser showed modest increases from 4.3°C to 6.3°C, the argon laser was found to have a thermal effect higher than 22°C. Furthermore, both lasers showed very high thermal effects with smaller spot sizes, up to 175°C for the argon laser. Their model, relying as it did on a black thermocouple that (unlike perilymph) could absorb light in these wavelengths, was criticized as overestimating the thermal effects, which spurred development of other investigational modalities. For example, Häusler and colleagues[16] used a saline-filled inner ear model equipped with thermosensitive rhodamine-coated polyurethane films to demonstrate that multiple argon laser pulses in the range commonly used for stapedotomy surgery, 1 to 2.5 W with 100 millisecond pulses, could be expected to increase the temperature in the irradiated zone about 1°C.

The erbium (Erb)-doped yttrium aluminium garnet (YAG) and yttrium-scandium-gallium-garnet (YSGG), also in the infrared range, exhibited the unique property of producing a loud bang on activation as bone was explosively vaporized. Unlike the visible lasers, however, infrared Erb laser energy is readily absorbed by water and thus concerns of thermal damage were replaced by concerns about the damage sound pressure levels could impart to the cochlea. Häusler and colleagues[17] found, for example, on early postoperative audiograms that midfrequency and high-frequency bone conduction thresholds could shift by up to 75 dB. Fortunately, they found that this recovered but nevertheless it was evidence that inner ear structures had been traumatized. Michaelides and Kartush,[18] using a Quest 155 Sound Level Meter (Oconomowoc, WI, USA) in a preserved human temporal bone preparation, measured peak sound pressure levels of 131 A-weighted dB (dBA) during the duration of the Erb laser's pulse. Although the pulse duration was on the order of picoseconds, the intensity of the exposure was sobering despite its brevity. In contrast, the KTP and CO_2 lasers exhibited peak sound pressure levels below 90 dBA.

The measurement of mechanical, acoustic, and thermal effects of lasers applied to the footplate has also undergone refinements. Whereas the earlier studies of Lesinski and colleagues[12,15] used a thermocouple, Kamalski and colleagues[19] have recently evolved a 3-modality protocol that reflects the state of the art. Their model dispenses with the use of whole or partial temporal bone preparations except for a fresh cadaveric human stapes. The vestibule is a slab of polyacrylamide gel with a 3 mm well filled with saline, over which a piece of dialysis membrane supports the cadaveric stapes. They document mechanical effects by using high-speed imaging at a frame rate of 400 per second under high-intensity light. Thermal effects are measured using a technique based on color Schlieren imaging, which measures changes in the refractive index of fluids mediated by temperature gradients. Finally, acoustic effects are measured by a hydrophone (Kingstate Omni, sensitivity -42 dB $\pm$ 3 dB, frequency range 25–20,000 Hz).

LASER DELIVERY SYSTEMS

The basic schema of laser light generation has experienced refinement over the years but the means by which this energy can be applied, as either a free beam or transmitted by a handheld fiber or waveguide, has also seen a great degree of innovation. Likewise, the argon laser of Perkins and Urban is now only 1 among many others: CO_2, thulium, Erb-YAG, Erb-YSGG, Holmium-YAG, KTP, diode laser, and so forth. All of these variants have features enabling a surgeon to apply advantages inherent to either the surgical task at hand or to individual preference. Some, like the Erb-YAG, were single indication devices not adaptable to surgery elsewhere in the body and thus are orphan technology. Others, like the femtosecond lasers used in ophthalmology, are not widely used in otosclerosis surgery; thus we shall mostly constrain discussion to the more market-penetrant lasers.

Visible lasers, such as the argon (2 wavelength peaks at 488 and 514 nm) and KTP laser (wavelength 532 nm), were among the first lasers used in stapes surgery. The KTP laser shares many properties with argon laser: both are visible in the blue-green range and were also the first to be adapted to use in a handpiece, transmitted via quartz silica fiber. Because KTP and argon light are in the range visible to humans, they can be used without an aiming beam, such as that initially incorporated for use by the CO_2 laser, which has a wavelength of 10,600 nm, in the infrared range, rendering it invisible.

As previously discussed, the first lasers to see widespread use in stapes surgery were delivered via microscope-mounted micromanipulators. A typical example was the HGM Argon Laser (HGM Medical Laser Systems, Inc, Salt Lake City, UT, USA). Because the energy was applied in the form of a highly focused, collimated, and coherent beam, concerns arose about how much potential damage could be caused to the delicate inner ear milieu once the footplate had been penetrated because these lasers exhibit negligible absorption by water. Another potential disadvantage was apparent in that the laser energy could only be delivered in the line of sight. This led to a demand to configure the laser into a handheld instrument and the industry responded with products such as the Argon Endo-Otoprobe (HGM Medical Laser Systems, Inc, Salt Lake City, UT, USA).

Horn and colleagues[20] reported on their use of a fiber-transmitted argon laser in 43 cases and noted numerous advantages over micromanipulator systems. The direction of the laser and its angle could be instantaneously changed and was no longer tethered to the viewing axis of the microscope. This property also obviated the tiny mirrors used for bank shots around structures, a technique that introduced a source of imprecision and thus the risk of complications.

Hodgson and Wilson[21] reviewed their use of the argon laser in 75 consecutive stapedotomies, using both the HGM micromanipulator and the Endo-Otoprobe. They reported adequate follow-up of 62 subjects and attained 87% closure of the air-bone gap (ABG) to within 10 dB, with only 1 subject experiencing total hearing loss. They did not subdivide the results into separate categories by delivery system but commented that they preferred the handheld configuration. Because the angle of divergence of the fiber-carried laser energy was much greater than that of the free beam, they observed that power density has a more rapid decrease when the working distance from the tip of the instrument is increased. It is an inherent property of fiber-optic laser delivery systems that the energy is defocused, noncollimated, noncoherent, and has a diffusion angle of 10°C to 14°C.[12]

EVOLUTION OF THE CARBON DIOXIDE LASER

Despite that for 3 decades it could only be delivered via free beam guided by micromanipulator, the CO_2 laser's property of high absorption in perilymph was in high demand among surgeons who thought this made it superior to the visible lasers. This property was held in common with the Erb lasers but without the attendant impulse sound pressure exposures. In 1999, the Lumenis Corporation (Tel Aviv, Israel) introduced an early innovation in laser delivery to the stapes: the development of the 1-shot technique. Instead of creating a rosette of laser craters on the footplate, this technique used a microprocessor scanning system (SurgiTouch Scanner) to create a perfectly circular 0.5 to 0.7 mm stapedotomy. Jovanovic and colleagues[22] reported excellent results in 188 subjects with a 3% incidence of reoperation for complications. Because this device reduced the total energy applied to the footplate, it could minimize the potential for damage to the membranous labyrinth.

Sergi and colleagues[23] provided indirect evidence of minimal effects on inner ear function when they gathered audiometric data 2 days after surgery and again at 1 month in a series of 58 subjects. Significant findings included no early or late decrease in bone conduction thresholds and a steadily improving ABG closure: 12 dB of improvement when comparing measurements 1 month postoperatively to thresholds obtained at 2 days.

The development of a handheld CO_2 laser, the BeamPath OTO fiber-enabled CO_2 laser system (OmniGuide Inc, Cambridge, MA, USA) was a major advance in otosclerosis surgery (**Fig. 2**). Surgeon preference had always tended toward this type of delivery system and accounted for the popularity of the visible laser systems despite the drawbacks these had from the standpoint of transmission of laser energy through perilymph. Additionally, there was no longer a need to fuss with calibration of the helium-neon aiming beam, and complications due to misalignment of the 2 beams were no longer a factor.

The refractive index of silica glass fibers renders it opaque to wavelengths greater than 2000 nm and thus the development of a handheld CO_2 laser had to await technological developments that surmounted this limitation. It was the telecommunications industry

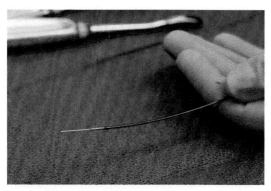

Fig. 2. CO_2 photonic crystal laser fiber implementation.

that first spurred the development of fiberoptic signals technology and the medium of the silica glass fiber. The theoretic basis that would lead to the development of waveguide technology, such as that found in the OmniGuide BeamPath CO_2 laser, which emerged around 1991 when the idea of photonic crystal was proposed.[24] Subsequently, it became possible to fabricate a photonic crystal fiber in which a lattice of microscopic holes oriented longitudinally along a hollow glass fiber traps light and guides it coaxially down the fiber. It was possible to propagate laser light using these microstructural modifications of polymer and chalcogenide glass fibers, thus liberating infrared lasers from the tyranny of refractive index differences. The BeamPath consists of "photonic bandgap fibers with each fiber having forty or more microscopic layers of alternating glass and polymer that form a reflective system known as a Bragg diffraction grating. The wavelength of light transmitted by this structure is a function of the thickness of the glass/polymer bi-layers, and may be varied."[25]

Early reporting of results using the new handpiece was encouraging. Vincent and colleagues[26] were able to report a trend, in 214 ears, toward smaller postoperative ABGs ($\leq$10 dB in 97% of CO_2 operated ears vs 92% in the KTP group) and a statistically significant 2.7 dB difference at 4 kHz in favor of the CO_2 group, with no sensorineural hearing loss. In a follow-up study,[27] the 315 subjects in the CO_2 group significantly showed a postoperative ABG of 10 dB or less 97% of the time, whereas in the KTP group (n = 334) equivalent results were achieved in 90%.

OUTCOMES OF LASER-ASSISTED STAPEDOTOMY

It is productive to review the findings of available systematic reviews and meta-analyses. Three such papers are germane to the topic. Fang and colleagues[28] sought to compare hearing outcomes and complications in cases of stapedotomy using laser in general to those cases in which a laser was not used. They identified 11 studies that met their criteria for reporting of hearing results (closure of preoperative ABG to within 10 dB) and 1614 subjects were analyzed. They also looked at complication rates and only 7 papers were included for that analysis, which encompassed 806 subjects. The laser group showed significantly better ABG closure, with a combined relative risk of 107 but no demonstrable difference in safety. Similarly, 8 studies were included in the paper by Wegner and colleagues,[29] which yielded 999 procedures for analysis. This study was unable to demonstrate superiority of any method over another with regard to hearing outcome. However, they did comment that footplate fracture and sensorineural hearing loss occurred more frequently in the conventional group. In a separate publication, they also performed a systematic review comparing the outcomes according to what kind of lasers were used.[30] Two studies ultimately met their criteria: the previously mentioned 2012 study by Vincent and colleagues[27] comparing the CO_2 handpiece to KTP laser and a study by Marchese and colleagues[31] comparing the 1-shot CO_2 laser to Erb-YAG. Although they found a risk difference of 28.1% in favor of the CO_2 laser with regard to ABG closure, they observed that the paucity of data was a severe limitation in drawing a firm conclusion (Video 1).

SUMMARY

The invention of the laser and its introduction into the surgical treatment of otosclerosis was a revolution within a revolution. In the 4 decades during which lasers have been used, the unique properties of this modality have enabled refinements of surgical technique that arguably have led to better hearing outcomes and safer surgeries. Technological innovation in laser research potentially could lead to the development of the ideal laser.

SUPPLEMENTARY DATA

Supplementary data related to this article can be found online at https://doi.org/10.1016/j.otc.2017.11.009.

REFERENCES

1. US Patent #2,929,922. Schawlow AL, Townes CH. Masers and Maser Communication Systems. March 22, 1960. US Patent #2,929,922. Available at: https://www.google.co.in/patents/US2929922. Accessed January 8, 2018.
2. Townes CH. A century of nature: twenty-one discoveries that changed science and the world. In: Garwin L, Lincoln T, editors. Chicago: University of Chicago Press; 2003. p. 107–12.
3. Shea JJ. A personal history of stapedectomy. Am J Otol 1998;19:2–12.
4. Perkins RC. Laser stapedotomy for otosclerosis. Laryngoscope 1980;90:228–41.
5. Plester D. Fortschritte in der Mikrosurgerie des Ohres in den letzte 10 Jahren. HNO 1970;18:33–40.
6. Shea JJ, Sanabria F, Smyth GDL. Teflon piston operation for otosclerosis. Arch Otolaryngol 1962;76:516–21.
7. Fisch U. Stapedotomy versus stapedectomy. Otol Neurotol 1982;4:112–7.
8. Silverstein H. Laser stapedotomy minus prosthesis (laser STAMP): a minimally invasive procedure. Am J Otol 1998;19:277–82.
9. Schomaker KT, Walsh JT, Flotte TJ, et al. Thermal damage produced by high irradiance continuous wave CO2 laser cutting of tissue. Lasers Surg Med 1990;10:74–84.
10. Strong MS, Jako GJ. Laser surgery in the larynx. Early clinical experience with continuous CO 2 laser. Ann Otol Rhinol Laryngol 1972;81:791–8.
11. Sataloff RT, Spiegel JR, Hawkshaw M, et al. Laser surgery of the larynx: the case for caution. Ear Nose Throat J 1992;71:593–5.
12. Lesinski SG. Lasers for otosclerosis – which one if any and why. Lasers Surg Med 1990;10:448–57.
13. Vollrath M, Schreiner C. The effects of the Argon laser on temperature within the cochlea. Acta Otolaryngol 1982;93:341–8.
14. Vollrath M, Schreiner C. Influence of argon laser stapedotomy on inner ear function and temperature. Otolaryngol Head Neck Surg 1983;91:251.

15. Lesinski SG, Palmer A. Lasers for otosclerosis: CO2 vs. Argon and KTP-532. Laryngoscope 1989;99(6 Pt 2 Suppl 46):1–8.
16. Häusler R, Messerli A, Romano V, et al. Experimental and clinical results of fiber-optic argon laser stapedotomy. Eur Arch Otorhinolaryngol 1996;253:193–200.
17. Häusler R, Schär PJ, Pratisto H, et al. Advantages and dangers of erbium laser application in stapedotomy. Acta Otolaryngol 1999;119:207–13.
18. Michaelides EM, Kartush JM. Implications of sound levels generated by otologic devices. Otolaryngol Head Neck Surg 2001;125:361–3.
19. Kamalski DMA, de Boorder T, Bitterman AJN, et al. Capturing thermal, mechanical, and acoustic effects of the diode (980 nm) laser in stapedotomy. Otol Neurotol 2014;35:1070–6.
20. Horn KL, Gherini S, Griffin GMJ. Argon laser stapedectomy using an endo-otoprobe system. Otolaryngol Head Neck Surg 1990;102:193–8.
21. Hodgson RS, Wilson DF. Argon laser stapedotomy. Laryngoscope 1991;101:230–3.
22. Jovanovic S, Schonfeld U, Scherer H. CO2 laser stapedotomy with the "one-shot" technique – clinical results. Otolaryngol Head Neck Surg 2004;131:750–7.
23. Sergi B, Scorpecci A, Parrilla C, et al. Early hearing assessment after "one shot" CO2 laser stapedotomy: is it helpful to predict inner ear damage and the functional outcome? Otol Neurotol 2010;31:1376–80.
24. Russell P. Photonic crystal fibers. Science 2003;299:358–62.
25. Gille, et al, inventors. Minimally invasive surgical system for CO2 lasers. United States Patent No. 8,894,636 B2. November 25, 2014. Available at: http://patft.uspto.gov/netacgi/nph-Parser?Sect1=PTO1&Sect2=HITOFF&d=PALL&p=1&u=%2Fnetahtml%2FPTO%2Fsrchnum.htm&r=1&f=G&l=50&s1=8894636.PN.&OS=PN/8894636&RS=PN/8894636. Accessed January 8, 2018.
26. Vincent R, Grolman W, Oates J, et al. A nonrandomized comparison of potassium titanyl phosphate and CO2 laser fiber stapedotomy for primary otosclerosis with the otology-neurotology database. Laryngoscope 2010;120:570–5.
27. Vincent R, Bitterman AJN, Oates J, et al. KTP versus CO2 laser fiber stapedotomy for primary otosclerosis: results of a new comparative series with the otology-neurotology database. Otol Neurotol 2012;33:928–33.
28. Fang L, Lin H, Zhang T, et al. Laser versus non-laser stapedotomy in otosclerosis: a systematic review and meta-analysis. Auris Nasus Larynx 2014;41:337–42.
29. Wegner I, Kamalski DMA, Tange RA, et al. Laser versus conventional fenestration in stapedotomy for otosclerosis: a systematic review. Laryngoscope 2014;124:1687–93.
30. Kamalski DMA, Wegner I, Tange RA, et al. Outcomes of different laser types in laser-assisted stapedotomy: a systematic review. Otol Neurotol 2014;35:1046–51.
31. Marchese MR, Scorpecci A, Cianfrone F. "One shot" CO2 versus Er:YAG laser stapedotomy: is the outcome the same? Eur Arch Otorhinolaryngol 2011;268:351–6.

Endoscopic Stapes Surgery

Brandon Isaacson, MD[a],*, Jacob B. Hunter, MD[a], Alejandro Rivas, MD[b]

KEYWORDS

- Otosclerosis • Endoscopic ear surgery • Stapedectomy • Stapedotomy
- Endoscope

KEY POINTS

- Transcanal endoscopic ear surgery provides a magnified, wide-field view of the entire middle ear even in the setting of a narrow external meatus or ear canal.
- Scutum removal during endoscopic stapes surgery is usually still required to access the oval window with instruments and for prosthesis placement.
- Stapes footplate work and prosthesis placement is often more challenging than microscopic stapes surgery given the lack of depth perception with the use of the endoscope.
- The efficacy of endoscopic stapes surgery seems to be equivalent to microscopic stapes surgery.
- No significant thermal or mechanical issues have been reported to date using the endoscope for stapes surgery.

 Video content accompanies this article at http://www.oto.theclinics.com.

INTRODUCTION

Rosen[1] introduced the stapes mobilization procedure for the management of otosclerosis in 1953. Since then, other surgical techniques have been described, including lateral semicircular canal fenestration, the stapedectomy, and the stapedotomy.[2–4] Traditionally, these surgical techniques were and have been performed with the use of an operating microscope.

Mer and colleagues[5] first described the use of an endoscope to visualize the structures of the middle ear in 1967. However, the last 2 decades have seen a dramatic

Disclosure: B. Isaacson is on the Advisory Board of Advanced Bionics and MED-EL, and is also a consultant for Stryker, Olympus, Storz, Advanced Bionics, and Medtronic. A. Rivas is associated with the Cochlear Corporation, Advanced Bionics, MED-EL, Olympus, and Grace Medical. J.B. Hunter has nothing to disclose.
[a] Department of Otolaryngology–Head and Neck Surgery, UT Southwestern Medical Center, 5323 Harry Hines Boulevard, Dallas, TX 75390, USA; [b] Department of Otolaryngology–Head and Neck Surgery, Vanderbilt University Medical Center, 1215 21st Avenue, Medical Center East, South Tower, 7th Floor, Nashville, TN 37232, USA
* Corresponding author. Department of Otolaryngology–Head and Neck Surgery, UT Southwestern Medical Center, 5323 Harry Hines Boulevard, Dallas, TX 75390-9035.
E-mail address: brandon.isaacson@utsouthwestern.edu

increase in the use of transcanal endoscopic ear surgery (TEES). TEES is now used to perform stapes surgery along with other otologic procedures, including tympanoplasty, cholesteatoma surgery, ossiculoplasty, and for the removal of middle ear and intracanalicular pathology.[6–13]

ADVANTAGES AND DISADVANTAGES OF TRANSCANAL ENDOSCOPIC EAR SURGERY

Supporters of TEES advocate that the endoscope might improve surgical outcomes as a result of improved visibility of the middle ear structures when compared with the microscope.[14] Specifically about stapes surgery, the wide angle of view allows for better visibility of the stapes and footplate, easy identification of anatomic or pathologic variations, the ability to visualize beyond the shaft of the surgical instruments, and close visualization and confirmation of prosthesis coupling. With these advantages, endoscopic stapes surgery provides similar audiologic results when compared with the microscopic technique as summarized by Hunter and Rivas in 2016.[15] Other potential surgical advantages include decreased scutum removal and reduced chorda tympani manipulation and injury.[16]

Disadvantages of TEES include the loss of stereopsis, one-handed surgery, and the potential risk of thermal injury to the inner ear resulting in sensorineural hearing loss and vestibular dysfunction secondary to the proximity of the light source. Analyzing these risks, Dundar and colleagues[17] measured oval window temperature changes during endoscopic stapedotomy in a guinea pig model. They concluded that the greatest risk comes with the use of a xenon light source in a 4-mm endoscope, whereas the least temperature elevation was found with the LED light source with a 3-mm endoscope.[17]

EQUIPMENT

The increased interest in TEES has stimulated the creation and adaptation of new endoscopes, special endoscopic equipment, and microinstruments designed to facilitate this type of surgery. The instruments and equipment required for TEES are listed in **Box 1**.

A high-definition monitor and 3-chip cameras provides ideal resolution and appropriate combination of contrast. Previous generation cameras create an oversaturation of the red color, which in turn decreases resolution in an already bloody field.

Rigid endoscopes frequently used for ear surgery are 2.7 mm, 3 mm, or 4 mm in diameter. A larger diameter endoscope provides increased illumination, and improved visual resolution of the operative field at the expense maneuverability within the narrow external auditory canal. The available working lengths include 18 cm, 14 cm, 11 cm, and 6 cm. Image stabilization, arm and hand fatigue, and an increased risk

---

Box 1
Equipment for endoscopic stapes surgery

- High-definition 3-chip camera
- High-definition monitor
- Rigid endoscopes 0°, 30°, 45°, 14 cm long, 3 mm in diameter
- Standard otologic instruments for stapes surgery
- Laser, micro drill, or hand drill

of damage to the endoscope are seen with longer working lengths. Collision and crowding between the camera and instrument hands becomes more of an issue with the shorter endoscopes. The 0° and 30° angled scopes are the most commonly used, followed by the 45° scope. Endoscopes with large angulations, such as the 70°, are difficult to master and can be disorienting, increasing the risk of damage to the ossicular chain.

The choice of length and diameter of the rigid endoscopes is surgeon dependent. The 3-mm diameter, 14-cm long endoscopes, in these authors' opinion, are the ideal size to provide a high-resolution view, a reduced risk of fatigue, and enough working room for instrumentation of the middle ear regardless of the size of the ear canal (EAC). Moreover, it is strong enough to withstand the forces that the surgeon might apply along the curvature of the canal. Last, the 0° and 30° endoscopes provide all the angulation needed for simple and complex stapes surgery cases.

The presence of an operating microscope in the operating room is essential when initially adopting TEES. The novice surgeon needs to be prepared to convert an endoscopic case into a microscopic case when excessive bleeding is encountered, or when the surgeon is in doubt about the depth of the stapes footplate, owing to the lack of depth perception from the endoscope.

The presence of a continuous video recording system not only is ideal for education of trainees, but it also enables the scrub nurse, anesthesiologist, and others to observe and follow the course of the operation.

New, customized designed instruments have been created and refined to provide access and manipulation of hidden structures when doing TEES. However, most endoscopic surgeries can be performed safely and efficiently with standard, updated otologic instrumentation, including stapes surgery.

PERIOPERATIVE CONSIDERATIONS

Hemostasis, patient positioning, anesthesia technique, and application of local anesthesia are especially important for any endoscopic ear surgery, including stapedectomy. Because TEES requires mastering a one-handed technique, hemostasis is of paramount importance; the surgeon is unable to suction during dissection because the nondominant hand is typically holding the endoscope.

To start, the choice of anesthesia is very important. Total intravenous anesthesia has proven to decrease bleeding in endoscopic sinus surgery studies.[18] Because total intravenous anesthesia produces less vasodilation compared with inhalation anesthesia, this allows to decrease both the mean arterial blood pressure and the heart rate of patients, decreasing their cardiac output. This in turn, decreases bleeding and improves visibility.

The head of the bed should be raised approximately 15° to 30° to increase venous return, while simultaneously extending the head to improve exposure of the stapes footplate and oval window.

Local anesthetic, approximately 1 mL of 1% lidocaine with 1:100,000 epinephrine is then injected into the EAC meatus just lateral to the osseocartilaginous junction. Either adjunctively or as an alternative means to achieve local vasoconstriction, cotton balls soaked in 1:1000 epinephrine are placed into the EAC for approximately 5 minutes, while the hairs of the outer EAC are cut to prevent smearing the endoscope lens.

Once the ear is prepped and draped, the surgeon should be in a comfortable working position during the prolonged holding of the endoscope. The monitor is aligned across from the surgeon and the patient's head at a comfortable height, with the scrub assistant positioned next to the monitor toward the patient's feet.

Once the endoscope is connected, the light intensity should not go higher than 60 to prevent a thermal injury to the inner ear. To optimize the image contrast during surgery, the settings of the camera include putting the enhancement in high and the contrast at peak. The image is then white balanced.

OPERATIVE CONSIDERATIONS

The wide-field, magnified view provided with the endoscope provides excellent visualization of the entire middle ear, even in the setting of a narrow external meatus and canal as compared with the view provided with a speculum. The main disadvantage of endoscopic stapes surgery is the lack of depth perception that makes footplate dissection more challenging. Endoscopic stapes surgery requires the same steps as with the microscope, with a few subtle modifications.

Superior and inferior canal incisions are performed starting just lateral and anterior to the pars flaccida and adjacent to the inferior annulus respectively. These canal incisions are then connected with an incision 8 mm lateral and parallel to the posterior annulus (**Fig. 1**). Bleeding from the canal incisions is readily controlled using cotton balls or cottonoid pledgets soaked in 1:1000 epinephrine that can also be used to facilitate flap elevation. The flap is then elevated down to the annulus that is then elevated out of the osseous annular sulcus (**Fig. 2**). Entering the middle ear in the notch of Rivinus or along the posterior inferior annulus facilitates the identification of the chorda tympani nerve to avoid avulsion or a stretch injury. The superior aspect of the flap is elevated up to the level of the malleus neck and lateral process to improve exposure of the posterior superior mesotympanum.

Visualization of the entire oval window niche, including the tympanic facial nerve, and the pyrimidal process is almost always achieved without any scutum removal using the 0° or angled endoscopes (**Fig. 3**). Despite the excellent wide field of view of the oval window niche with the endoscope, removal of at least some of the posterior scutum is almost always required so that instruments can access the oval window and for eventual prosthesis placement (**Fig. 4**). Scutum removal with a curette requires

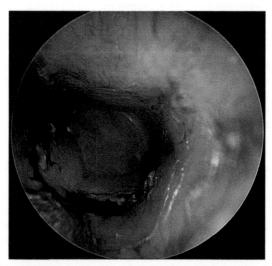

Fig. 1. Canal incisions are demonstrated in a right ear demonstrating 6 and 12 o'clock incisions that have been connected with a lateral incision parallel to the annulus.

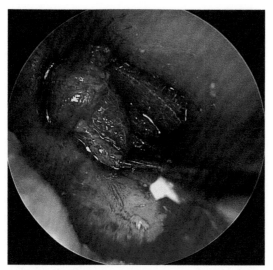

Fig. 2. The tympanomeatal flap has been elevated down to the osseous annulus using epinephrine soaked cottonoid pledgets.

more caution given the lack of depth perception with the endoscope. Thermal injuries of the middle ear and the chorda tympani nerve are possible given the proximity of the light source to the operative field. Frequent irrigation, and withdrawal and reinsertion of the endoscope for cleaning and defogging reduce the risk of thermal injury with endoscopic ear surgery. The lateral chain and stapes are palpated to assess for location and degree of fixation. A measuring rod is used to estimate the distance between the medial aspect of the incus long process and the stapes footplate either before or after the superstructure is removed depending on if the oval window niche is narrow (**Fig. 5**). An appropriate length stapes prosthesis is then selected.

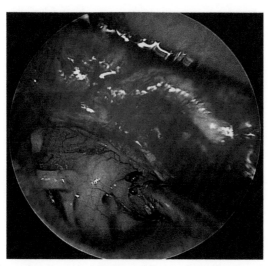

Fig. 3. The middle ear has been exposed providing a view of stapes, incus, malleus, and pyramidal process without scutum removal using a 0°, 3-mm diameter endoscope.

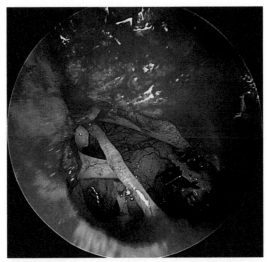

Fig. 4. The posterior scutum has been removed, exposing the tympanic facial nerve and the entire oval window niche, using a 0°, 3-mm diameter endoscope.

The incudostapedial joint is divided with a joint knife or a small right angled micro pick followed by division of the stapedius tendon. The posterior stapes crus is then divided with crurotomy scissors, a micro drill, or with a laser (**Fig. 6**). A distinct advantage of using the endoscope for stapes surgery is the ability to visualize and divide the anterior crus of the stapes, especially in the setting limited footplate fixation. Malleus or incus fixation can also be readily addressed with the endoscope with a more limited atticotomy if identified at the time of surgery. The stapes superstructure is then removed (**Fig. 7**). The mucosa adjacent to the oval window niche can be ablated with the laser or removed if a stapedectomy is being performed. If a partial or total

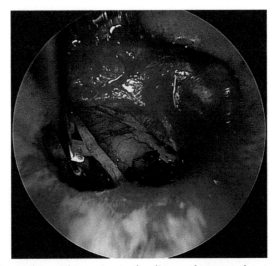

Fig. 5. A measuring rod is used to estimate the distance between the stapes footplate and the long process of the incus.

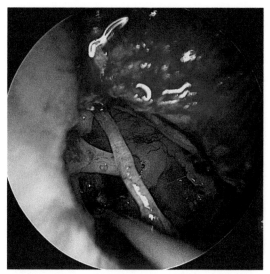

Fig. 6. The stapedius tendon and posterior crus are divided with a laser.

stapedectomy is being performed, a tissue graft (perichondrium, vein, fascia, fat) is harvested and placed onto the promontory inferior to the oval window before addressing the stapes footplate.

A laser or hand drill is then used to perform a stapedotomy at which point a piston type prosthesis can be placed followed by a blood patch or tissue seal (**Fig. 8**). A partial or total stapedectomy can also be performed removing some or all the footplate (**Fig. 9**). The tissue graft on the promontory can then be immediately positioned over the oval window to seal off the vestibule (**Fig. 10**). The previously selected stapes prosthesis is then placed between the incus long or lenticular process and the oval

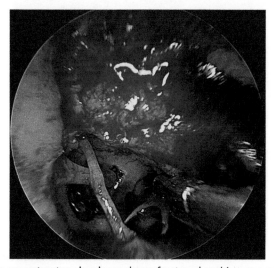

Fig. 7. The stapes superstructure has been down-fractured and is removed.

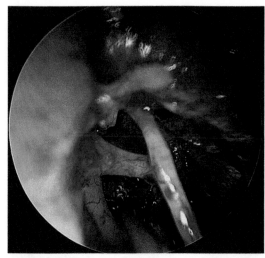

Fig. 8. A Rosette pattern is created in the central portion of the stapes footplate using a laser.

window (**Fig. 11**). The round window reflex can be assessed quite readily with the endoscope to confirm appropriate prosthesis coupling. The tympanomeatal flap is then used to cover the exposed posterior osseous canal, which is then covered with a layer of antibiotic-soaked Gelfoam or ointment (**Fig. 12**, Video 1).

AUDIOLOGIC OUTCOMES

The initial studies describing outcomes after endoscopic stapes surgery consisted of few patients with minimal data. Tarabichi[9] reported on 13 patients who underwent

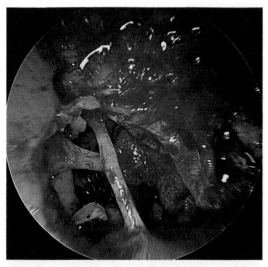

Fig. 9. The posterior half of the stapes footplate has been removed and is seen on the pyramidal process and distal tympanic facial nerve.

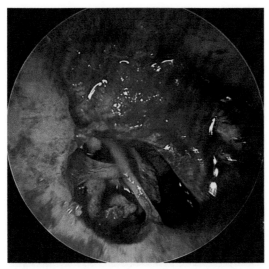

Fig. 10. A tragal perichondrial graft us used to seal the oval window.

stapedectomies, with only 7 patients having at least 1 year of follow-up, 6 of whom had closure of their air–bone gap (ABG) to less than 10 dB of hearing loss. Poe reported on 5 patients who underwent endoscopic laser stapedioplasties; however, these 5 patients were among 34 patients who underwent primary surgery for otosclerosis, and whose outcomes were not reported separately.[12]

In 2011, Nogueira Junior and colleagues[16] reported on the first substantial study regarding endoscopic stapedotomies. They assessed 15 patients, reporting that the oval window niche, the tympanic segment of the facial nerve, and the pyramidal

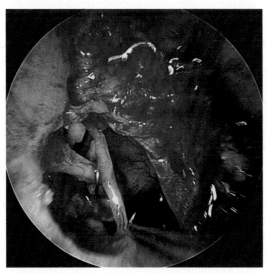

Fig. 11. A notched, titanium bucket handle prosthesis is placed between the perichondrium and the incus lenticular process.

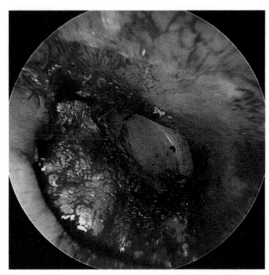

Fig. 12. The tympanomeatal flap is positioned back over the posterior canal wall.

process were all able to be visualized without bone removal with a 0° endoscope in 8 of 15 patients, compared with 12 of 15 patients when using a 30° endoscope.[16] With reduced need for bone removal, only 3 of 15 patients required manipulation of the chorda tympani.[16] Despite improved visualization, these investigators commented on increased difficulty in placing the stapes prosthesis.[16] At postoperative day 15, all patients had subjective improvement in their hearing, whereas 14 of 15 had "audiogram improvements," with the mean speech reception threshold improving to 25 dB of hearing loss.[16]

In 2012, Sarkar and colleagues[19] reported the results of 30 patients who underwent endoscopic stapedotomies, with a mean preoperative ABG of 41.5 dB of hearing loss, significantly improving to 10.1 dB of hearing loss at 3 months postoperatively. In addition, 93% of patients had their ABG close to less than 15 dB of hearing loss.[19] Migirov and Wolf[20] also reported the outcomes of 8 consecutive patients who underwent endoscopic stapedotomies with at least 6 months of follow-up. The authors highlighted the lack of bony removal, using a curved 0.5-mm diameter diamond burr for the fenestra, and the improved comfort of a right-handed surgeon performing surgery on right ears, with the mean air-conduction threshold improving to 30.6 dB of hearing loss postoperatively, compared with 64 dB of hearing loss preoperatively, and 6 of 8 patients having closure of the ABG to less than 10 dB of hearing loss.[20]

In 2014, Naik and Nemade[21] reported their experience with 20 endoscopic stapedotomies, two of which were revision cases. These investigators obtained postoperative audiometry at 6 weeks, noting complete ABG closure in 55% of patients, mild conductive hearing loss of up to 20 dB in 30% of patients, and mixed hearing losses in 2 patients, one of which was a revision case.[21] Dursun and colleagues[22] reported on the outcomes of 31 ears who underwent endoscopic stapes procedures, with closure of the postoperative ABG to less than 10 dB in 61.3% of patients, and less than 20 dB in 86.8%. Surmelioglu and colleagues[23] compared 22 endoscopic and 24 microscopic stapedotomies, with mean postoperative ABGs of 9.3 dB and 13.5 dB, respectively, which were not significantly different.

In the largest single surgeon's endoscopic stapes surgery experience to date, Sproat and colleagues[24] compared 34 patients who had undergone endoscopic stapedotomies with the same surgeon's prior 47 microscopic stapedotomies. They found no differences in group or prosthesis type when comparing postoperative ABGs.[24] Audiometrically, 79% of patients in both groups had their ABG close to less than 10 dB of hearing loss.[24]

Hunter and colleagues[10] reported on the outcomes of 50 patients who underwent endoscopic stapes surgery between 4 tertiary otologic referral centers. Although all centers exclusively used endoscopes, 3 different surgical techniques were used: laser stapedotomy, drill stapedotomy, and laser stapedectomy.[10] The authors reported that scutum anatomy prevented prosthesis placement with a straight and curved alligator in 77.1% and 67.3% of cases, respectively.[10] Furthermore, 94.0% of cases required manipulation of the chorda tympani nerve, leading to nerve transection in 12.0%.[10] With an average follow-up of 13.4 months (range, 0.76–57.4 months), the mean postoperative ABG was 11.2 dB of hearing loss.[10] When each surgical technique was analyzed, each demonstrated a significant improvement in the ABG, although no differences were noted between techniques.[10]

Emphasizing the learning curve with the endoscope, Iannella and Magliulo[25] compared 20 endoscopic stapedotomies with 20 microscopic stapedotomies with an endaural incision. They found no significant differences between closure of the postoperative ABG to less than 20 dB of hearing loss, postoperative pain, and chorda tympani mobilization and injuries.[25] Specifically, 95% of endoscopic patients had their ABG close to less than 20 dB of hearing loss, as compared with 90% in the control group.[25] Comparing the operative times between groups, there was no difference in the overall time after 10 cases and or at least 8 months of experience had been gained with the endoscopic technique.[25]

A summary of the published studies for endoscopic stapes surgery is summarized in **Table 1**.

PATIENT OUTCOMES

In Japan, patients tend to have narrow and curved external auditory canals, with stapes surgery routinely performed via a posterior or anterior auricular incision.[26] Thus, Kojima and colleagues[26] compared 15 ears who underwent endoscopic stapedotomies with 41 ears who underwent microscopic procedures. Noting the proclivity to perform anterior or posterior auricular incisions in Japanese patients with otosclerosis when using a microscope, Kojima and colleagues[26] asked each endoscopic patient 6 hours after their surgery to rate the severity of their pain between 3 categories. Although 93.3% of endoscopic patients reported either "almost no pain" or "mild pain requiring no analgesics," 4 patients had undergone bilateral procedures, with an anterior or posterior auricular incision and microscope used in one ear, and an endoscopic approach on the contralateral ear.[26] In those 4 patients, all of them reported "irritating pain for 2 to 3 days" with an anterior or posterior auricular incision, and all of them had no pain with the use of the endoscope.[26]

In 2015, in the only other endoscopic stapes surgery study that assessed patient outcomes, Daneshi and Jahnadideh[27] compared 19 endoscopic stapedotomies with 15 microscopic stapedotomies, fixing the tympanomeatal flap with tissue adhesive in the endoscopic group, as compared with packing the external auditory canal. Reporting a reduced need for bone removal in the endoscopic cases, as well as a reduced need for head turning in patients with difficult anatomy, such as those with cervical osteoarthritis or short necks, the surgical time in the endoscopic group was

Table 1
Summary of the published studies for endoscopic stapes surgery

Author, Year	N	Procedure	Follow-up (mo)	Audiometric Outcomes	Chorda Tympani Comments	Surgical Time
Tarabichi,[9] 1999	13	Stapedectomy	≥12	ABG <10 dB 85.7%	N/A	N/A
Poe,[12] 2000	5	Stapedioplasty	N/A	N/A	N/A	N/A
Marchioni et al,[28] 2016	6	Stapedectomy and stapedotomy	N/A	ABG <10 dB 83.3%, 100.0% <20 dB	N/A	N/A
Nogueira Junior et al,[16] 2011	15	Stapedotomy	1–1.3	ABG <25 dB 93.3%	Manipulated in 20.0%	N/A
Migirov and Wolf,[20] 2013	8	Stapedotomy	≥6	ABG <10 dB 75.0%, 100.0% <20 dB	100.0% preservation rate	N/A
Sarkar et al,[19] 2013	30	Stapedotomy	3	ABG <10 dB 56.0%, 100.0% <20 dB	N/A	N/A
Daneshi and Jahandideh,[27] 2015	19	Stapedotomy	N/A	ABG <10 dB 57.9%, 93.7% <20 dB	100.0% preservation rate	31.8
Kojima et al,[26] 2014	15	Stapedotomy	8.6	ABG <10 dB 86.7%, 93.3% <20 dB	No postoperative dysgeusia	53.0
Hunter et al,[10] 2016	50	Stapedectomy and stapedotomy	13.4	ABG <20 dB 90.0%	88.0% preservation rate	77.4

Abbreviations: ABG, air–bone gap; N/A, not applicable.

significantly shorter as compared with the microscopic group, at 31.8 minutes versus 54.3 minutes, respectively.[27] In addition, the authors used a visual analog scale to ask all patients if they were satisfied with their ear surgery about 6 hours after the procedure.[27] Using a 100-mm long horizontal line for the visual analog scale, they found that the endoscopic group indicated a significantly higher satisfaction as compared with the control group, 78.8 versus 62.9 mm.[27]

COMPLICATIONS

As for complications, few have been reported. In 2014, Naik and Nemade[21] reported on 1 incus dislocation, and Dursun and colleagues[22] reported a tympanic membrane perforation rate of 9.7%, with 2 patients who had transient facial nerve paralysis, thought to be secondary to the local anesthetic. They also had 1 patient with a perilymphatic gusher, controlled with inserting the prosthesis, supported by soft tissue, and undergoing lumbar punctures on consecutive days, with the leak stopping on postoperative day 3.[22] Kojima and colleagues[26] reported 1 case of delayed facial paralysis 10 days postoperatively, resolving within 1 month, with no postoperative dysgeusia in their endoscopic patients, compared with 11.4% of patients in the microscope cohort. Similarly, Surmelioglu and colleagues[23] reported no differences in dizziness between endoscopic and microscopic stapedotomies, although dysgeusia, assessed at 6 months postoperatively, was recorded in 4.5% of endoscopic patients as compared with 33% of microscopic patients. Sproat and colleagues[24] found no differences in intraoperative complications, postoperative sensorineural hearing loss, or dysgeusia. Hunter and colleagues[10] reported an 8.0% tympanic membrane perforation rate, 4.0% with floating footplates, and 2.0% with incus subluxation.

In a cohort of patients with a high risk of complications, using the improved visualization with the endoscope, Marchioni and colleagues[28] published their exclusive endoscopic management of stapes malformations in 17 patients, 6 of whom underwent either a stapedotomy or stapedectomy depending on the intraoperative findings. Although these patients had stapes malformations, the mean ABG improved from 36.3 dB of hearing loss to 7.8 dB of hearing loss postoperatively.[28] Of the 6 patients, 1 patient had a "low intraoperative gusher," controlled with positioning the prosthesis, bovine perichondrium, and fibrin glue, with complete preservation of hearing and closure of the ABG to 5 dB.[28]

SUMMARY

TEES is a viable alternative for managing stapes fixation. The main advantages of TEES are the magnified, wide-field of view and improved illumination as compared with that provided with a microscope using a speculum. Single-handed instrumentation, and prosthesis placement, as well the lack of depth perception, are important disadvantages of endoscopic stapes surgery.

Between 56.0% and 86.7% of patients had closure of their ABGs to less than 10 dB of hearing loss. The authors are unaware of any permanent facial nerve injuries, and the incidence of postoperative dizziness is comparable with microscopic procedures. However, postoperative dysgeusia and pain scores seem to be improved in endoscopic stapes surgeries as compared with microscopic approaches. Nonetheless, further prospective studies with larger patient populations are warranted.

SUPPLEMENTARY DATA

Supplementary data related to this article can be found online at https://doi.org/10.1016/j.otc.2017.11.011.

REFERENCES

1. Rosen S. Mobilization of the stapes to restore hearing in otosclerosis. N Y State J Med 1953;53(22):2650–3.
2. Lempert J. An analytical survey of the evolutionary development of the fenestration operation. Ann Otol Rhinol Laryngol 1950;59(4):988–1019.
3. Shea JJ Jr. A personal history of stapedectomy. Am J Otol 1998;19(5 Suppl):S2–12.
4. Perkins R, Curto FS Jr. Laser stapedotomy: a comparative study of prostheses and seals. Laryngoscope 1992;102(12 Pt 1):1321–7.
5. Mer SB, Derbyshire AJ, Brushenko A, et al. Fiberoptic endotoscopes for examining the middle ear. Arch Otolaryngol 1967;85(4):387–93.
6. Hunter JB, Zuniga MG, Sweeney AD, et al. Pediatric endoscopic cholesteatoma surgery. Otolaryngol Head Neck Surg 2016;154(6):1121–7.
7. Marchioni D, Alicandri-Ciufelli M, Rubini A, et al. Exclusive endoscopic transcanal transpromontorial approach: a new perspective for internal auditory canal vestibular schwannoma treatment. J Neurosurg 2017;126(1):98–105.

8. Ozgur A, Dursun E, Erdivanli OC, et al. Endoscopic cartilage tympanoplasty in chronic otitis media. J Laryngol Otol 2015;129(11):1073–7.

9. Tarabichi M. Endoscopic middle ear surgery. Ann Otol Rhinol Laryngol 1999; 108(1):39–46.

10. Hunter JB, Zuniga MG, Leite J, et al. Surgical and audiologic outcomes in endoscopic stapes surgery across 4 institutions. Otolaryngol Head Neck Surg 2016; 154(6):1093–8.

11. Thomassin JM, Korchia D, Doris JM. Endoscopic-guided otosurgery in the prevention of residual cholesteatomas. Laryngoscope 1993;103(8):939–43.

12. Poe DS. Laser-assisted endoscopic stapedectomy: a prospective study. Laryngoscope 2000;110(5 Pt 2 Suppl 95):1–37.

13. Killeen DE, Wick CC, Hunter JB, et al. Endoscopic management of middle ear paragangliomas: a case series. Otol Neurotol 2017;38(3):408–15.

14. Bennett ML, Zhang D, Labadie RF, et al. Comparison of middle ear visualization with endoscopy and microscopy. Otol Neurotol 2016;37(4):362–6.

15. Hunter JB, Rivas A. Outcomes following endoscopic stapes surgery. Otolaryngol Clin North Am 2016;49(5):1215–25.

16. Nogueira Junior JF, Martins MJ, Aguiar CV, et al. Fully endoscopic stapes surgery (stapedotomy): technique and preliminary results. Braz J Otorhinolaryngol 2011; 77(6):721–7.

17. Dundar R, Bulut H, Guler OK, et al. Oval window temperature changes in an endoscopic stapedectomy. J Craniofac Surg 2015;26(5):1704–8.

18. Kelly EA, Gollapudy S, Riess ML, et al. Quality of surgical field during endoscopic sinus surgery: a systematic literature review of the effect of total intravenous compared to inhalational anesthesia. Int Forum Allergy Rhinol 2013;3(6):474–81.

19. Sarkar S, Banerjee S, Chakravarty S, et al. Endoscopic stapes surgery: our experience in thirty two patients. Clin Otolaryngol 2013;38(2):157–60.

20. Migirov L, Wolf M. Endoscopic transcanal stapedotomy: how I do it. Eur Arch Otorhinolaryngol 2013;270(4):1547–9.

21. Naik C, Nemade S. Endoscopic stapedotomy: our view point. Eur Arch Otorhinolaryngol 2016;273(1):37–41.

22. Dursun E, Ozgur A, Terzi S, et al. Endoscopic transcanal stapes surgery: our technique and outcomes. Kulak Burun Bogaz Ihtis Derg 2016;26(4):201–6.

23. Surmelioglu O, Ozdemir S, Tarkan O, et al. Endoscopic versus microscopic stapes surgery. Auris Nasus Larynx 2017;44(3):253–7.

24. Sproat R, Yiannakis C, Iyer A. Endoscopic stapes surgery: a comparison with microscopic surgery. Otol Neurotol 2017;38(5):662–6.

25. Iannella G, Magliulo G. Endoscopic versus microscopic approach in stapes surgery: are operative times and learning curve important for making the choice? Otol Neurotol 2016;37(9):1350–7.

26. Kojima H, Komori M, Chikazawa S, et al. Comparison between endoscopic and microscopic stapes surgery. Laryngoscope 2014;124(1):266–71.

27. Daneshi A, Jahandideh H. Totally endoscopic stapes surgery without packing: novel technique bringing most comfort to the patients. Eur Arch Otorhinolaryngol 2016;273(3):631–4.

28. Marchioni D, Soloperto D, Villari D, et al. Stapes malformations: the contribute of the endoscopy for diagnosis and surgery. Eur Arch Otorhinolaryngol 2016;273(7): 1723–9.

Advanced Otosclerosis
Stapes Surgery or Cochlear Implantation?

Adrien A. Eshraghi, MD, MSc*, Kadri Ila, MD, Emre Ocak, MD, Fred F. Telischi, MEE, MD

KEYWORDS

- Advanced otosclerosis • Cochlear implant • Stapedotomy • Hearing loss
- Facial nerve stimulation

KEY POINTS

- Diagnosis of advanced otosclerosis may be challenging, requiring a comprehensive patient history combined with an audiologic evaluation and imaging.
- The treatment dilemma is selecting stapedotomy and hearing aid over cochlear implantation to be more helpful.
- Cochlear implant surgery may be challenging in these patients, sometimes requiring drill out of the promontorium to detect lumen of basal turn. The insertion of an electrode may also encounter some resistance.
- Facial nerve stimulation may be observed after cochlear implant surgery, which may require deactivation of some electrodes.

 Video content accompanies this article at http://www.oto.theclinics.com.

DEFINITION OF ADVANCED OTOSCLEROSIS

Otosclerosis is an abnormal process of the otic and labyrinthine capsules that involves continuous osteolysis and osteogenesis of the bone. Although otospongiotic lesions typically occur during the active phase of otosclerosis, newly formed and more compact lamellar bones dominate during the late inactive phase of otosclerosis.[1] During the active phase, a reddish tint called Schwartze sign can also appear through the tympanic membrane. Schwartze sign can aid in the diagnosis of otosclerosis and is related to the promontorium vascularity that is associated with the active otospongiotic focus of otosclerosis.[2] Otosclerosis usually occurs during the postlingual period between the second and fifth decade of life.[3] It also typically affects the area adjacent to the oval window and causes conductive hearing loss through stapes fixation.[4] It has

Disclosure: Dr. A.A. Eshraghi has research grant from Medel Corporation. Dr. F.F. Telischi has surgical advisory funding from Medel and Cochlear Corporation. Drs. K. Ila and E.Ocak have nothing to disclose.
Department of Otolaryngology, University of Miami Miller School of Medicine, 1600 Northwest 10th Avenue, Miami, FL 33136, USA
* Corresponding author. 1600 Northwest 10th Avenue, Room 3160, RMSB, Miami, FL 33136.
E-mail address: aeshraghi@med.miami.edu

been reported that 96% of affected patients have otosclerosis foci that are located in the anterior part of the oval window, and round window niche involvement also occurs in 30% of clinical otosclerosis.[5] In a series of advanced otosclerosis that was treated by cochlear implant (CI) surgery, round window membrane ossification was detected in 60%, and scala tympani ossification was identified in 30% of the patients.[1]

Once started, hearing loss usually worsens in otosclerosis patients. Hearing loss is initially observed at low frequencies and later at higher frequencies (**Fig. 1**). Studies show that 10% of otosclerosis patients with conductive hearing loss also develop sensorineural hearing loss (SNHL).[6] In 1961, House and Sheehy[7] defined advanced otosclerosis as hearing loss in air conduction (AC) threshold by 85 dB with nonmeasurable bone conduction (BC) (probably because of limitations in audiometry at that time).[7] There is no universally accepted definition for advanced otosclerosis.[8] Recently, the term advanced otosclerosis is used when a patient with otosclerosis has severely decreased speech recognition.[9] Calmels and colleagues[10] described advanced otosclerosis by its audiologic and radiologic criteria. The audiologic criteria for diagnosis was the detection of dissyllabic words less than 30% of the speech discrimination (SD) score at 70 dB, with a well-equipped hearing aid and a blank audiogram.

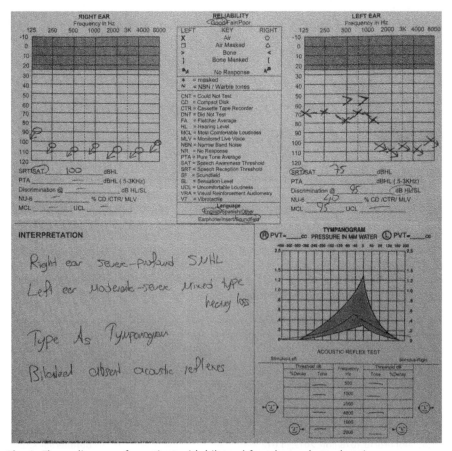

Fig. 1. The audiogram of a patient with bilateral far-advanced otosclerosis.

Because the diagnosis and treatment of the disease can be challenging, comprehensive evaluation of those challenges will help in making more appropriate decisions.

HISTOPATHOLOGY OF ADVANCED OTOSCLEROSIS

As the otosclerosis progresses, conductive hearing loss can become mixed with SNHL by affecting the spiral ligament and the otic capsule.[11] SNHL occurs when ionic homeostasis of the cochlea is disrupted due to atrophy and hyalinization in the stria vascularis and spiral ligament. As a result, loss of hair cells, hair cell dysfunction, and loss of spiral ganglion can occur. SNHL can also be caused by the release of lytic enzymes from the otosclerotic foci into the perilymph.[12] Histologically, the effect of otosclerosis on spiral ganglion cell survival is relatively small when compared with other causes of SNHL.[13] It has also been reported that otosclerosis focus on the lateral wall of the cochlea can result in the degeneration of the spiral ligament and stria vascularis during advanced otosclerosis.[1]

SNHL can also transpire when the otosclerotic focus involves the cochlear endosteum. Cochlear otosclerosis has classically been defined as a phenomenon whereby the otosclerotic focus is in the otic capsule and affects the cochlear endosteum, causing mixed-type or SNHL. According to histopathological studies, the footplate is usually fixed in cochlear otosclerosis.[2]

In a temporal bone study, it was found that the number of spiral ganglion cells in cochlear otosclerosis was sufficient for electrical stimulation.[14] Sato and colleagues[15] demonstrated that the loss of outer hair cells and spiral ganglion cells was significantly higher when cochlear otosclerosis was adjacent to the round window than when cochlear otosclerosis was adjacent to the oval window. Their study also revealed that the area of the spiral ligament adjacent to the oval window was significantly smaller in patients with cochlear otosclerosis when compared with the healthy control group.

Histopathologic studies have determined that the most common area of cochlear ossification is in the basal turn of the scala tympani. Complete round window obliteration can be seen in patients with advanced otosclerosis by ossification of the intracochlear foci that extends to the basal turn and results in a remodeled labyrinth.[1]

RADIOLOGIC IMAGING AND CLASSIFICATION SYSTEMS FOR ADVANCED OTOSCLEROSIS

Clinical history, audiologic tests, previous otosclerosis surgery, and high-resolution computed tomography (CT) scans can aid in the diagnosis of advanced otosclerosis.[16] Because of the recent prevalence of cochlear implantation, SD scores have been more commonly used than pure-tone thresholds for the diagnosis of advanced otosclerosis.[17]

Temporal bone CT and/or MRI can aid in the detection of advanced otosclerosis (**Fig. 2**). CT imaging studies have reported that SNHL correlated with the severity of otosclerosis.[18] High-resolution CT can detect oval window abnormalities in 80% to 90% of otosclerosis cases.[11] Bone densitometry can show the disease severity and help to measure the grade of otospongiosis.[18] On CT scan, the presence of pericochlear lucency is specific to cochlear otosclerosis. This finding is usually referred to as a ring or double halo (**Fig. 3**).[19] Rings emerge in cases whereby the pericochlear confluent foci surround the cochlear lumen.[20] On MRI, a ring with an intermediate signal is usually detected in the pericochlear area, with mild to moderate enhancement of the gadolinium in T1-weighted images.[21] MRI can also detect cochlear duct patency.[18] The MRI fast-spin T2-weighted sequence is particularly useful during

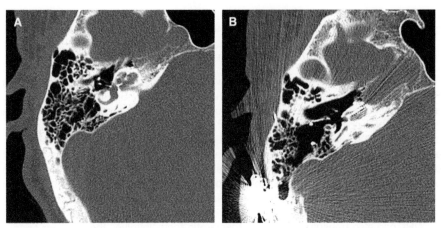

Fig. 2. (*A*) Axial CT of temporal bone, patient with right retrofenestral cochlear otosclerosis and stapes prostheses in place. (*B*) Axial CT of temporal bone for the same patient after cochlear implantation.

evaluations of cochlear patency (eg, fibrosis, ossification, intralabyrinthine schwannomas).[21] It has also been stated that T2-weighted MRI scans are superior to CT scans during assessments of luminal patency.[22]

Rotteveel and colleagues[20] described a classification system for advanced otosclerosis based on CT evaluation of the otic capsule involvement (**Table 1**). Kabbara and colleagues[12] described another classification system based on radiologically detected otosclerotic lesions. In Kabbara's system, stage 1 lesions were characterized by limited footplate and pericochlear lesions without endosteum involvement; stage 2 lesions were characterized by significant pericochlear and endosteum involvement, and stage 3 lesions were characterized by full obliteration of the round window and/or basal turn ossification associated with pericochlear lesions.

TREATMENT MODALITIES OF ADVANCED OTOSCLEROSIS

Although various methods have been used to treat advanced otosclerosis in recent years, no standard guideline for its treatment has been established. The following

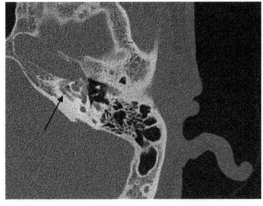

Fig. 3. Double halo and narrowed basal turn in a patient with left retrofenestral otosclerosis (type 2a based on Rotteveel classification system).

| Table 1 | | |
Classification of otosclerosis based on the computered tomography scans		
	Otosclerotic Lesions of the Otic Capsule	**No. of Ears (%)**
Type 1[a]	Solely fenestral involvement (thickened footplate and/or narrowed or enlarged windows)	7 (7)
Type 2	Retrofenestral with or without fenestral involvement	55 (52)
Type 2a	Double ring effect	26 (25)
Type 2b	Narrowed basal turn	4 (4)
Type 2c	Double ring and narrowed basal turn	25 (23)
Type 3	Severe retrofenestral (unrecognizable otic capsule), with or without fenestral involvement	27 (25)

[a] In 17 (16%), ears no signs of otosclerosis were detected.

From Rotteveel LJ, Proops DW, Ramsden RT, et al. Cochlear implantation in 53 patients with otosclerosis: demographics, computed tomographic scanning, surgery, and complications. Otol Neurotol 2004;25:946; with permission.

treatment options are in recent use: (1) hearing aids without surgery, (2) hearing aids with stapes surgery, (3) the direct acoustic cochlear stimulation implant, and (4) cochlear implantation.[17,23,24]

The advantages of stapedotomy include lower cost, local anesthesia, better natural sound, and minimally invasive surgical approaches. However stapedotomy does not treat SNHL. So patients should be selected in terms of significant conductive component with potential for improved speech understanding. Severe retrofenestral sclerosis and speech recognition scores of less than 30% are associated with poor results. Less retrofenestral involvement and speech recognition scores of more than 50% are associated with better results.[4] Because of claims of electronic stimulation reduction and inadequate neural elements in patients with otosclerosis, cochlear implantation was once considered to be contraindicated.[1] However, treating advanced otosclerosis with CIs can yield satisfactory results. Some disadvantages of cochlear implantation include high cost, need for experienced implant teams, and difficulties during electrode insertion because of sclerosis and spongiosis. Programming the CI can be challenging because of the progression of otosclerosis.[17]

STAPES SURGERY AND/OR HEARING AIDS

Lachance and colleagues[8] studied 16 patients with advanced otosclerosis who were candidates for cochlear implantation but had undergone stapes surgery and used hearing aids instead of CI. The study revealed that 94% of the patients were satisfied by the surgery and were able to use the phone postoperatively. One year after operation, 87% of the patients claimed that their hearing had improved sufficiently and that they had no need for cochlear implantation. Air-conduction threshold pure-tone average improvement was identified in all patients, and average gains in hearing were found to be 33 dB. As a result, the investigators claimed that stapes surgery was a safe and effective procedure for patients who had suffered profound hearing loss due to advanced otosclerosis.

Van Loon and colleagues[9] asserted that the stapedotomy should be performed before considering cochlear implantation in patients with advanced otosclerosis. They also claimed that if the results of an initial stapedotomy are unsatisfactory, a contralateral stapedotomy should be performed.

COCHLEAR IMPLANTATION

Cochlear implantation has benefited from many technological advances, and its indication has been expanded significantly in recent years, including the application to severe-profound hearing losses related to otosclerosis.[25,26] There has been an increase in the use of cochlear implantation for the treatment of advanced otosclerosis. Castillo and colleagues[11] revealed that CIs improved the hearing of 100% of the patients with advanced otosclerosis. In a contemporary review by Merkus and colleagues[17] for the treatment of advanced otosclerosis, results with a wide range of success with both stapedotomy and cochlear implantation surgery were reported. Speech perception after cochlear implantation was found to vary between 45% and 98%, and improvement in speech perception after cochlear implantation ranged from 34% to 94%. By comparison, speech perception after stapedotomy varied between 38% and 75%, and improvement in speech perception after stapedotomy ranged at a slightly poorer rate of 17% to 75%. Merkus and colleagues[17] proposed a treatment algorithm where the choice of surgical treatment should be based on SD rates and CT findings of each individual patient. They proposed a treatment algorithm.

Matterson and colleagues[27] demonstrated that implantation at a younger age and a shorter duration of hearing loss can be an advantage for early postoperative speech recognition. However, no long-term improvements have been reported in the implanted ears of patients with otosclerosis that have been affected by hearing loss for shorter periods of time. Although Matterson and colleagues[27] claimed that the rehabilitation of implanted ears that have been deafened for long periods of time can take several months, comparable standards of hearing are expected to be achieved within 6 months with therapy. Therefore, it is recommended that ears with worse hearing be chosen initially for cochlear implantation because of results suggesting that the implantation of either ear can lead to equivalent speech perception in the longer term.

Abdurehim and colleagues[4] revealed that cochlear implantation improved speech recognition significantly more than stapedotomy in their meta-analysis study. The study also reported that the quality of postoperative speech recognition was similar between successful stapedotomy and well-fitted hearing aids and CIs. In addition, the meta-analysis revealed that previously failed stapedotomy did not affect the speech recognition of patients with advanced otosclerosis who had been fitted with CIs.

Calmels and colleagues[10] performed stapedotomy and CI surgeries on patients with advanced otosclerosis. For the stapedotomy group, although postoperative recognition of dissyllabic words at 70 dB was significantly better than preoperative recognition, there were no significant differences between preoperative and postoperative BC thresholds. For the cochlear implantation group, postoperative BC thresholds and SD at 70 dB were significantly better than preoperative scores. In sum, the BC thresholds and SD values were reported to be statistically better in the cochlear implantation group.

According to the algorithm proposed by Merkus and colleagues,[17] patients could be divided into 3 main groups according to their maximum SD scores. Group 1 SD scores were less than 30%; group 2 SD scores were 30% to 50%, and group 3 SD scores were 50% to 70%. Because group 1 patients typically had severe SNHL, the most effective treatment of this group was cochlear implantation. For group 2 patients who exhibited severe retrofenestral otosclerosis in their CT scans (Rotteveel grade system type 2C or 3), cochlear implantation was typically recommended. In cases where group 2 patients had less advanced otosclerosis by imaging and air-bone gaps that were greater than 30 dB, stapedotomy was recommended. Group 3 patients underwent the same management as group 2 except that hearing aid fittings were recommended when patients' air-bone gaps were less than 30 dB.

Despite this interesting algorithm that emphasizes the benefit of cochlear implantation, we still recommend to our patients with advanced otosclerosis to consider stapes surgery with hearing aid as a first option. Indeed, the outcome of auditory stimuli at this time is still better than electrical stimuli in terms of SD and musical appreciation. If the outcome of stapedotomy is not satisfactory in terms of subjective hearing and audiologic testing, then CI can be pursued (**Fig. 4**). No treatment bridges are burned by considering stapes surgery initially and, given the cost difference, resource management issues may be satisfied as well. Advanced otosclerosis classifications and most treatment algorithms are based primarily on audiologic measurements and imaging. Pure or primary retrofenestral otosclerosis may be best managed with CI, but neither audiology nor imaging can identify these uncommon cases with certainty, so that the authors' recommendation to most patients with far-advanced otosclerosis is to consider stapes surgery first.

SURGICAL TECHNIQUE AND CHALLENGES OF COCHLEAR IMPLANTATION IN OTOSCLEROSIS

Cortical mastoidectomy, posterior tympanotomy, and electrode insertion through the round window or via cochleostomy are standard techniques of cochlear implantation. The landmarks for CIs, such as the promontory and round window niche, may be altered due to bony remodeling in otosclerosis patients, thereby making the identification of scala tympani difficult. In these cases, basal turn obliteration often occurs, and

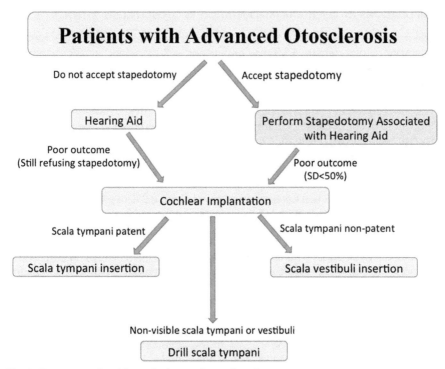

Fig. 4. Treatment algorithm of advanced otosclerosis.

drilling the promontorium may be required to detect the lumen of the basal turn.[1] It has been reported that cochlear ossification does not affect the audiologic results of cochlear implantation.[11]

Matterson and colleagues[27] reported that 11 of 59 otosclerosis patients with profound SNHL had some degree of obliteration in the scala tympani. Their study identified the involvement of the round window in 2 patients, proximal 3 to 5 mm scala tympani in 5 patients, and complete ossification of the basal turn in 4 patients.[28] Semaan and colleagues[22] identified intraoperative ossification in 29.4% of patients with advanced otosclerosis. Interestingly, preoperative CT scans revealed that 60% of these patients did not present findings that were consistent with otosclerosis. Therefore, the study concluded that cochlear drilling may be necessary in cases whereby the basal turn has been obliterated and the surgeon must be prepared for drilling despite lack of imaging findings. Obliteration of the scala tympani may occur in 2% to 25% of patients with advanced otosclerosis, and electrode insertion via scala vestibuli may be necessary.[17]

Marchioni and colleagues[1] described an endoscopic-assisted cochlear implantation technique for advanced otosclerosis in 3 patients with CT scan evidence of round-window obliteration. In this study, the fustis was used to identify the landmark of the round window. After finding and following the fustis endoscopically, drilling was performed on the promontory near the anterior portion of the fustis where the fenestral region was located. These investigators thought that the endoscopic approach aided in the correct identification of the round window by allowing better visualization of the related perifenestral anatomic landmarks, including the fustis, the funiculus, and the concamerata area. CI in an advanced otosclerosis case is illustrated in Video 1.

COMPLICATIONS OF COCHLEAR IMPLANTATION IN OTOSCLEROSIS PATIENTS

Facial nerve stimulation (FNS) during CI use occurs with some regularity in patients with advanced otosclerosis. FNS may be a minor, self-resolving, or major complication that can usually be resolved by reprogramming or deactivation of the problematic electrodes in a multichannel CI.[19] However, when many electrodes require deactivation, the performance of the device may be negatively impacted. In some cases, FNS cannot be resolved through deactivation and reimplantation may be necessary.[19] FNS is thought to occur because of current leaks, especially in cases where the electrode array has been partially inserted. It has been asserted that electrode design can influence the incidence of FNS, with perimodiolar configurations less leaky and, therefore, less likely to cause FNS.[29] The effect of electrode design on FNS in advanced otosclerosis has not been confirmed using rigorous clinical trials.

The incidence of FNS has been reported to vary from 0.9% to 14.9% in the general CI population. In a study that based its findings on reports from a large database on cochlear implantation, incidence of FNS was found to be 2.71% in adults and 0.94% in children.[30] FNS is most commonly associated with otosclerosis, cochlear malformation, and temporal bone fractures. Symptoms of FNS include tingling, visible facial spasms, and facial pain.[31] According to a relevant study, FNS, when it occurs, begins on average approximately 6.8 months after cochlear implantation.[32]

FNS affects many patients with advanced otosclerosis who have undergone cochlear implantation.[33] Marshall and colleagues[18] compared 30 patients with advanced otosclerosis treated with CIs and 30 patients without otosclerosis who had CI as control. FNS occurred in 17% of the patients in the otosclerotic group, whereas none of the patients in the control group had FNS. Treatment of these patients required deactivation of one or more of the electrodes in their implants. This study also showed that there was no difference between the radiologic extent of otosclerosis and the performance with CIs.

The risk for FNS in grade 3 (diffuse confluent retrofenestral involvement) advanced ososclerosis is significant and may be related to electrode configuration.[18] Flook and colleagues[29] reported that 21 patients who had undergone cochlear implantation with perimodiolar electrodes developed no FNS, but 6 of 14 (43%) patients with straight electrodes did develop FNS. In addition, Matterson and colleagues[27] indicated that none of 24 patients who had undergone cochlear implantation with contour electrodes experienced FNS, whereas 14 of 35 patients with straight electrodes experienced FNS.

Reprogramming or deactivation of the electrodes that cause FNS can aid in the treatment of FNS. Another treatment modality for refractory FNS after cochlear implantation is the injection of botulinum toxin.[30] Gold and colleagues[30] reported the benefit of oral fluoride treatment in cases refractory to the previously described options.

Cochlear ossification or pericochlear hypodensity findings on imaging can be associated with incorrect or partial electrode placement.[18] As otosclerosis progresses, demineralization can cause the formation of cavitation around the cochlea with resultant perilymphatic gusher during cochleostomy.[12]

Rotteveel and colleagues[20] reported that the insertion of a multichannel electrode array was problematic for 10 of 53 of the patients with advanced otosclerosis in their study. Three of these patients experienced misplacement, and 7 of them experienced partial insertion of the electrode array. In this study, perimodiolar implants were used on 10 patients, and nonmodiolus hugging devices were used on 43 patients. Although FNS was identified in 1 of the patients with a perimodiolar implant (10%), it was detected in 19 of the patients with nonmodiolus implants (44%). Kabbara and colleagues[12] stated that advanced otosclerotic lesions can result in significant difficulties during surgery. On the other hand, Semaan and colleagues[22] revealed that complete electrode insertion was achieved in all 34 of the patients in their study with advanced otosclerosis who had received CIs.

Other untoward symptoms can appear after CI in far-advanced otosclerosis. In their series, Sainz and colleagues[34] reported that 2 of 15 (13.3%) patients with advanced otosclerosis experienced progressive episodes of intense tinnitus, dizziness, and headaches after cochlear implantation. All patients were treated with the deactivation of the offending electrodes. In another series, Semaan and colleagues[22] reported that 2 of 30 patients with advanced otosclerosis experienced new tinnitus after cochlear implantation.

Vestibular problems can also be identified in patients with advanced otosclerosis. Vertigo can be recurrent, positional, or spontaneous. Benign positional vertigo may be associated with advanced otosclerosis, and vestibular problems can be detected regardless of cochlear involvement.[2]

THE DIRECT ACOUSTIC COCHLEAR IMPLANT

The direct acoustic cochlear implant (DACI) device (Codacs, Cochlear Ltd, Sydney, Australia, not US Food and Drug Administration approved) is a new type of hearing implant. This system transfers acoustic energy directly to the inner ear via an implantable electromagnetic transducer.[24] It is designed for patients with severe to profound mixed hearing loss.[35] Recently, DACI has been applied successfully in the treatment of advanced otosclerosis.[28]

Kludt and colleagues[35] compared the outcomes of 25 patients implanted with DACI and 54 implanted with CI. All patients in the study were potential candidates for both devices. The word-recognition score in quiet was significantly better in the DACI group for average preoperative BC less than 60-dB hearing loss. Speech in noise intelligibility was also significantly better in patients implanted with DACI for all tested groups. These results indicate that patients with sufficient cochlear reserve perform significantly better with DACI than the CI in terms of speech in noise intelligibility and word recognition score in quiet. Lenarz and colleagues[36] included 15 otosclerosis patients with severe to profound mixed hearing loss in their study. They reported that the DACI device is quite beneficial for patients with severe to profound mixed hearing loss. Busch and colleagues[37] compared conventional hearing aids to DACI in otosclerosis patients with severe to profound hearing loss. The results indicated that hearing improvement, speech intelligibility, and satisfaction of patients with the DACI was significantly better than with conventional hearing aids. The investigators stated that the indication for DACI should be a BC threshold between 40 and 80-dB hearing loss and AC threshold higher than 60-dB hearing loss. Larger clinic trials with this device are required to reach definitive conclusions.

SUMMARY

Challenges of advanced otosclerosis are both diagnostic and therapeutic. The diagnosis of advanced otosclerosis with surgically manageable severe to profound mixed hearing loss versus profound primary SNHL may be difficult and is based on history, audiologic testing, and imaging findings. An initial trial of stapes surgery with hearing aid is appropriate for most patients, with cochlear implantation reserved for those who refuse stapedotomy despite poor hearing aid outcome, or patients who failed stapedotomy and hearing aid combined.

SUPPLEMENTARY DATA

Supplementary data related to this article can be found online at https://doi.org/10. 1016/j.otc.2017.11.012.

REFERENCES

1. Marchioni D, Soloperto D, Bianconi L, et al. Endoscopic approach for cochlear implantation in advanced otosclerosis: a case report. Auris Nasus Larynx 2016; 43:584–90.

2. Cureoglu S, Baylan MY, Paparella MM. Cochlear otosclerosis. Curr Opin Otolaryngol Head Neck Surg 2010;18:357–62.

3. Rama-López J, Cervera-Paz FJ, Manrique M. Cochlear implantation of patients with far-advanced otosclerosis. Otol Neurotol 2006;27:153–8.

4. Abdurehim Y, Lehmann A, Zeitouni AG. Stapedotomy vs cochlear implantation for advanced otosclerosis: systematic review and meta-analysis. Otolaryngol Head Neck Surg 2016;155:764–70.

5. Chole RA, McKenna M. Pathophysiology of otosclerosis. Otol Neurotol 2001;22: 249–57.

6. Muñoz-Fernández N, Morant-Ventura A, Achiques MT, et al. Evolution of otosclerosis to cochlear implantation. Acta Otorrinolaringol Esp 2012;63:265–71.

7. House HP, Sheehy JL. Stapes surgery: selection of the patient. Ann Otol Rhinol Laryngol 1961;70:1062–8.

8. Lachance S, Bussières R, Côté M. Stapes surgery in profound hearing loss due to otosclerosis. Otol Neurotol 2012;33:721–3.

9. van Loon MC, Merkus P, Smit CF, et al. Stapedotomy in cochlear implant candidates with far advanced otosclerosis: a systematic review of the literature and meta-analysis. Otol Neurotol 2014;35:1707–14.

10. Calmels MN, Viana C, Wanna G, et al. Very far-advanced otosclerosis: stapedotomy or cochlear implantation. Acta Otolaryngol 2007;127:574–8.

11. Castillo F, Polo R, Gutiérrez A, et al. Cochlear implantation outcomes in advanced otosclerosis. Am J Otolaryngol 2014;35:558–64.

12. Kabbara B, Gauche C, Calmels MN, et al. Decisive criteria between stapedotomy and cochlear implantation in patients with far advanced otosclerosis. Otol Neurotol 2015;36:e73–8.

13. Rotteveel LJ, Snik AF, Cooper H, et al. Speech perception after cochlear implantation in 53 patients with otosclerosis: multicentre results. Audiol Neurootol 2010; 15:128–36.

14. Psillas G, Kyriafinis G, Constantinidis J, et al. Far-advanced otosclerosis and cochlear implantation. B-ENT 2007;3:67–71.

15. Sato T, Morita N, Cureoglu S, et al. Cochlear otosclerosis adjacent to round window and oval window: a histopathological temporal bone study. Otol Neurotol 2010;31:574–9.

16. Quaranta N, Bartoli R, Lopriore A, et al. Cochlear implantation in otosclerosis. Otol Neurotol 2005;26:983–7.

17. Merkus P, van Loon MC, Smit CF, et al. Decision making in advanced otosclerosis: an evidence-based strategy. Laryngoscope 2011;121:1935–41.

18. Marshall AH, Fanning N, Symons S, et al. Cochlear implantation in cochlear otosclerosis. Laryngoscope 2005;115:1728–33.

19. Polak M, Ulubil SA, Hodges AV, et al. Revision cochlear implantation for facial nerve stimulation in otosclerosis. Arch Otolaryngol Head Neck Surg 2006;132: 398–404.

20. Rotteveel LJ, Proops DW, Ramsden RT, et al. Cochlear implantation in 53 patients with otosclerosis: demographics, computed tomographic scanning, surgery, and complications. Otol Neurotol 2004;25:943–52.

21. Toung JS, Zwolan T, Spooner TR, et al. Late failure of cochlear implantation resulting from advanced cochlear otosclerosis: surgical and programming challenges. Otol Neurotol 2004;25:723–6.

22. Semaan MT, Gehani NC, Tummala N, et al. Cochlear implantation outcomes in patients with far advanced otosclerosis. Am J Otolaryngol 2012;33:608–14.

23. Eshraghi AA, Nazarian R, Telischi FF, et al. The cochlear implant: historical aspects and future prospects. Anat Rec (Hoboken) 2012;295:1967–80.

24. Häusler R, Stieger C, Bernhard H, et al. A novel implantable hearing system with direct acoustic cochlear stimulation. Audiol Neurootol 2008;13:247–56.

25. Eshraghi AA, Gupta C, Ozdamar O, et al. Biomedical engineering principles of modern cochlear implants and recent surgical innovations. Anat Rec (Hoboken) 2012;295:1957–66.

26. Eshraghi AA, Ahmed J, Krysiak E, et al. Clinical, surgical, and electrical factors impacting residual hearing in cochlear implant surgery. Acta Otolaryngol 2017; 137:384–8.

27. Matterson AG, O'Leary S, Pinder D, et al. Otosclerosis: selection of ear for cochlear implantation. Otol Neurotol 2007;28:438–46.

28. Lenarz T, Verhaert N, Desloovere C, et al. A comparative study on speech in noise understanding with a direct acoustic cochlear implant in subjects with severe to profound mixed hearing loss. Audiol Neurootol 2014;19:164–74.

29. Flook EP, Broomfield SJ, Saeed S, et al. Cochlear implantation in far advanced otosclerosis: a surgical, audiological and quality of life review of 35 cases in a single unit. J Int Adv Otol 2010;7:35–40.

30. Gold SR, Miller V, Kamerer DB, et al. Fluoride treatment for facial nerve stimulation caused by cochlear implants in otosclerosis. Otolaryngol Head Neck Surg 1998; 119:521–3.

31. Seyyedi M, Herrmann BS, Eddington DK, et al. The pathologic basis of facial nerve stimulation in otosclerosis and multi-channel cochlear implantation. Otol Neurotol 2013;34:1603–9.

32. Rayner MG, King T, Djalilian HR, et al. Resolution of facial stimulation in otosclerotic cochlear implants. Otolaryngol Head Neck Surg 2003;129:475–80.

33. Fernandez-Vega S, Quaranta N, Bartoli R, et al. Management of facial nerve stimulation in otosclerosis by revision cochlear implantation. Audiol Med 2008;6: 155–60.

34. Sainz M, Garcia-Valdecasas J, Ballesteros JM. Complications and pitfalls of cochlear implantation in otosclerosis: a 6-year follow-up cohort study. Otol Neurotol 2009;30:1044–8.

35. Kludt E, Büchner A, Schwab B, et al. Indication of direct acoustical cochlea stimulation in comparison to cochlear implants. Hear Res 2016;340:185–90.

36. Lenarz T, Zwartenkot JW, Stieger C, et al. Multicenter study with a direct acoustic cochlear implant. Otol Neurotol 2013;34:1215–25.

37. Busch S, Kruck S, Spickers D, et al. First clinical experiences with a direct acoustic cochlear stimulator in comparison to preoperative fitted conventional hearing aids. Otol Neurotol 2013;34:1711–8.

Medical Management of Otosclerosis

Norma de Oliveira Penido, MD, PhD[a],*, Andy de Oliveira Vicente, MD, PhD[b]

KEYWORDS

- Otosclerosis • Otospongiosis • Hearing loss • Computed tomography • MRI
- Sodium alendronate • Sodium fluoride

KEY POINTS

- Otosclerosis/otospongiosis is a primary osteodystrophy of the otic capsule that affects genetically predisposed individuals and leads to progressive hearing loss.
- The onset of hearing loss occurs around the third or fourth decade of life, and mixed and sensorineural hearing loss may also occur.
- Imaging studies (high-resolution computed tomography scan and MRI) have played an important role in the diagnosis and therapeutic approach of otosclerosis and in assisting with differential diagnosis.
- The medical management of otosclerosis patients is aimed at preventing, or at least slowing, disease progression while attempting to restore auditory thresholds.
- The use of sodium fluoride and bisphosphonates has become necessary in cases of active lesions to limit the progressively degenerative activity of otospongiosis.

CONCEPT

Otosclerosis/otospongiosis is a primary osteodystrophy of the otic capsule characterized by the resorption and disordered formation of new, harder, bone growth caused by a metabolic disorder on the endochondral layer of the labyrinth bone.[1] The etiology of this disease is complex and indefinite, probably resulting from the interactions among genetic, infectious, hormonal, immunologic, and environmental factors.[2] Otosclerosis affects genetically predisposed individuals and leads to progressive hearing loss. Therapeutic options to arrest or slow the progress of the disease exist but are limited.[3]

HISTOPATHOLOGY FINDINGS

Histologically, otospongiosis/otosclerosis can be defined as pleomorphic inflammatory osteodystrophy, characterized by an initial (spongiotic) phase in which there is

Disclosure Statement: The authors have nothing to disclose.
[a] Department of Otorhinolaryngology–Head and Neck Surgery, Universidade Federal de São Paulo, Escola Paulista de Medicina, Rua Mário Whateley 109/72, São Paulo, São Paulo 05083140, Brazil; [b] Otorhinolaryngology Department, Hospital Especializado CEMA, Rua do Oratório, 1369 - Mooca, São Paulo-SP, 03117-000, Brazil
* Corresponding author.
E-mail address: nopenido@terra.com.br

Otolaryngol Clin N Am 51 (2018) 441–452
https://doi.org/10.1016/j.otc.2017.11.006
0030-6665/18/© 2017 Elsevier Inc. All rights reserved.

oto.theclinics.com

an increase of perivascular spaces, osteoclastic bone resorption, hypercellularity, immature bone formation in the endochondral layer of the otic capsule, and a late (sclerotic) phase with decreased cellularity, obliteration of the blood vessels, and remineralization, with formation of dense sclerotic bone as reparative process.[1]

Otosclerosis, in most cases, reaches isolated tiny regions of the otic capsule without causing any symptoms (histologic form). However, under certain circumstances, it may compromise the stapediovestibular joint and lead to progressive conductive hearing loss. In some other cases, the disease may be more aggressive and injure inner ear sensorineural structures, thus producing mixed or even sensorineural hearing loss (clinical form). Otospongiotic lesions may structurally alter the endosteum and the cochlear neuroepithelium without causing fixation of the stapes footplate, causing a pure sensorineural hearing loss disproportionate to the patient's age. This type of lesion has been termed *cochlear otosclerosis* (**Fig. 1**). Injury to the inner ear neuroepithelium probably is caused by several factors that may be associated or occur in isolation, including the following: release of cytotoxic enzymes (trypsin, antitrypsin, collagenases) in labyrinthine fluids; formation of abnormal vascular shunts with consequent cochlear venous congestion and arterial ischemia; involvement of the cochlear and vestibular aqueducts; involvement of the cochlear endosteum; vascular striae atrophy; hyalinization of the spiral ligament; and degeneration of cochlear neurons, especially those located in the basal turn.[1]

CLINICAL FEATURES

The onset of symptoms usually occurs around the third or fourth decades of life, but there are reports that the first manifestations of the disease occurred in children younger than 6 years or in adults older than 54 years.[2] North American estimates suggest that otosclerosis is the leading cause of acquired hearing loss, affecting 15 million people.[4] Otosclerosis is bilateral in 70% to 85% of patients, and its clinical picture accompanied a progressive conductive hearing loss and tinnitus in more than 70% of cases. Mixed and sensorineural hearing loss (SNHL) may also occur, depending on the evolution and degree of disease activity. Progressive SNHL occurs in 75% of the patients, regardless of whether they undergo surgical treatment. It is estimated that 9% of patients with otosclerosis will have profound sensorineural hearing loss.[5] Vestibular symptoms can be observed in up to 20% of the patients (otosclerotic inner syndrome) and, in the more advanced cases, there may be a picture of endolymphatic hydrops.[6]

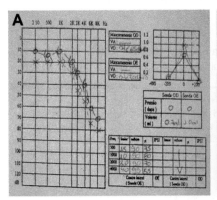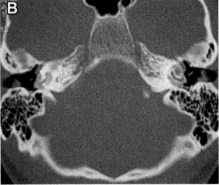

Fig. 1. Audiogram with pure sensorineural hearing loss (*A*) and axial section of HRCT shows pericochlear luscence. Double halo signal (*B*) in a case of cochlear otosclerosis.

Usually the physical examination of patients with otosclerosis does not find significant alterations that are important for diagnosis. Although otoscopy is normal in most cases, the otolaryngologist should be attentive to the presence of hyperemia on the promontory, seen through the translucent tympanic membrane, (Schwartze sign) that can be erroneously interpreted as serous otitis media (**Fig. 2**).

DIAGNOSIS

The diagnosis of otosclerosis is usually clinical, based on the findings of anamnesis, physical examination, and audiometric evaluation. However, this type of evaluation is not able to provide a definitive diagnosis of the disease or identify the degree of involvement of the otic capsule. Imaging studies can play a role in the diagnosis.

High-resolution computed tomography (HRCT) is the imaging modality of choice.[7,8] The fenestral focus, located in the region anterior to the oval window, can be found in more than 80% of patients with otosclerosis (**Fig. 3**). HRCT evidence of footplate thickening (**Fig. 4**), and obliterative involvement of the round window (**Fig. 5**), may guide treatment approach.[7,9] Retrofenestral focus, identified by pericochlear lucency or hypodensity (double halo sign), is associated with cochlear otosclerosis (**Fig. 6**). Endosteal involvement of the cochlea (**Fig. 7**) and internal auditory canal (**Fig. 8**) and vestibular labyrinth may be related to sensorineural hearing losses and vestibular symptoms such as vertigo.

MRI has demonstrated its applicability in the diagnosis of active otospongiotic lesions. The affected otic capsule is hypointense or isointense in T1 and hyperintense after administration of gadolinium (**Fig. 9**). The involvement of the endosteum of the cochlea by otospongiosis can also be evidenced by MRI (**Fig. 10**) even more accurately than in HRCT, because MRI more effectively shows the limits of the membranous labyrinth.[10] MRI may find an application as an objective evaluation method of therapeutic drug efficacy (**Fig. 11**).[11]

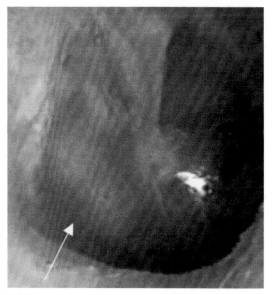

Fig. 2. Schwartze sign.

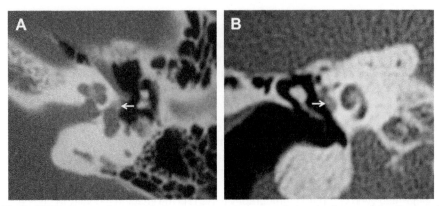

Fig. 3. HRCT shows a fenestral lesion in the most commonly involved area of the temporal bone region anterior to the oval window. Axial section (*A*) and coronal section (*B*).

THERAPY

The therapeutic approach for otosclerosis patients is aimed at preventing, or at least limiting, disease progression and restoring auditory thresholds. No curative medical therapy exists for otosclerosis. The use of medications has been investigated for cases of active otosclerosis to limit the progressively degenerative activity of the disease. The enzymatic theory, more widely accepted in the literature, attempts to explain the lesions in the inner ear caused by otospongiosis. The use of inhibitors of bone metabolism aims to preserve hearing thresholds (sensorineural component) and improve symptoms such as tinnitus and vertigo. Options for the medical treatment of otosclerosis include sodium fluoride and bisphosphonates.[12]

The indication to medical treatment depends on each specific case. Otolaryngologists may consider prescribing medication therapy in patients with signs of greater activity, such as presence of Schwartze sign, onset or worsening of tinnitus and/or vertigo, and progressive deterioration of the sensorineural component of hearing. The following criteria have been suggested: hearing loss of 2 dB per year in the speech frequencies;

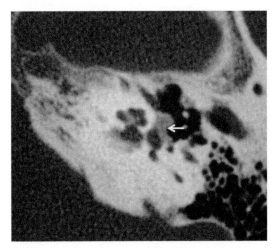

Fig. 4. Axial section of HRCT shows presence of footplate thickening.

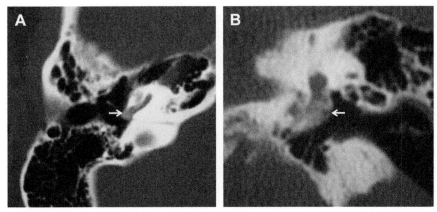

Fig. 5. Axial (*A*) and coronal (*B*) sections of HRCT show obliterative focus on the round window.

hearing loss of greater than 5 dB in any frequency, unexplained, progressive SNHL disproportionate to the patient's age, particularly with a positive family history of otosclerosis.[12] Medication may also be introduced, with evidence in the imaging studies (HRCT or MRI) of demineralization foci that involve the cochlear endosteum, even in the absence of clinical-audiometric clues of active disease, with the purpose to inactivate the otospongiotic lesions and prevent future cochleovestibular dysfunction.[13]

Sodium Fluoride

Sodium fluoride is the most widely prescribed treatment of this condition. Clinical studies found that a lower dose of 3 to 10 mg/d is sufficient for the enzymatically less-active stapedial fixation. With a cochlear component, presumably there is more enzymatic activity with the spread of hydrolytic and proteolytic enzymes in the cochlear fluids; hence, a dose of greater than 20 mg is suggested. The treatment is continued for 3 to 9 months. For patients with a progressive cochlear component, 20 mg/d is given for up to 2 years. After this period, a dose of 15 mg/d is administered until the otosclerotic focus becomes inactive as determined by stable bone

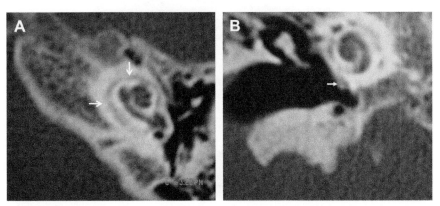

Fig. 6. Axial (*A*) and coronal (*B*) sections of HRCT show presence of retrofenestral lesion with pericochlear luscence without endosteal involvement of the cochlea.

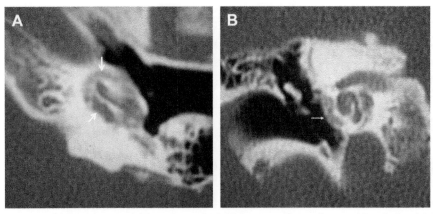

Fig. 7. Axial (*A*) and coronal (*B*) sections of HRCT show presence of precochlear lesion with endosteal involvement and cavitation of the cochlea.

conduction thresholds. For pure cochlear otospongiosis, 3 to 10 mg/d is given for years thereafter.[12] A retrospective review of 10,441 patients suggested that sodium fluoride treatment slowed, but did not release, stapedial fixation. Presumably, this is because doses of 45 mg or less only act on otospongiotic phase of lysis to prevent pseudohaversian bone formation. Larger doses of fluoride actually increase stapedial fixation based on older literature.[14] This conversion of otospongiosis to mature sclerosis occurs as a result of reduced enzyme activity derived from otospongiosis and from diminished rate of osteoblast-induced bone remodeling. The primary effect seems to be to contain bone resorption by mononuclear cells, whereas the novel bone formation effect may be of minor importance.[15] It is thought that sodium fluoride slows or stops the progression of sensorineural hearing loss by neutralizing and inactivating the hydrolytic and proteolytic enzymes that are toxic to hair cells rather than changing an active otospongiotic lesion to an inactive otosclerotic lesion.[16] Double-blind controlled clinical trials using sodium fluoride have shown stabilization of hearing thresholds.[17]

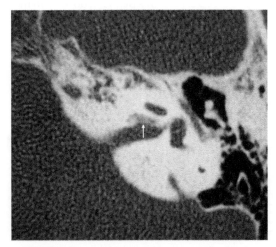

Fig. 8. Axial section of HRCT shows presence of lesion in the fundus of internal auditory meatus.

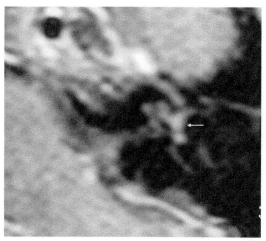

Fig. 9. MRI T1-weighted images with paramagnetic contrast show fenestral lesion at region anterior to the oval window.

The most frequent side effect of sodium fluoride treatment is gastrointestinal, including nausea, vomiting, gastritis, and peptic ulcer disease that can be relieved by the use of the enteric coated preparation or by gastric buffer. Other side effects include arthralgias, painful plantar fasciitis, and, rarely, nephrolithiasis. The use of this therapy is contraindicated in patients with impaired renal function because excretion of sodium fluoride may be reduced with resulting toxic levels. Sodium fluoride can pass easily through the placenta and is secreted into the milk. Thus, it may have a deleterious effect on the rapidly growing fetus and infants being breastfed. Pregnant and breastfeeding women should eliminate or decrease the dose of sodium fluoride. In children less than 12 years of age, the dosage should be reduced according to their weight because of the increase in bone volume in this age group and should be prescribed only in consultation with the pediatrician. After puberty, the adult dose may be initiated.

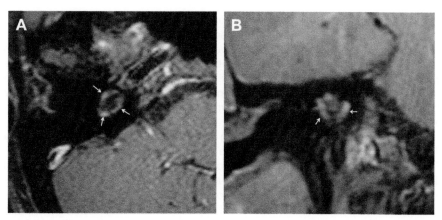

Fig. 10. MRI T1-weighted images with paramagnetic contrast show axial (*A*) and coronal (*B*) sections of perichochlear lesions.

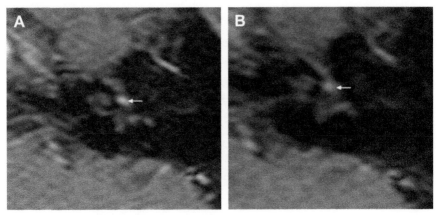

Fig. 11. MRI pretreatment with alendronate (*A*) and posttreatment (*B*) show decrease of signal intensity in region anterior to the oval window.

Bisphosphonates

The discovery that bisphosphonates could inhibit bone resorption was made in 1960 after attempts to identify agents that were similar to pyrophosphates, physiologic regulators of calcification and bone resorption. Early-generation bisphosphonates (clodronate and etidronate) were poorly tolerated because of frequency of dosing and side effects. Formulations with higher concentration and different routes of administration were developed, allowing for more convenient weekly, monthly, or annual dosing. Newer generations of bisphosphonates containing a primary nitrogen atom in an alkyl chain, such as pamidronate and alendronate, may be 10 to 100 times more potent than etidronate and clodronate, whereas derivatives of these compounds, which contain tertiary nitrogen such as ibandronate and olpadronate, are generally more potent in inhibiting bone resorption. Among the most potent latest generation bisphosphonates that inhibit bone resorption are those containing the nitrogen atom in a heterocyclic ring such as risedronate and zoledronate, the latter with potency up to 1000 times that of etidronate, with the best tolerability profile and the advantage of intravenous administration.[18,19]

Bisphosphonates have replaced the sodium fluoride in the treatment of osteodystrophy, such as Paget disease, osteogenesis imperfecta, and osteoporosis, because of their improved antiresorptive properties and a higher affinity with bone tissue. Following this line of therapy, bisphosphonates have begun to be used to treat otosclerosis. These drugs interact with osteoclast metabolism to induce osteoclast apoptosis, therefore inhibiting bone resorption. By that same mechanism, the production of toxic enzymes secondary to abnormal bone metabolism is reduced.

Alendronate, a bisphosphonate similar in action to etidronate, is recommended in a daily dose of a 10-mg tablet; risedronate is recommended at a dose of 5 mg/d. Formulations with a higher concentration of alendronate and risedronate have been developed with a more convenient, once-a-week dosing of 70 and 35 mg, respectively. The bisphosphonates that present formulations for intravenous use are Clodronate, Pamidronate, and zoledronate at doses of 1500 mg (monthly), 90 mg (monthly), and 4 mg (annual), respectively, for infusion over 4 hours for both clodronate and pamidronate and over 15 minutes for zoledronate (**Table 1**).[12,13,18,19]

Table 1
Medications, posology, and side effects in the treatment of cochlear otospongiosis

	Drugs	Dose	Frequency	Administration Routes	Side Effects
Sodium Fluoride	Fluoride	20–40 mg	Daily	Oral	Epigastralgia, nephrolithiasis, arthritis
B I P H O S P H O N A T E S	Alendronate	10 mg	Daily	Oral	Epigastralgia, esophagitis, mandible necrosis, teratogenicity
		70 mg	Weekly		
	Risedronate	5 mg			
		35 mg			
	Zoledronate	4-5 mg	Yearly	Intravenous	

Data from Refs.[12,13,18,19]

A double-blind prospective study to assess disodium etidronate in treating progressive hearing loss in otospongiosis patients observed the group given etidronate tended to have their hearing thresholds stabilized.[20] Another randomized, controlled, double-blind study found that treatment with either fluoride at 20 mg daily or alendronate at 10 mg/d for 6 months resulted in maintenance of hearing thresholds and stabilization of hearing loss.[13] In the same group of patients, using MRI, it was possible to detect the decrease of the enzymatic activity of the otospongiotic lesions.[11] In these studies, no significant side effects of alendronate for treatment of otosclerosis were reported at a weekly dosing of up to 70 mg.

Third-generation heterocyclic bisphosphonates, such as risedronate and zoledronate, have been reported for the treatment of otosclerosis-related sensorineural hearing loss with promising results in one study, which was retrospective in a small group of patients.[21] Commentary to the article suggested that higher dosing may have been even more successful. In the author's own opinion, when properly dosed with a combination of risedronate and etidronate, a more beneficial effect was achieved on inner ear function than using either alone. Although patients may be referred to medical specialists, bisphosphonates are safe enough to be prescribed by otolaryngologists.[22]

Weekly oral bisphosphonate treatment may be safer and more prudent than annual parenteral use, as one may have more control over the side effects of this therapy because of the possibility of therapy suspension in oral cases, which would not be possible in the parenteral option. This type of therapeutic approach with weekly oral doses has been shown to be sufficient to inactivate otospongiosis lesions as can be demonstrated in imaging (**Fig. 12**), and it can also stabilize the auditory thresholds in most cases. In some cases even an improvement of 10 to 15 dB can be observed in the annual posttreatment audiometric follow-up.

Possible adverse effects of bisphosphonates
One of the major problems in the use of bisphosphonates is patient lack of adherence to treatment, mainly because of the high cost of medication and adverse effects in

A

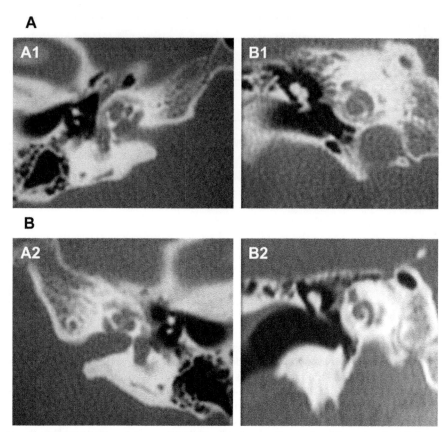

B

Fig. 12. (A) Axial (A1) and Coronal (B1) CT scans show active pericochlear otosclerotic focus. (B) Axial (A2) and Coronal (B2) CT scans show inactive pericochlear otosclerotic focus after treatment with bisphosphonate (alendronate).

some cases. In 2008, the US Food and Drug Administration (FDA) issued an alert highlighting the possibility of severe and even disabling pain in bones, joints, and muscles in patients using bisphosphonates. Prolonged use of alendronate sodium, for longer than 3 years, has been associated with an increase in atypical femoral fractures, which occur in the absence of trauma and correspond to less than 1% of femoral or hip fractures.[23] In 2011, the European Medicines Agency extended the cautionary alert to these adverse effects for all classes of bisphosphonates when used for the treatment of osteoporosis.[24] Gastrointestinal disorders can be severe and manifest as esophagitis or peptic ulcer. Another adverse reaction that has alerted regulatory agencies worldwide is jaw osteonecrosis. However, it should be emphasized that patients with this type of complication have well-established local jaw issues (such as exodontia, periapical lesions, irradiated bone areas, sclerosing bone diseases) and are carriers of underlying diseases such as generalized malignancies, uncontrolled diabetes, and alcoholism. Systemically healthy patients rarely have osteonecrosis. Lack of understanding of its mechanism of action leads to the generation of myths and controversies in bisphosphonate therapy; however, current prospective randomized studies have found safety for the proper management of this therapy in cases of otosclerosis.

Medical management of otosclerosis is essential for the prevention or reduction of disease progression, and drug therapy should be considered for all patients with clinical manifestations of otospongiosis. Fluoride-based medications, and bisphosphonates, are currently the most indicated remedies that may be associated with hearing rehabilitation procedures or the use of hearing aids. This therapeutic approach improves around 80% of patient's symptoms, or at least prevents symptoms worsening, and presents small side effects, which can be minimized by decreasing the medication dose or by using enteric coated tablets.

REFERENCES

1. Ramsay HA, Linthicum FH Jr. Mixed hearing loss in otosclerosis: indication for long-term follow-up. Am J Otol 1994;15(4):536–9.
2. Niedermeyer HP, Arnold W. Etiopathogenesis of otosclerosis. ORL J Otorhinolaryngol Relat Spec 2002;64(2):114–9.
3. Causse JR, Causse JB. Otospongiosis as a genetic disease. Early detection, medical management and prevention. Am J Otol 1984;5(3):211–23.
4. Niedermeyer HP, Arnold W, Schwub D, et al. Shift of the distribution of age in patients with otosclerosis. Acta Otolaryngol 2001;121:197–9.
5. Stankovic KM, McKenna MJ. Current research in otosclerosis. Curr Opin Otolaryngol Head Neck Surg 2006;14(5):347–51.
6. Gros A, Vatovec J, Sereg-Bahar M. Histologic changes on stapedial footplate in otosclerosis. Correlations between histologic activity and clinical findings. Otol Neurotol 2003;24(1):43–7.
7. Vicente Ade O, Yamashita HK, Albernaz PL, et al. Computed tomography in the diagnosis of otosclerosis. Otolaryngol Head Neck Surg 2006;134(4):685–92.
8. Valvassori GE. Imaging of the otosclerosis. Otolaryngol Clin North Am 1993;26(3):359–71.
9. Swartz JD, Faerber EN, Wolfson RJ, et al. Fenestral otosclerosis: significance of preoperative CT evaluation. Radiology 1984;151(3):703–7.
10. Stimmer H, Arnold W, Schwaiger M, et al. Magnetic resonance imaging and high-resolution computed tomography in the otospongiotic phase of otosclerosis. ORL J Otorhinolaryngol Relat Spec 2002;64(6):451–3.
11. De Oliveira Vicente A, Chandrasekhar SS, Yamashita HK, et al. Magnetic resonance imaging in the evaluation of clinical treatment of otospongiosis: a pilot study. Otolaryngol Head Neck Surg 2015;152:1119–26.
12. Uppal S, Bajaj Y, Coatesworth AP. Otosclerosis 2: the medical management of otosclerosis. Int J Clin Pract 2009;63:1526–30.
13. De Oliveira Vicente A, Yamashita HK, Cruz OLM, et al. The effectiveness of audiometric evaluation in drug treatment for otospongiosis. Braz J Otorhinolaryngol 2012;78(2):73–9.
14. Causse JR, Shambaugh GE, Causse B, et al. Enzymology of otospongiosis and NaF therapy. Am J Otol 1980;1:206–14.
15. Petrovic AG, Stutzmann JJ, Shambaugh GE Jr. Experimental studies on pathology and therapy of otospongiosis. Am J Otol 1985;6:43–50.
16. Parahy C, Linthicum FH Jr. Otosclerosis and otospongiosis: clinical and histological comparisons. Laryngoscope 1984;94:508–12.
17. Bretlau P, Salomon G, Johnsen NJ. Otospongiosis and sodium fluoride: a clinical double-blind, placebo-controlled study on sodium fluoride treatment in otospongiosis. Am J Otol 1989;10(1):20–2.

18. El-Rayes BF, LoRusso PM. The role of bisphosphonates in the treatment of skeletal complications of breast cancer. Am J Cancer 2004;3(6):369–75.
19. Tanakol R, Yarman S, Bayraktaroglu T, et al. Clodronic acid in the treatment of postmenopausal osteoporosis. Clin Drug Investig 2007;27(6):419–33.
20. Kennedy DW, Hoffer ME, Holliday M. The effects of etidronate disodium on progressive hearing loss from otosclerosis. Otolaryngol Head Neck Surg 1993; 109(3 Pt 1):461–7.
21. Quesnel AM, Seton M, Saumil NM, et al. Third generation bisphosphonates for treatment of sensorineural hearing loss in otosclerosis. Otol Neurotol 2012; 33(8):1308–14.
22. Brookler KH, Gilston N. Letters to the editor. Re: third-generation bisphosphonates for treatment of sensorineural hearing loss in otosclerosis. Otol Neurotol 2013;34(4):778–9.
23. FDA. Information for healthcare professionals: bisphosphonates. USA, 2008. Available at: https://www.fda.gov/Drugs/DrugSafety/PostmarketDrugSafetyInformation forPatientsandProviders/ucm124165.htm. Accessed January 17, 2018.
24. European Medicines Agency. Questions and answers on the review of bisphosphonates and atypical stress fracture. 2011. Available at: https://www.google.ca/url?sa=t&source=web&rct=j&url=http://www.ema.europa.eu/docs/en_GB/document_library/Referrals_document/Bisphosphonates_31/WC500105287.pdf&ved=0ahUKEwjLjZChjqHYAhVn4oMKHQO-AnEQFggeMAA&usg=AOvVaw2v BEQfts_hASZstH_J9ALO. Accessed January 17, 2018.

Prevention and Management of Complications in Otosclerosis Surgery

Patrick J. Antonelli, MD

KEYWORDS

- Otosclerosis • Stapedectomy • Stapedotomy • Complication • Hearing loss
- Dizziness

KEY POINTS

- Complications are uncommon with stapes surgery.
- Preoperative evaluation may allow for the prevention of some complications.
- Intraoperative complications may be avoided with proper surgical techniques.
- Most early postoperative complications usually can be managed medically.
- Revision surgery may be necessary to achieve optimal long-term outcomes.

PREOPERATIVE ISSUES

Complications may be avoided by performing a thorough preoperative evaluation. This effort is largely to identify conditions that may either mimic otosclerosis or may be present in conjunction with otosclerosis and are more likely to lead to suboptimal outcomes[1] or complications (**Box 1**). A history of lifelong hearing loss raises the potential for congenital dysplasia, most commonly an enlarged vestibular aqueduct,[2] and other congenital anomalies.[3] Autophony and sound- or pressure-induced vertigo suggests semicircular canal dehiscence.[4] The tympanic membrane should be carefully inspected for subtle evidence of atelectasis or cholesteatoma. The presence of myringosclerosis may suggest tympanosclerotic fixation of any of the ossicles. In addition to a comprehensive head and neck examination, which may reveal branchial arch anomalies, the skeletal system should be briefly surveyed for other markers of syndromic hearing loss (eg, digit anomalies with NOG mutations).[5] Audiometry may reveal patterns of hearing loss that are atypical for otosclerosis. Acoustic reflexes may be intact in the presence of an air-bone gap due to semicircular canal dehiscence.[6] The use of preoperative imaging, specifically, high-resolution computed

Disclosure Statement: The author has nothing to disclose.
Department of Otolaryngology, University of Florida, 1345 Center Drive, M2-228 MSB, PO Box 100264, Gainesville, FL 32610-0264, USA
E-mail address: pa@ufl.edu

Otolaryngol Clin N Am 51 (2018) 453–462
https://doi.org/10.1016/j.otc.2017.11.015
0030-6665/18/© 2017 Elsevier Inc. All rights reserved.

> **Box 1**
> **Clinically significant conditions that may mimic otosclerosis or may be found in conjunction with otosclerosis**
>
> - Ossicular pathology
>   - Malleus fixation
>   - Incus fixation
>   - Incus necrosis
>   - Congenital footplate fixation
>
> - Tympanosclerosis
>
> - Cholesteatoma
>
> - Persistent stapedial artery
>
> - Inner ear dysplasia
>   - Large vestibular aqueduct/Mondini dysplasia
>   - X-linked gusher
>
> - Anomalous facial nerve
>
> - Semicircular canal dehiscence, superior or posterior
>
> - Paget's disease
>
> - Osteogenesis imperfecta

tomography (CT), can identify such anomalies. Imaging is generally considered unnecessary for patients with a presentation typical of otosclerosis (eg, adult onset of progressive hearing loss with a large air-bone gap and otherwise normal history, examination, and audiometric testing).

INTRAOPERATIVE ISSUES
Bleeding

The surgical approach generally begins with injection of an anesthetic agent with the vasoconstrictor, epinephrine. The author favors xylocaine 1% with epinephrine 1:100,000, as this is widely available and it provides both sufficient anesthesia and vasoconstriction to carry out stapedotomy.[7] Many surgeons favor higher concentrations of epinephrine; but these require either compounding by the pharmacy or mixing by operating room staff, which increase the chance of errors, resulting in potentially life-threatening cardiac events.[8] If the injection is performed too quickly or patients are moving, the solution may pass between the skin and the periosteum, creating blebs that may compromise visualization and lead to more oozing of blood during the procedure. Bleeding from bone and mucosa is common, but usually limited, following the atticotomy. Otosclerotic bone and the overlying mucosa may be particularly hyperemic during active phases of bone turnover (otospongiosis).

Intraoperative bleeding can usually be controlled by topical application of epinephrine (eg, 1:20,000) on a gelatin sponge. Preparing such concentrated solutions only after canal injections have been completed reduces the risk of their injection. Hemostasis should be obtained before opening the oval window. Placing a delicate stapes prosthesis into a stapedotomy in the presence of significant bleeding can prove challenging. Concerns have been raised about the potential of blood in the inner ear to compromise outcomes.[9]

A persistent stapedial artery can present particularly brisk bleeding if not recognized and properly managed. The application of microbipolar electrocautery, laser energy (in a diffused mode), and bone wax can be used to manage small-caliber arteries and allow completion of the stapedectomy.[10] If the artery has more than a nominal diameter, it is best left intact until it is known that this is not critical for the central nervous system circulation.

Tympanic Membrane Perforation

Unfavorable anatomy, such as external auditory canal stenosis and exostoses, limited neck range of motion, and delicate tissue (eg, with advanced patient age), increase the risk of violating the tympanomeatal flap. If this breech is small, it can generally be handled by reinforcing the area with a small piece of fibrofatty tissue and a small amount of gelatin sponge. If the native tissue is suspect or the defect in the drum is substantial, consideration should be given to staging the stapedotomy following the drum repair. Failure to visualize the annulus—and enter middle ear deep to this— and use of a cutting bur with the atticotomy seem to be the main avoidable causes.

Chorda Tympani Injury (Dysgeusia)

Simply exposing the chorda tympani to the intense light of the operating microscope can lead to its desiccation. Thus, transient dysgeusia is common.[11] The chorda tympani is particularly vulnerable to damage during the atticotomy, fenestrating or removing the footplate, and securing the prosthesis on the incus (especially, crimping). The author removes less bone around the chorda tympani than earlier in his career, as he can work around this nerve as long as the entirety of the footplate is visible with the scope positioned either cranial or caudal to the chorda. If the chorda tympani sustains appreciable trauma, there is less likelihood of long-term dysgeusia if the nerve is transected.[12]

Incus Subluxation

This complication may occur at any stage in the procedure, but the risk seems to be greatest during the atticotomy and with securing the prosthesis on the incus (eg, crimping). The atticotomy should be done by removing heavy bone, lateral to the scutum first. Once this is done, the thin, remaining bone overlying the incus can be removed with less force, in a more controlled fashion, using a pick or curette. Micro-drills probably reduce the risk of this complication but can still occur if the drill catches an edge of the scutum and the bur jumps in an uncontrolled manner. Fenestrating the footplate and crimping a stapes piston on the incus before superstructure removal results in lower rates of subluxation than doing this after.[13] Historically, subluxation has been managed by repositioning the incus and placing the stapes prosthesis, as the incus can refix to the malleus and good hearing results can occur.[14] With the availability of bone cement, the author would favor the use of cement between the incus and malleus as a more certain means of achieving ossicular continuity.

Facial Nerve Injury

The facial nerve's normal location at the cranial aspect of the oval window places it at risk of injury during stapedectomy. Fortunately, this is extremely unlikely,[15] even in the presence of a prolapsed, dehiscent facial nerve,[16] which increases the risk of iatrogenic injury.[17] Most cases of immediate-onset facial palsy result from the local anesthetic and resolve spontaneously in a matter of a few hours. Collateral damage to the nerve from the laser stapedotomy is possible.[18] The facial nerve can be traumatized simply by forcibly removing a thick footplate. In such cases, the footplate should be thinned with a microdrill before fenestration or footplate removal. In cases of obliterative otosclerosis, the facial nerve may not be readily visible. Drilling a trough parallel to the facial nerve, beginning at the level of the crura, generally allows the oval window to be identified and the vestibule opened safely. In revision cases, when the crura are absent, the facial nerve location can generally be determined by identifying the round window niche and the cochleariform process. In the author's experience, the bone in the oval window in such cases is generally softer and more chalk-like than the normal otic capsule, facilitating fenestration and avoiding trauma to the facial nerve. With prolapsed facial nerves, the author finds it helpful to leave much of the crura intact, removing only the upper portion of the arch and capitulum with a laser and perform a stapedotomy with a microdrill in such cases. The crura maintain a channel for both the drill and the prosthesis. If necessary, access can be improved by drilling down the lip of the promontory.[19] Stapedectomy is contraindicated if the nerve bifurcates around the superstructure.

Floating Footplate

If the oval window annulus is nominally fixed with otosclerosis, attempts to fenestrate or remove the footplate may lead to mobilization of the footplate. Placement of a control hole in the footplate or completing the fenestration before superstructure removal facilitates footplate extraction in such cases.[13] Performing the stapedotomy with a laser can reduce the force placed on the oval window annulus, thereby allowing for the prevention and management of this uncommon complication. In the presence of a very thick footplate and a relatively minimally involved annulus, known as a biscuit footplate, it can be helpful to create a control hole at the annulus before attempting to take down the superstructure or perform the stapedotomy. If a floating footplate occurs, placing a tissue graft, followed by a stapes prosthesis usually leads to good hearing results.[20] Attempting to remove a floating footplate may result in the remaining stapes sinking into the vestibule, with possible adverse consequences to hearing. If the footplate or other parts of the stapes sink completely into the vestibule, no attempt should be made for extraction, as a high likelihood of sensorineural hearing loss (SNHL) will ensue.

Pneumo-Labyrinth

A small amount of air is routinely found in the labyrinth postoperatively.[21] Overly aggressive use of suction and the application of a gelatin sponge around a fenestrated oval window can lead to marked loss of perilymph (ie, a dry vestibule), which increases the rate of both hearing loss and vestibular complaints. In the author's experience, mild cases may self-correct, including by the oozing of blood into the vestibule. If it is dry, placing a Barber or Rosen needle at the edge of the stapedotomy and instilling a drop of saline onto the needle will replenish the perilymph, generally with good results.

Perilymph Gusher and Oozer

In rare circumstances, reported as 1 in 200 before the availability of CT imaging,[22] stapes footplate fenestration may lead to brisk flow of perilymph (actually, cerebrospinal fluid). Preoperative imaging may demonstrate dysplasia of the internal auditory canal and cochlea, consistent with X-linked gusher, or they may be read as normal.[23] Careful inspection of the internal auditory canal fundus, both in axial and coronal planes, may be needed to demonstrate the anomalous connection between the subarachnoid space and the perilymph (**Fig. 1**). Management of the gusher requires calm and patience. After the cerebrospinal fluid flow has abated, a fibrous tissue graft can be placed over the stapedotomy and a prosthesis placed in the usual fashion. Although the author has placed different prostheses in such cases, including relatively weak fluoroplastic-platinum pistons, he favors the rigidity of a titanium bucket-handle

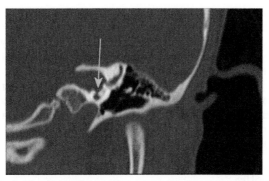

Fig. 1. CT, coronal plane, of a patient with a surgically proven perilymph gusher that was initially interpreted as normal. This image reveals a defect in the bony partition between the fundus of the internal auditory canal and the basal turn of the cochlea (*arrow*).

prosthesis. The fibrous tissue graft can be further supported with a gelatin sponge. Some surgeons advocate the placement of lumbar drains. Overaggressive drainage may lead to undesirable outcomes, such as pneumocephalus.[24] In the author's experience, lumbar drains have proven to be unnecessary in the treatment of perilymph gushers.

Perilymph oozers are similarly due to congenital dysplasia. Based primarily on the author's experience—primarily from cochlear implants, as this is considered a contraindication to stapedectomy—these are most commonly found in patients with large vestibular aqueducts and modiolar deficiencies (eg, Mondini dysplasia). Although these are normally readily seen on CT, common problems, such as motion artifact or suboptimal techniques (eg, thick cuts), can lead them to be missed. Surgeons should read their own CTs and not rely on radiologists to detect these anomalies.

Hearing results with both gushers and oozers are worse than expected. Although some cases have closure of the air-bone gap, these are more the exception than the rule. SNHL is more common.

Vertigo

When stapedotomy is performed without general anesthesia, patients may complain of vertigo. If excessive local anesthetic is injected into the ear canal, or raising the tympanomeatal flap is delayed, the local anesthetic agent may diffuse into the inner ear, creating an acute vestibular imbalance and vertigo. This complication is very uncommon. It is also surprisingly uncommon for patients to describe vertigo simply as a result of the cooling effect of suctioning the middle ear. The author has only observed this after suctioning aggressively to keep bone cement dry on the incus during a revision procedure. Patients will more commonly describe vertigo with laser stapedotomy and placing a bucket-handle prosthesis. The former is due to transient heating of the vestibule and will pass fairly quickly. Placing the bucket-handle prosthesis requires passing the prosthesis under the lenticular process, leading to a brief, slight overpenetration of the piston into the vestibule. It is a clear reminder of the limited tolerance some patients have to prosthesis length. The author has witnessed prostheses placed too deep into the vestibule. In most cases, patients have not reported vertigo. This complication is usually prevented by a tissue graft over the stapedotomy before placing the prosthesis.

As mentioned earlier, in the process of removing a portion or all of the stapes footplate, bone fragments may become mobilized and fall into the vestibule, which increases the likelihood of postoperative vertigo and disequilibrium. No attempt should be made to remove these fragments, which may more severely injure the membranous labyrinth. Resulting vestibular complaints generally clear within a month or two. Such events are less likely when the stapedotomy is performed with a microdrill and, more so, with a laser.

Concerns have been raised about the potential injury of the saccule by visible light laser energy (eg, potassium titanyl phosphate and argon).[25] The energy from these lasers is absorbed by pigmented tissues, as found in the saccule, and not by clear fluid, as occurs with carbon dioxide laser energy. These concerns have not been borne out in clinical practice.

POSTOPERATIVE ISSUES
Surgical Site Infection

These infections are remarkably uncommon following stapedectomy, and antimicrobial therapy does not reduce these further.[26] Most commonly, infection may present as acute otitis externa. Acute otitis media and suppurative labyrinthitis are quite rare.[26] Meningitis has been reported.[27] Prophylactic antibiotics have never been shown to be efficacious.[26,28]

Labyrinthitis

The normal healing response to stapedectomy involves a low level serofibrinous labyrinthitis.[29] As a result, most patients will report some degree of dizziness, especially with rapid head movements, immediately following the procedure.[30,31] This dizziness will usually clear in the first few postoperative days. Further improvement is generally seen over the first week in most patients. A small but significant subset of patients will worsen again around 5 to 7 days postoperatively. This worsening may be accompanied by a transient loss of hearing. If the healing response is extreme, marked hearing loss, tinnitus, and dizziness can ensue. This process can extend throughout the labyrinth and extend intracranially.[32] The mainstay of treatment is steroids.[33] Patients are not as acutely ill as would be expected with suppurative labyrinthitis. As it can be difficult to exclude bacterial involvement on clinical grounds, systemic antibiotics typically are given.

Historically, the term *reparative granuloma* has been used to describe such cases of extreme healing, manifest as severe hearing loss and disequilibrium. Findings include edema and hyperemia of the skin flap. It was reported to be one of the most common complications in the early decades of stapes surgery.[34] The recommended treatment was surgical replacement of the oval window tissue graft and prosthesis. These recommendations were not, however, supported by clinical trials or histopathologic findings; they predated the current imaging modalities. In nearly 25 years, the author has yet to see a case that truly fits this description. The author suspects that if reparative granulomas were truly distinct from severe serofibrinous labyrinthitis, they may have been due to outdated practices, such as contamination of the middle ear with talcum powder from surgical gloves or the use of contaminated gelatin sponge.[35,36]

Sensorineural Hearing Loss

SNHL is probably the most common, serious complication following stapedectomy. Anacusis has been reported at nearly 2% with stapedectomy, less with stapedotomy.[37] Other series have reported permanent SNHL of more than 15 dB at less than 0.5%.[38] Less severe forms are more common.[39] Transient high-frequency SNHL is very common.[40] The risk of SNHL is greater with revision procedures and with drill-outs for obliterative otosclerosis.[41] Low-frequency SNHL, without other man-ifestations of Meniere's disease, and histologic evidence of *endolymphatic hydrops* have been reported in around 10% of patients after stapedectomy.[42] *Sympathetic hearing loss* (ie, in the contralateral ear) is possible and more common with revision stapedectomy.[43] Rarely will concomitant conditions, such as acoustic neuroma, become manifest only after stapedectomy. Sudden SNHL or conductive hearing loss that develops with trauma (esp, barotrauma) long after a stapedectomy may warrant consideration of a *perilymph fistula* and surgical exploration. These rare occurrences are thought to be more common with total footplate removal with subop-timal oval window grafts, but reports are conflicting.[44–46] The only apparent consensus risk factor was the use of a gelatin sponge to seal the oval window, a practice that seems to have long since been abandoned.

Conductive Hearing Loss

When this is observed following stapedectomy, it is important to understand whether there was initial improvement. If the hearing improved initially, then worsened again—primarily due to an air-bone gap—many possibilities must be considered. The primary concerns are prosthesis displacement, regrowth of bone in the oval window, and incus necrosis.[47] Iatrogenic cholesteatoma (ie, middle ear without drum defect) may present in this fashion.[48] If the hearing never improved, causes may include prosthesis displacement, malleus or incus fixation, semicircular canal dehiscence, round window obliteration, and incus subluxation. CT can be helpful to elucidate the underlying problem in such cases.[49–52] Some patients with relatively minimal air-bone gaps may complain of sound distortion, like a blown speaker. This distortion is due to a loose connection between the incus and the stapes prosthesis (also known as loose wire syndrome).[53]

Vestibular Dysfunction

Vestibular complaints are not uncommon with otosclerosis, even in the absence of stapes surgery.[54] Vertigo and disequilibrium are very common in the early postoper-ative period, as described earlier.[31] Stapedectomy may precipitate or unmask latent vestibular pathology, such as benign paroxysmal positional vertigo. Persistent vestib-ular complaints resulting from surgery may result from a prosthesis that is impacting the saccule (ie, too long or medially displaced). If a long prosthesis remains in conti-nuity with the incus, patients may complain of dizziness with hiccupping, burping, yawning, popping the ears, and with specific acoustic stimuli. Sensitivity to the pros-thesis length seems, however, to be highly variable.[55] Replacement with a shorter prosthesis is highly successful, especially when done with awake patients providing feedback.

Facial Palsy

Facial motor palsy may develop in a delayed fashion in less than 1% of patients following uncomplicated stapedectomy.[56] This complication occurs around a week postoperatively and is thought to be due to iatrogenic reactivation of varicella zoster or herpes simplex viruses. Prompt treatment with systemic corticosteroids and anti-viral agents results in uniformly good outcomes.

Atelectasis and Cholesteatoma

Performing an atticotomy in patients with compromised eustachian tube function may result in the development of atelectasis and cholesteatoma.[57,58] Although this compli-cation has been limited to isolated case reports, the author's experience suggests that it is underappreciated. Because opening the vestibule in the presence of a cholesteatoma is fraught with the risk of SNHL and dizziness,[59] it is preferable to avoid this complication. Stapedectomy should be avoided in patients with poor tubal function. If for some reason this is required (eg, far advanced otosclerosis), consideration should be given to bolstering the atticotomy defect with cartilage.

SUMMARY

Serious complications resulting from surgery for otosclerosis are relatively uncommon. Many undesirable stapedectomy issues may be avoided by a thorough preoperative evaluation and meticulous operative technique. Informed management, that is, knowing when to reoperate and when to manage medically, can optimize outcomes when complications do arise.

REFERENCES

1. Massey BL, Hillman TA, Shelton C. Stapedectomy in congenital stapes fixation: are hearing outcomes poorer? Otolaryngol Head Neck Surg 2006;134:816–8.
2. Antonelli PJ, Nall AV, Lemmerling MM, et al. Hearing loss with cochlear modiolar defects and large vestibular aqueducts. Am J Otol 1998;19:306–12.
3. Merchant SN, Rosowski JJ. Conductive hearing loss caused by third-window lesions of the inner ear. Otol Neurotol 2008;29:282–9.
4. Merchant SN, Rosowski JJ, McKenna MJ. Superior semicircular canal dehiscence mimicking otosclerotic hearing loss. Adv Otorhinolaryngol 2007;65: 137–45.
5. Cremers CW, Admiraal RJ, Huygen PL, et al. Progressive hearing loss, hypoplasia of the cochlea and widened vestibular aqueducts are very common features in Pendred's syndrome. Int J Pediatr Otorhinolaryngol 1998;45:113–23.
6. Hong RS, Metz CM, Bojrab DI, et al. Acoustic reflex screening of conductive hearing loss for third window disorders. Otolaryngol Head Neck Surg 2016;154: 343–8.
7. Gessler EM, Hart AK, Dunlevy TM, et al. Optimal concentration of epinephrine for vasoconstriction in ear surgery. Laryngoscope 2001;111:1687–90.
8. Wanamaker HH, Arandia HY, Wanamaker HH. Epinephrine hypersensitivity-induced cardiovascular crisis in otologic surgery. Otolaryngol Head Neck Surg 1994;111:841–4.
9. Radeloff A, Unkelbach MH, Tillein J, et al. Impact of intrascalar blood on hearing. Laryngoscope 2007;117:58–62.
10. Govaerts PJ, Marquet TF, Cremers WR, et al. Persistent stapedial artery: does it prevent successful surgery? Ann Otol Rhinol Laryngol 1993;102:724–8.
11. Guder E, Bottcher A, Pau HW, et al. Taste function after stapes surgery. Auris Nasus Larynx 2012;39:562–6.
12. Michael P, Raut V. Chorda tympani injury: operative findings and postoperative symptoms. Otolaryngol Head Neck Surg 2007;136:978–81.
13. Szymanski M, Golabek W, Morshed K, et al. The influence of the sequence of surgical steps on complications rate in stapedotomy. Otol Neurotol 2007;28:152–6.
14. Golabek W, Szymanski M, Siwiec H, et al. Incus subluxation and luxation during stapedectomy. Ann Univ Mariae Curie Sklodowska Med 2003;58:302–5.
15. Blake DM, Svider PF, Carniol ET, et al. Malpractice in otology. Otolaryngol Head Neck Surg 2013;149:554–61.
16. Neff BA, Lippy WH, Schuring AG, et al. Stapedectomy in patients with a prolapsed facial nerve. Otolaryngol Head Neck Surg 2004;130:597–603.

17. Welling DB, Glasscock ME 3rd, Gantz BJ. Avulsion of the anomalous facial nerve at stapedectomy. Laryngoscope 1992;102:729–33.
18. Lescanne E, Moriniere S, Gohler C, et al. Retrospective case study of carbon dioxide laser stapedotomy with lens-based and mirror-based micromanipulators. J Laryngol Otol 2003;117:256–60.
19. Lippy WH, Berenholz LP, Schuring AG, et al. Promontory drilling in stapedectomy. Otol Neurotol 2002;23:439–41.
20. Lippy WH, Fucci MJ, Schuring AG, et al. Prosthesis on a mobilized stapes footplate. Am J Otol 1996;17:713–6.
21. Bajin MD, Mocan BO, Sarac S, et al. Early computed tomography findings of the inner ear after stapes surgery and its clinical correlations. Otol Neurotol 2013;34: 639–43.
22. Ginsberg IA, Hoffman SR, Stinziano GD, et al. Stapedectomy–in depth analysis of 2405 cases. Laryngoscope 1978;88:1999–2016.
23. McFadden MD, Wilmoth JG, Mancuso AA, et al. Preoperative computed tomography may fail to detect patients at risk for perilymph gusher. Ear Nose Throat J 2005;84(770):772–4.
24. Flood LM, Kemink JL, Kartush JM. Pneumocephalus following treatment of a stapes gusher. Am J Otol 1985;6:508–11.
25. Gantz BJ, Jenkins HA, Kishimoto S, et al. Argon laser stapedotomy. Ann Otol Rhinol Laryngol 1982;91:25–6.
26. Leonard JR. Prophylactic antibiotics in human stapedectomy. Laryngoscope 1967;77(4):663–80.
27. Nielsen TR, Thomsen J. Meningitis following stapedotomy: a rare and early complication. J Laryngol Otol 2000;114:781–3.
28. Govaerts PJ, Raemaekers J, Verlinden A, et al. Use of antibiotic prophylaxis in ear surgery. Laryngoscope 1998;108:107–10.
29. Hohmann A. Inner ear reactions to stapes surgery (animal experiments). In: Schuknecht HF, editor. Otosclerosis, vol. 11. Boston (MA): Little, Brown and Company; 1962. p. 305–17.
30. Hirvonen TP, Aalto H. Immediate postoperative nystagmus and vestibular symptoms after stapes surgery. Acta Otolaryngol 2013;133(8):842–5.
31. Ozmen AO, Aksoy S, Ozmen S, et al. Balance after stapedotomy: analysis of balance with computerized dynamic posturography. Clin Otolaryngol 2009;34: 212–7.
32. Watts E, Powell HR, Saeed SR, et al. Post-stapedectomy granuloma: a devastating complication. J Laryngol Otol 2017;131:557–60.
33. Elies W, Hermes H. Early complications following stapedectomy–surgical or conservative treatment? HNO 1990;38(2):67–70 [in German].
34. Kaufman RS, Schuknecht HF. Reparative granuloma following stapedectomy: a clinical entity. Ann Otol Rhinol Laryngol 1967;76:1008–17.
35. Dawes JD, Cameron DS, Curry AR, et al. Post-stapedectomy granuloma of the oval window. J Laryngol Otol 1973;87:365–78.
36. Burtner D, Goodman ML. Etiological factors in poststapedectomy granulomas. Arch Otolaryngol 1974;100:171–3.
37. Kursten R, Schneider B, Zrunek M. Long-term results after stapedectomy versus stapedotomy. Am J Otol 1994;15:804–6.
38. Vincent R, Sperling NM, Oates J, et al. Surgical findings and long-term hearing results in 3,050 stapedotomies for primary otosclerosis: a prospective study with the otology-neurotology database. Otol Neurotol 2006;27:S25–47.

39. Ishai R, Halpin CF, Shin JJ, et al. Long-term incidence and degree of sensorineural hearing loss in otosclerosis. Otol Neurotol 2016;37:1489–96.
40. Bauchet St Martin M, Rubinstein EN, Hirsch BE. High-frequency sensorineural hearing loss after stapedectomy. Otol Neurotol 2008;29:447–52.
41. Vincent R, Rovers M, Zingade N, et al. Revision stapedotomy: operative findings and hearing results. A prospective study of 652 cases from the otology-neurotology database. Otol Neurotol 2010;31:875–82.
42. Ishai R, Halpin CF, McKenna MJ, et al. How often does stapedectomy for otosclerosis result in endolymphatic hydrops? Otol Neurotol 2016;37:984–90.
43. Richards ML, Moorhead JE, Antonelli PJ. Sympathetic cochleolabyrinthitis in revision stapedectomy surgery. Otolaryngol Head Neck Surg 2002;126:273–80.
44. Moon CN Jr. Perilymph fistulas complicating the stapedectomy operation. A review of forty-nine cases. Laryngoscope 1970;80:515–31.
45. Lesinski SG. Causes of conductive hearing loss after stapedectomy or stapedotomy: a prospective study of 279 consecutive surgical revisions. Otol Neurotol 2002;23:281–8.
46. Lin KF, Selesnick S. Stapedotomy with adipose tissue seal: hearing outcomes, incidence of sensorineural hearing loss, and comparison to alternative techniques. Otol Neurotol 2016;37:851–8.
47. Lesinski SG, Stein JA. CO2 laser stapedotomy. Laryngoscope 1989;99(6 Pt 2 Suppl 46):20–4.
48. von Haacke NP, Wilson JA, Murray JA, et al. Cholesteatoma following stapedectomy. J Laryngol Otol 1987;101:708–10.
49. Whetstone J, Nguyen A, Nguyen-Huynh A, et al. Surgical and clinical confirmation of temporal bone CT findings in patients with otosclerosis with failed stapes surgery. AJNR Am J Neuroradiol 2014;35:1195–201.
50. Mikulec AA, McKenna MJ, Ramsey MJ, et al. Superior semicircular canal dehiscence presenting as conductive hearing loss without vertigo. Otol Neurotol 2004;25:121–9.
51. Picavet V, Govaere E, Forton G. Superior semicircular canal dehiscence: prevalence in a population with clinical suspected otosclerosis-type hearing loss. B-ENT 2009;5:83–8.
52. Wieczorek SS, Anderson ME Jr, Harris DA, et al. Enlarged vestibular aqueduct syndrome mimicking otosclerosis in adults. Am J Otol 2013;34:619–25.
53. McGee TM. The loose wire syndrome. Laryngoscope 1981;91:1478–83.
54. Freeman J. Otosclerosis and vestibular dysfunction. Laryngoscope 1980;90:1481–7.
55. Yehudai N, Masoud S, Most T, et al. Depth of stapes prosthesis in the vestibule: baseline values and correlation with stapedectomy outcome. Acta Otolaryngol 2010;130:904–8.
56. Shea JJ Jr, Ge X. Delayed facial palsy after stapedectomy. Otol Neurotol 2001;22:465–70.
57. Ferguson BJ, Gillespie CA, Kenan PD, et al. Mechanisms of cholesteatoma formation following stapedectomy. Am J Otol 1986;7:420–4.
58. Eviatar A, Jamal H. Cholesteatoma induced by stapedectomy. Arch Otolaryngol 1983;109:413–4.
59. Palva T, Karja J, Palva A. Opening of the labyrinth during chronic ear surgery. Arch Otolaryngol 1971;93:75–8.

Revision Surgery for Otosclerosis

Apoorva T. Ramaswamy, MD, Lawrence R. Lustig, MD*

KEYWORDS

- Otosclerosis • Revision • Stapedectomy • Stapedotomy • Prosthesis
- Complications

KEY POINTS

- Revision surgery for otosclerosis is fraught with the risk of complications, including failure to improve hearing, inner ear damage, dead ear, and facial nerve damage.
- Primary indications for revision are persistent air bone gap, intractable vertigo, and facial nerve complication.
- Audiogram, computed tomography, and the previous operative report can be important in surgical planning.
- Preoperative preparation of equipment including laser, bone cement, and necessary prosthetics is critical.
- Local anesthesia with sedation can provide immediate feedback during challenging cases.

BACKGROUND

Revision surgery for the treatment of otosclerosis is fraught with difficulty for the ear surgeon. In previous years, the risk of severe inner ear damage with sensorineural hearing loss ranged from 0.4% to 20%, while 32.7% to 66% of patients achieved closure of air-bone gap defined either as less than 10 dB or less than 20 dB.[1–14] Over the last 2 decades, partially because of changes in methodology as outlined below and the consolidation of expertise within high-volume centers, the outcomes have improved but continue to be worse than those of primary surgery.[15,16] Today, less than 20-dB air bone gap results are achieved in 71% to 96.3%, and 0% to 2% of patients go on to have profound sensorineural hearing loss, or a dead ear,

Disclosure Statement: Disclosure of any relationship with a commercial company that has a direct financial interest in subject matter or materials discussed in article or with a company making a competing product.
The authors have nothing to disclose.
Department of Otolaryngology–Head and Neck Surgery, Columbia University Medical Center, 180 Fort Washington Avenue, 8th Floor, New York, NY 10032, USA
* Corresponding author.
E-mail address: lrl2125@cumc.columbia.edu

Otolaryngol Clin N Am 51 (2018) 463–474
https://doi.org/10.1016/j.otc.2017.11.014
0030-6665/18/© 2017 Elsevier Inc. All rights reserved.

postoperatively.[17–24] These challenges partly stem from a selection bias for more severe disease, but a revision surgeon must also adapt each surgery to the previous surgeon's handiwork. The primary management of otosclerosis has evolved greatly over the last 6 decades since Shea first described modern stapedectomy with a Teflon implant. Thus, complete evaluation of a revision patient requires a robust system that minimizes intraoperative surprises and optimizes postoperative results with techniques and equipment tailored to each case.[25] Below, the initial evaluation, preoperative planning, and intraoperative techniques are detailed with review of the available evidence for each step.

INITIAL EVALUATION

The initial challenge facing an otologist with a patient presenting with poor outcomes from primary otosclerosis surgery is in understanding the nature and etiology of the patient's complaints.

Patient Presentation[26]

- Early presentation
  - Failure of improved hearing
  - Severe vertigo
  - Severe tinnitus
- Later presentation
  - Progressive hearing loss
  - Loose wire syndrome
  - Aural fullness
  - Dysgeusia

Physical examination can help evaluate additional conditions such as semicircular canal dehiscence or cholesteatoma, which would require a change in treatment plan. An audiologic evaluation is also essential for understanding the etiology of the patient's concerns.

Causes of immediate conductive hearing loss or poor response to primary surgery include

- Failure of initial prosthesis placement
- Excessive tissue graft
- Reparative granuloma
- Incorrect diagnosis such as third mobile window syndrome or ossicular fixation from the malleus or incus[26]

Causes of progressive conductive loss

- Displacement of the prosthesis
- Inappropriate prosthesis length
- Incus erosion
- Allergy to the prosthetic substance, typically nickel-titanium (Nitinol)
- Footplate refixation
- Ongoing otosclerosis[12,26–29]

In any case, an observation period of up to 6 weeks after the initial surgery can be important in assessing severity and stability of symptoms. At follow-up, it is important to discuss the risks and benefits of potential surgery with the patient. In particular, this conversation should assess the feasibility of the patient's expectations.

The primary indications for revision surgery are

- Hearing loss with an air-bone gap greater than 25 dB
- Persistent intractable vertigo
- Facial nerve complication requiring intervention[30]

A patient who presents with one of these indications and does not have signs of a complicating condition, such as semicircular canal dehiscence or cholesteatoma or with severe cochlear otosclerosis with minimal air-bone gap, may be offered revision surgery.

SURGICAL PLANNING

If available, the prior operative note is critical in helping identify potential anomalies or surgical pitfalls that may be encountered, including a dehiscent facial nerve.
Important points to look out for in the operative report include

- Mobility of the remaining ossicular chain
- Type of footplate opening
- Type of prosthesis (material, length, diameter)
- Additional grating material used (fat, fascia, vein, perichondrium)

However, in evaluating previous surgical reports, a 26-year retrospective review from Schimanski and colleagues[26] found that fewer than 40% of reports contained all above data. Consequently, understanding previous trends in otosclerosis management, communication with the previous surgeon, and knowledge of the common complications with different surgical interventions are paramount for the surgeon planning a revision intervention.

Aside from history, physical examination, audiologic examination, and review of the previous operative report, temporal bone computed tomography (CT) scan preoperatively can assist in planning. The utility of CT was recently studied by Whetstone and colleagues[31] who analyzed 22 scans of patients presenting after failed stapes surgery, comparing radiologic findings with intraoperative findings at revision. They showed the feasibility of preoperatively identifying common causes of primary surgical failure: piston migration, incus necrosis, and vestibular penetration on temporal bone CT. Others have emphasized the importance of providing relevant clinical history to the radiologist to allow an appropriate interpretation of the results of the study. For example, a 2013 study of early CT findings after stapes surgery found pneumolabyrinth, canonically a sign of perilymphatic fistula, to be a common finding in the early postoperative period, yet does not necessarily herald a bad outcome. Despite having excellent clinical surgical outcomes, all patients who underwent CT scan on the first postoperative day had evidence of pneumolabyrinth that all resolved by postoperative day 7.[32] Further, results of the CT have to be interpreted with caution, as studies have found that CT can systematically overestimate depth of penetration of the prosthesis into the vestibule.[33]

In preparing for a revision case for otosclerosis, a surgeon must consider

- Method of anesthesia
- Approach
- Equipment needs and preferences, including laser, bone cement, and alternative prostheses that may be needed

A 2013 systematic review of local versus general anesthesia in primary stapes surgery found no differences in postoperative outcomes in either group.[24] However, to date, there have been no studies that have specifically examined local versus general anesthesia in revision cases.[24] An advantage of local anesthesia with mild sedation in revision cases is the immediate feedback obtained for violation of crucial structures, including the inducement of vertigo. Further it affords the ability to test hearing while the patient is still on the table and allows the surgeon to make necessary adjustments. One downside of local sedation, however, is the inability to use facial nerve monitoring. Further, an uncooperative patient may make local anesthesia with sedation quite challenging.

The intraoperative findings during revision surgery for otosclerosis fall in to several categories: surgeon related, prosthesis related, disease related, and unclear etiology.[19,21,23,26,34,35]

Surgeon-related findings include

- Incorrect prosthesis length
- Insufficient footplate opening size
- Scarring of the oval window niche from excessive graft use
- Attic fixation from bone dust
- Poor fixation of the prosthesis to the incus[26]

A prosthesis that is too long has the much-feared consequence of vertigo and inner ear damage. In this scenario, patients typically complain of dizziness with loud noise or dizziness with Valsalva-type maneuvers or coughing or sneezing. In customized implants, such as the Schuknecht prosthesis, the most common finding is a prosthesis that is too short, resulting in an air-bone gap, presumably because of a primary surgeon's systematic desire to avoid inner ear damage. Poor movement of the prosthesis can result from a narrow footplate opening, a finding that can occur with any type of prosthesis associated with stapedotomy. At primary surgery, connective tissue sleeves are often used around the prosthesis for stabilization or for covering larger stapedotomies or stapedectomies. However, when too large, thick, or numerous, these can contribute to scarring and adhesions in the oval window niche. Similarly, bone fragments left in the middle ear during primary surgery can result in attic fixation of the incus. Lastly, a prosthesis can become dislocated from the incus or cause a "rattling" tinnitus from being too loosely attached at time of primary surgery. This may result from improper crimping of a wire prosthesis or erosion of the incus at the site of prosthesis fixation caused by overly aggressive crimping or excessive use of the laser on self-crimping prostheses.

Prosthesis related complications include

- Incus erosion
- Incus necrosis
- Granuloma formation[26]

Incus erosion and incus necrosis are common causes of long-term hearing loss after stapedectomy, found in 12.5% to 32% of revision cases (**Fig. 1**).[7–9,11,13,14] Theories for why this occurs vary but include overly zealous crimping, loss of blood supply, or a poorly fit prosthesis causing inflammation and bone erosion over time. Reparative granuloma is a rare postoperative phenomenon, occurring from 0.07% to 5% of the time, depending on the type of piston inserted at the primary surgery. This poorly understood entity is thought to be a foreign body tissue reaction. Gel foam and fat have been most commonly implicated in their development. See **Table 1** for outline of intraoperative findings at revision surgery from large case series.

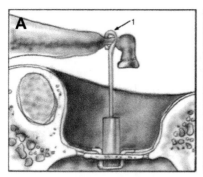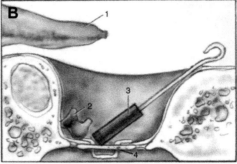

Fig. 1. (*A*) Incus erosion. (*B*) Incus necrosis. (*From* Roberson J Jr. Avoidance and management of complications of otosclerosis surgery. In: Brackmann DE, Shelton C, Arriaga MA, editors. Otologic surgery. 3rd edition. Philadelphia: Elsevier; 2010. p. 257–71; with permission.)

SURGICAL TECHNIQUE

To best identify and address all possible issues at revision surgery, a systematic approach is essential, although the exact order of steps can be varied by physician preference.

1. Generally, a transcanal approach provides sufficient visualization for the procedure. An endaural incision can improve access in narrower ear canals.
2. At visualization of the middle ear, periprosthetic fibroses are first divided to allow assessment of prosthesis placement. Lesinski and Stein,[36] among others, found that lasers allow atraumatic vaporization of adhesions in revision cases that facilitates adequate visualization and diagnosis of abnormalities.[21,37,38] The safety of each has been shown, but no studies have found clinical reasons to favor either CO_2, potassium-titanyl-phosphate-(KTP) or argon for the obliteration of fibroses.[38–41]
3. Attention is then turned to the ossicular chain. Using palpation and direct visualization, the mobility and integrity of the chain and each of its constituents are verified. At this point, fixation of the malleus or incus or of the prosthetic itself can be identified. The other classes of common findings at this step include displaced or loose prosthesis or necrosis of the incus.
4. Next, the stapes footplate is examined after again atraumatically dividing surrounding adhesions.
5. The existing prosthesis is then removed.
6. Once the prosthesis is removed, its length can be assessed. Prediction of appropriate prosthesis length has been the subject of extensive inquiry, as it can be difficult to assess on imaging as discussed above, and the manner of attaching the prosthesis can also change the effective length of the prosthesis. A combination of visual assessment with measuring rod and knowledge of one's own technique is the primary mode of estimating appropriate length. New technologies are being developed to eliminate error from this step; however, none are common in clinical practice.[42–47]
7. Next, the stapedotomy (if applicable) is examined with a trephine to ensure appropriate size to fit the chosen prosthesis; it is modified as needed. Atraumatically accomplishing this step is critical, and for this reason many favor using lasers again for this step.[17,21,37,48,49] However, older studies have argued for the safety of the microdrill, and advocates of this methodology remain.[23,50]

Table 1
Findings on revision surgery

Study	N	Incus Erosion/ Necrosis	Displaced Prosthesis	Adhesions	Otosclerosis	Prosthesis Length	Loose Prosthesis	Perilymph Fistula	Unclear/ Misc	Granuloma	Footplate Opening	Lateral Ossicular Chain Fixation
Schimanski et al,[26] 2011	343	10.76	1.45	1.74	0.29	5.52	2.03	0.87	3.78	11.63	2.91	0.87
Stucken et al,[21] 2012	26	15.4	42.3	30.8	N/A	15.4	3.8	N/A	N/A	N/A	N/A	N/A
Kanona et al,[23] 2017	49	24.5	24.5	28.6	16.3	6.1	6.1	N/A	N/A	N/A	20.4	6.1
Ozuer et al,[19] 2012	84	17.8	40.4	10.7	2.4	14.3	3.6	3.5	N/A	3.5	5.9	2.4
Bakhos et al,[34] 2010	89	49.0	24.0	25.0	N/A	8.0	4.0	8.0	7.0	N/A	12.0	N/A
Gros et al,[35] 2005	63	N/A	48.2	13.1	N/A	N/A	N/A	N/A	37.7	N/A	N/A	N/A
Lippy et al,[16] 2003	522	24.7	58.1	N/A	2.7	5.1	N/A	N/A	9.2	N/A	10.6	7.5

Abbreviation: N/A, not applicable.

8. The next step entails insertion of the new prosthesis. There are many options of prosthetics that vary based on material, attachment method, size, and shape. Surgeons must be facile with not only with their preferred prosthetic but also those tailored to address common issues found during revision surgery. The presence of incudal necrosis or erosion is an important factor for this step. This finding can pose a challenge for the revision surgery, as the anatomy of the incus is now altered. There are several options for dealing with this when encountered. One option is to use a longer wire prosthesis that attaches to the incus higher up on the long process. A second option is to use bone cement to rebuild the long process of the incus to allow placement of the prosthesis in its usual location. A third option is to use a modified buckethandle prosthesis that cups the residual incus. This prosthesis typically requires a graft over the stapedotomy. If there is too much erosion of incus to allow the fitting of any prosthesis, a final option is to bypass the incus and attach the prosthesis directly to the malleus See **Table 2** for an overview of available prostheses (**Fig. 2**).

9. The stapedotomy is then sealed with material of choice. Fat, perichondrium, fascia, venous blood, and vein grafts have all been used in this step. Many studies have compared each methodology, with good results found with each and no conclusive results, particularly in the limited case of revisions.[20,51–68] However, Szymanski and colleagues[39,40] did find that the use of a sealant, in their case vein graft, can limit thermal injury to the vestibule during revision cases using lasers, both KTP and CO_2.

10. The tympanomeatal flap is then replaced, and if the patient is under local anesthesia, hearing is checked using a tuning fork (512 Hz preferred). If the hearing is not improved, the tympanomeatal flap should be raised and the steps above repeated.

If the hearing is improved, then the surgeon can apply appropriate packing material with antibiotic drops in external auditory canal. If not, the steps above may be repeated. Conversely, if the surgeon feels this is too dangerous or futile, then the surgery is stopped, accepting the conductive hearing loss, as a residual conductive hearing loss is infinitely superior to a dead ear.

POSTOPERATIVE CARE

Postoperatively, the patient is discharged home with a limited number of pain medications, and steroids can be considered at this step for cochlear protection. In a guinea pig study, Kiefer and colleagues[69] found that topical and intracochlear corticosteroids could improve hearing after a stapedectomy. In a 1974 study, Hendershot[70] found that although long-acting corticosteroids prolonged the reformation of the oval window resulting in vestibular symptoms, short-acting steroids could be used to prevent

Table 2
Reconstruction options for incus complications

Reconstruction	Appropriate Situations
Bone cement	Incus erosion
Lippy modified prosthesis	Incus necrosis
Malleovestibular prosthesis	Incus necrosis
Total ossicular replacement prosthesis	Incus erosion or necrosis with poor anatomy

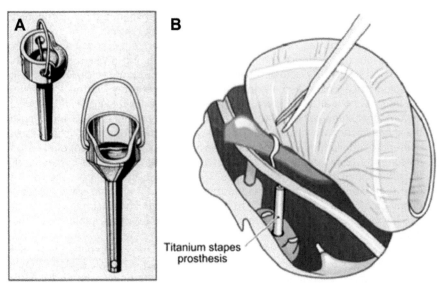

Fig. 2. (A) Lippy modified prosthetic for incus necrosis. (B) Malleus to footplate prosthesis. Fisch Titanium stapes prosthesis (diameter, 0.4 mm). (*From* [A] Lippy WH, Schuring AG. Prosthesis for the problem incus in stapedectomy. Arch Otolaryngol 1974;100(3):237–9; with permission; and [B] Microsurgery of the temporal bone – the Zurich dissection guidelines. p. 31. Fig. 61b; and Fisch U, Linder T. Temporal bone dissection–the Zurich guidelines. Tuttlingen (Germany): Endopress; 2006. p. 61; with permission.)

serous labyrinthitis.[70] However, in a more recent randomized controlled trial of 95 patients, Riechelmann and colleagues[71] found that prescribing prednisolone did not improve postoperative hearing, although it was associated with increased vertigo. Other postoperative considerations include activity restrictions on bending, lifting, and straining for 2 to 4 weeks postoperatively.

SUMMARY

Revision stapedectomy can be one of the most challenging surgeries faced by the ear surgeon. Maximizing success involves adequate preoperative evaluation and being prepared for all potential scenarios intraoperatively with appropriate equipment and prostheses available. Recognizing the limits of one's surgical abilities is also critical. In the end, it is important for the surgeon to always remember throughout the procedure that an aidable ear, even with a large conductive hearing loss, is an infinitely better outcome than an ear with a profound sensorineural hearing loss from iatrogetic injury.

REFERENCES

1. Han WW, Incesulu A, McKenna MJ, et al. Revision stapedectomy: intraoperative findings, results, and review of the literature. Laryngoscope 1997;107:1185–92.
2. Hammerschlag PE, Fishman A, Scheer AA. A review of 308 cases of revision stapedectomy. Laryngoscope 1998;108:1794–800.
3. Lesinski SG. Revision stapedectomy. Curr Opin Otolaryngol Head Neck Surg 2003;11:347–54.

4. Lesinski SG. Causes of conductive hearing loss after stapedectomy or stapedotomy: a prospective study of 279 consecutive surgical revisions. Otol Neurotol 2002;23:281–8.
5. Crabtree JA, Britton BH, Powers WH. An evaluation of revision stapes surgery. Laryngoscope 1980;90:224–7.
6. Derlacki EL. Revision stapes surgery: problems with some solutions. Laryngoscope 1985;95:1047–53.
7. Farrior J, Sutherland A. Revision stapes surgery. Laryngoscope 1991;101: 1155–61.
8. Glasscock ME 3rd, McKennan KX, Levine SC. Revision stapedectomy surgery. Otolaryngol Head Neck Surg 1987;96:141–8.
9. Langman AW, Lindeman RC. Revision stapedectomy. Laryngoscope 1993;103: 954–8.
10. Lippy WL, Schuring AG. Stapedectomy revision of the wire-Gelfoam prosthesis. Otolaryngol Head Neck Surg 1983;91:9–13.
11. Palva T, Ramsay H. Revision surgery for otosclerosis. Acta Otolaryngol 1990;110: 416–20.
12. Pearman K, Dawes JD. Post-stapedectomy conductive deafness and results of revision surgery. J Laryngol Otol 1982;96:405–10.
13. Sheehy JL, Nelson RA, House HP. Revision stapedectomy: a review of 258 cases. Laryngoscope 1981;91:43–51.
14. Somers T, Govaerts P, de Varebeke SJ, et al. Revision stapes surgery. J Laryngol Otol 1997;111:233–9.
15. Lippy WH, Wingate J, Burkey JM, et al. Stapedectomy revision in elderly patients. Laryngoscope 2002;112:1100–3.
16. Lippy WH, Battista RA, Berenholz L, et al. Twenty-year review of revision stapedectomy. Otol Neurotol 2003;24:560–6.
17. Albers AE, Schonfeld U, Kandilakis K, et al. CO(2) laser revision stapedotomy. Laryngoscope 2013;123:1519–26.
18. Hudson SK, Gurgel RK, Shelton C. Revision stapedectomy with bone cement: are results comparable to those of standard techniques? Otol Neurotol 2014;35: 1501–3.
19. Ozuer MZ, Olgun L, Gultekin G. Revision stapes surgery. Otolaryngol Head Neck Surg 2012;146:109–13.
20. Berenholz LP, Burkey JM, Lippy WH. The use of cartilage in revision stapedectomy. Otol Neurotol 2014;35:1187–90.
21. Stucken EZ, Brown KD, Selesnick SH. The use of KTP laser in revision stapedectomy. Otol Neurotol 2012;33:1297–9.
22. Pitiot V, Hermann R, Tringali S, et al. Revision stapes surgery for lysis of the long process of the incus: comparing hydroxyapatite bone cement versus malleovestibulopexy and total ossicular replacement prosthesis. Eur Arch Otorhinolaryngol 2016;273:2515–21.
23. Kanona H, Bhutta MF, Lavy J. Our approach to revision stapes surgery and the outcomes from 49 procedures at a UK tertiary centre. Clin Otolaryngol 2017; 42(4):931–5.
24. Wegner I, Bittermann AJ, Zinsmeester MM, et al. Local versus general anesthesia in stapes surgery for otosclerosis: a systematic review of the evidence. Otolaryngol Head Neck Surg 2013;149:360–5.
25. Shea JJ Jr. The teflon piston operation for otosclerosis. Laryngoscope 1963;73: 508–9.

26. Schimanski G, Schimanski E, Berthold MR. Diagnostic findings in stapes revision surgery–a retrospective of 26 years. Otol Neurotol 2011;32:373–83.
27. Shah N. Revision stapedectomy for late conductive deafness. J Laryngol Otol 1974;88:207–12.
28. Dawes JD, Curry AR. Types of stapedectomy failure and prognosis of revision operations. J Laryngol Otol 1974;88:213–26.
29. Harris JP, Gong S. Comparison of hearing results of nitinol SMART stapes piston prosthesis with conventional piston prostheses: postoperative results of nitinol stapes prosthesis. Otol Neurotol 2007;28:692–5.
30. Lippy WH, Schuring AG. Stapedectomy revision following sensorineural hearing loss. Otolaryngol Head Neck Surg 1984;92:580–2.
31. Whetstone J, Nguyen A, Nguyen-Huynh A, et al. Surgical and clinical confirmation of temporal bone CT findings in patients with otosclerosis with failed stapes surgery. AJNR Am J Neuroradiol 2014;35:1195–201.
32. Bajin MD, Mocan BO, Sarac S, et al. Early computed tomography findings of the inner ear after stapes surgery and its clinical correlations. Otol Neurotol 2013;34:639–43.
33. Bozzato A, Struffert T, Hertel V, et al. Analysis of the accuracy of high-resolution computed tomography techniques for the measurement of stapes prostheses. Eur Radiol 2010;20:566–71.
34. Bakhos D, Lescanne E, Charretier C, et al. A review of 89 revision stapes surgeries for otosclerosis. Eur Ann Otorhinolaryngol Head Neck Dis 2010;127:177–82.
35. Gros A, Vatovec J, Zargi M, et al. Success rate in revision stapes surgery for otosclerosis. Otol Neurotol 2005;26:1143–8.
36. Lesinski SG, Stein JA. Stapedectomy revision with the CO2 laser. Laryngoscope 1989;99:13–9.
37. McGee TM, Diaz-Ordaz EA, Kartush JM. The role of KTP laser in revision stapedectomy. Otolaryngol Head Neck Surg 1993;109:839–43.
38. Wiet RJ, Kubek DC, Lemberg P, et al. A meta-analysis review of revision stapes surgery with argon laser: effectiveness and safety. Am J Otol 1997;18:166–71.
39. Szymanski M, Mills R, Abel E. Transmission of heat to the vestibule during revision stapes surgery using a KTP laser: an in vitro study. J Laryngol Otol 2003;117:349–52.
40. Szymanski M, Morshed K, Mills R. Experimental study on heat transmission to the vestibule during CO2 laser use in revision stapes surgery. J Laryngol Otol 2007;121:5–8.
41. Szymanski M, Morshed K, Mills RP. The use of CO(2) laser in revision stapes surgery: experimental studies on heat transmission to the vestibule. Adv Otorhinolaryngol 2007;65:250–4.
42. Edwards WG. Functional middle ear reconstruction: experience with prostheses and tissue graft. Aust N Z J Surg 1980;50:356–60.
43. Huttenbrink KB. Biomechanics of stapesplasty: a review. Otol Neurotol 2003;24:548–57 [discussion: 557–9].
44. Kaftan H, Blaurock M, Kaftan S. Design-dependent calculation of the prosthesis length in malleostapedotomy. Ann Otol Rhinol Laryngol 2015;124:728–33.
45. Kaftan H, Bohme A, Martin H. Is the prosthesis length in malleostapedotomy for otosclerosis revision surgery predictable? Otol Neurotol 2014;35:1150–5.
46. Lee J, Nadol JB Jr, Eddington DK. Factors associated with incomplete insertion of electrodes in cochlear implant surgery: a histopathologic study. Audiol Neurootol 2011;16:69–81.

47. Marchica CL, Saliba I. The relationship between stapes prosthesis length and rate of stapedectomy success. Clin Med Insights Ear Nose Throat 2015;8:23–31.
48. Lesinski SG, Newrock R. Carbon dioxide lasers for otosclerosis. Otolaryngol Clin North Am 1993;26:417–41.
49. Sakamoto T, Kikuta S, Kikkawa YS, et al. Differences in postoperative hearing outcomes and vertigo in patients with otosclerosis treated with laser-assisted stapedotomy versus stapedectomy. ORL J Otorhinolaryngol Relat Spec 2015;77:287–93.
50. Sedwick JD, Louden CL, Shelton C. Stapedectomy vs stapedotomy. Do you really need a laser? Arch Otolaryngol Head Neck Surg 1997;123:177–80.
51. Bailey HA Jr. Stapedectomy with vein graft and polyethylene prosthesis. J Ark Med Soc 1962;58:409–15.
52. Benecke JE Jr, Gadre AK, Linthicum FH Jr. Chondrogenic potential of tragal perichondrium: a cause of hearing loss following stapedectomy. Laryngoscope 1990;100:1292–3.
53. Bittermann AJ, Vincent R, Rovers MM, et al. A nonrandomized comparison of stapes surgery with and without a vein graft in patients with otosclerosis. Otol Neurotol 2013;34:827–31.
54. Colman BH. Stapedectomy. Observations on 100 cases using an adipose tissue graft and steel-pin prosthesis. Acta Otolaryngol 1964;57:97–112.
55. Das UC, Ross A, Chary G. Annular ligament reconstruction - a better technique in the surgical treatment of stapes fixation. Indian J Otolaryngol Head Neck Surg 2004;56:88–90.
56. Farrior JB. Stapes surgery: pathologic indications for the bypass operations and the vein graft. Trans Am Acad Ophthalmol Otolaryngol 1960;64:248–63.
57. Goodhill V. Articulated polyethylene prosthesis with perichondral graft in stapedectomy. Rev Laryngol Otol Rhinol (Bord) 1961;82:305–20.
58. Hall IS. Preliminary experience with the vein graft operation for otosclerosis. J Laryngol Otol 1959;73:475–8.
59. Holden HB, Hood WG, Taylor LR. Stapedectomy with polystrut and fat graft reconstruction–a survey and analysis of the results of 200 cases. J Laryngol Otol 1967;81:593–600.
60. Igarashi M, Guilford FR, Alford BR. Bilateral vein graft stapedectomy. Human temporal bone study. Acta Otolaryngol 1970;69:94–9.
61. Kamal SA. Vein graft in stapes surgery. Am J Otol 1996;17:230–5.
62. Lin KF, Selesnick S. Stapedotomy with adipose tissue seal: hearing outcomes, incidence of sensorineural hearing loss, and comparison to alternative techniques. Otol Neurotol 2016;37:851–8.
63. Moon CN Jr. Stapedectomy with vein graft and metal prosthesis: one year's experience. Va Med Mon (1918) 1964;91:375–9.
64. Moon CN Jr. Stapedectomy, connective tissue graft and the stainless steel prosthesis. Laryngoscope 1968;78:799–807.
65. Perkins R, Curto FS Jr. Laser stapedotomy: a comparative study of prostheses and seals. Laryngoscope 1992;102:1321–7.
66. Salib RJ, Oates J. KTP laser fine fenestra stapedotomy with vein graft interposition in the surgical management of otosclerosis. Surgeon 2003;1:269–72.
67. Schuknecht HF. Stapedectomy and graft-prosthesis operation. Acta Otolaryngol 1960;51:241–3.
68. Strong MS, Vaughan CW. Partial stapedectomy and vein graft replacement; one year follow-up on 100 consecutive cases of otosclerosis. Arch Otolaryngol 1964;80:249–55.

69. Kiefer J, Ye Q, Tillein J, et al. Protecting the cochlea during stapes surgery: is there a role for corticosteroids? Adv Otorhinolaryngol 2007;65:300–7.
70. Hendershot EL. Corticosteroid therapy in stapedectomy: a clinical study. Laryngoscope 1974;84:1346–51.
71. Riechelmann H, Tholen M, Keck T, et al. Perioperative glucocorticoid treatment does not influence early post-laser stapedotomy hearing thresholds. Am J Otol 2000;21:809–12.

Potential of Robot-Based Surgery for Otosclerosis Surgery

Yann Nguyen, MD, PhD[a,b,*], Daniele Bernardeschi, MD, PhD[a,b],
Olivier Sterkers, MD, PhD[a,b]

KEYWORDS

- Stapes • Otology • Robotics • Planning • Stapedotomy • Minimally invasive

KEY POINTS

- Robot-based devices have the potential to improve accuracy of the surgical gesture.
- Prototypes have proved the feasibility of achieving some of the key steps of stapedotomy with success on temporal bones models.
- The functional outcomes, potential improvements, and medicoeconomic efficiency of robot-based devices remain to be demonstrated.

 Video content accompanies this article at http://www.oto.theclinics.com.

INTRODUCTION

Otosclerosis surgery requires complex procedures and surgical gestures to be carried out in a confined surgical workspace. When it comes to planning surgical treatment for otosclerosis, one should always propose a hearing aid fitting as an alternative for hearing rehabilitation. Otosclerosis surgery is very demanding, because a high percentage of success with no complications is expected by the patient. Consequently, when the procedure is performed by experienced surgeons, excellent outcomes are expected, with a hearing improvement and a postoperative air–bone gap of less than 10 dB in more than 90% of cases. Immediate postoperative complications of the surgery

Disclosure: Y. Nguyen, D. Bernardeschi, and O. Sterkers received financial and technical support from Collins Medical for the design and conception of the RobOtol device. Financial support was also provided by the French National Institute of Health and Medical Research (Inserm), as well as by the University Pierre et Marie Curie.
[a] Sorbonne Université, Inserm, UMR-S 1159 "Minimally Invasive Robot-based Hearing Rehabilitation", 16 Rue Henri Huchard, 75018 Paris, France; [b] Otolaryngology Department, Unit of Otology, Auditory Implants and Skull Base Surgery, AP-HP, GHU Pitié-Salpêtrière, 43 bd de l'hôpital, 75013 Paris, France
* Corresponding author. Bâtiment Castaigne Groupe hospitalier, Pitié Salpêtrière 47-83 boulevard de l'Hôpital, Paris 75651 cedex, France.
E-mail address: yann.nguyen@inserm.fr

Otolaryngol Clin N Am 51 (2018) 475–485
https://doi.org/10.1016/j.otc.2017.11.016
0030-6665/18/© 2017 Elsevier Inc. All rights reserved.

include invalidating vertigo or worsening of the auditory threshold. Worsening of the auditory threshold can result from an abnormal positioning of the prosthesis, a dry labyrinth, an intralabyrinthine hemorrhage, or a perilymph fistula. In the worst cases, this can lead to sensorineural hearing loss that can be partial or total and irreversible. Even though these complications are rare, their rates may vary with the experience of the surgeon.[1,2]

Some technical refinements have been proposed and progressively adopted by the otological community to lower the complication rate and achieve a minimal postoperative air–bone gap. Subsequently, stapedotomy instead of stapedectomy was proposed to lower sensorineural hearing loss. The mechanical stapedotomy using a drill or a trephine was further secured with the use of a laser alone[3] or in combination with a microdrill[4] to improve reproducibility from one procedure to another. Development has also focused on piston prostheses to obtain thinner devices so as to allow a good exposure of the footplate during placement and easy crimping of the incus with a clipping system or nitinol prostheses that only requires heating and no crimping to achieve contact with the incus.[5] Moreover, it has been shown in some stapes fixation training models that more experienced surgeons would apply less mechanical constraints on the ossicular chain during prosthesis manipulation.[6]

In this context, it seems that one of the limitations to further improving the safety and results of otosclerosis surgery is the surgeon's dexterity and experience. Thus, it has been proposed to use robot-based devices to enhance the quality of the surgical gesture. This article discusses the main contributions in the field of robot-based devices for otosclerosis surgery.

A ROBOT-BASED DEVICE FOR OTOSCLEROSIS SURGERY: RATIONALE

Otosclerosis surgery is conventionally performed through a small endaural incision or more frequently through a transcanal approach guided by the view from an operating microscope. Such an approach raises constraints that are commonly encountered in middle ear surgery. First, the surgery is performed in a deep workspace through a narrow approach restricted by the diameter of the external auditory canal and speculum. Under these conditions, even a small amount of bleeding can affect field exposure. Second, the surgeon holds the tools oriented along an axis collinear with exposure of the surgical field; thus, she or he may interfere with his visual field. Even though he is not working blindly, he may lose the stereoscopic view if one of the oculars of the microscope is hidden and, thus, she or he may lose depth perception. Third, the procedure is performed on millimetric structures, and low forces of less than 1 N are used to achieve the surgical tasks.

In addition, otosclerosis can also be considered to be a simpler procedure compared with other middle ear surgeries. First, the approach is repeated from 1 patient to another. Second, the lesions are mostly located in the oval window region and the extent of disease does not change the surgical strategy apart from in the case of well-advanced otosclerosis. Third, the anatomy is not often modified by the disease from 1 patient to another. Fourth, even though their order can be modified according to each surgeon's technique, the steps performed during the procedure are always the same: raising the tympanomeatal flap, lowering the scutum, sectioning the posterior tendon and crura, stapedotomy, piston placement and crimping, and folding the tympanomeatal flap down. For these reasons, a high level of success is expected when the surgical procedure is performed.

However, the current technique has 2 limitations to guaranteeing a reproducible quality of surgical gesture. First, the conventional technique with a tool holder relies on the benefits and drawbacks of the human hand. Second, exposure of the middle ear structures and especially the round window depends on the external auditory anatomy.

The human hand is versatile. It combines 22° of freedom to achieve various positions and orientations. The arm adds 6 additional degrees of freedom and the hand can be placed with redundant positions of the arm. Furthermore, the hand is given tactile sensitivity that can be used by the surgeon to appreciate tool–organ interactions. However, when it comes to performing a gesture with high accuracy such as microsurgery, the human faces limitations. Four kinds of involuntary motion have been described in microsurgery[7] and this description can be applied to middle ear surgery. Tremor is a rhythmic and sinusoidal (range of <0.2 mm) motion (wrist 8–12 Hz, fingers 17–30 Hz). The consequence of tremor is that the tip of the tool oscillates around the target position. Drift is a low-frequency motion with a higher amplitude (>0.5 mm) that is nonsinusoidal. The consequence of drift is that, after a few seconds, the tip of the tool is translated instead of remaining stationery. Jerk is a sudden reflexive or spasmodic muscular movement; it can be related to a lack of experience or tiredness. Finally, undershoot or overshoot represent the lack of accuracy while trying to reach a target point during a displacement. These involuntary motions can be reduced with training. Thus, tremor compensation techniques such as wrist and instrument support can enhance gesture accuracy within certain limits. If one may want to go to further in accuracy control, the use of robot-based devices offers a promising solution.

Hence, research and efforts conducted into the design and manufacture of a robot-based device for otosclerosis surgery rely on the assumption that a more accurate gesture during surgery will lead to lower complication rates and improved surgical hearing outcomes. Robots as tool holders offer many advantages over the human hand. Their motion accuracy and resolution are higher. A steady position can be maintained without the effects of tiredness. Their surgical environment can be enriched with all kinds of sensors, such as computer-assisted navigation, nerve monitoring, force sensing, and chemical sensors. However, their autonomy and capacity to adapt to a modification of the surgical scenario are limited by current technology on one hand and ethical reasons on the other. Different approaches with various architectures and command schemes have been developed during the past 20 years in the domain of otosclerosis surgery. This experience with advantages and drawbacks is discussed by considering the control mode that has been envisioned by their authors.

STATE-OF-THE-ART OF ROBOTS PREVIOUSLY REPORTED FOR OTOSCLEROSIS SURGERY
Comanipulated Systems

In comanipulated systems, the surgeon and robot hold the tool conjointly. This offers advantages such as immediate and intuitive ergonomics as the gesture is preserved. Thus, such systems can be rapidly embraced by surgeons who have varying degrees of openness to new technologies. Furthermore, eye–hand synchronization is preserved. The resistance of the device can be programmed to offer total transparency with a total weight-balancing correction or, in contrast, to offer filtering to suppress tremor or force feedback to improve stabilization or even prevent access to preoperatively planned restricted zones (these virtual restrictions can be set up by coupling the robot-based device to a navigation system). This force feedback can also be used to improve tactile sensations. The main disadvantages of such a system are that displacement can only be scaled as one-to-one and exposure of the surgical field is impaired by both the robot and the surgeon's hand.

The first robot to be evaluated for a task in otosclerosis surgery was the Steady Hand. It has 7° of freedom and was evaluated by surgeons for microsurgical gestures.[8] It has been tested in various applications such as retinal vessel cannulation,[9] footplate fenestration, or control of cochlear implant insertion.[10] For otosclerosis surgical tasks, it has been shown to improve the positional accuracy of footplate fenestration with a micropick with lower cumulated forces required to achieve the stapedotomy.[11] Performance comparisons in groups of surgeons with various levels of experience showed that Steady Hand assistance would have increased benefits in less experienced surgeons compared with seniors.[12]

The second device is a handheld device called the Micron. It has 3 piezo actuators that compensate for hand tremor to improve control of the tip of the mounted tool. Its small size makes it less affordable but easier to replace when necessary compared with conventional robots. It was evaluated in a stapes fenestration task with either a micropick or a CO_2 fiber laser.[13] It was shown that, when the tremor cancellation system was activated, the gesture accuracy increased for stapedotomy positioning, and that less time was spent in nondesired areas around the target point.[14]

Teleoperated Systems

Teleoperated robot-based systems are composed of a master arm that is controlled by the surgeon and a slave arm that functions as an effector for tool–organ interactions. The benefits of such an assembly are to offer the surgeon the choice to stay remote from the surgical field. Thus, the surgeon's comfort is increased, she or he does not need to be dressed in sterile clothing, and she or he can be rapidly replaced if necessary. Advanced coupling modes between the 2 arms can be achieved to obtain command filtering for tremor suppression, force feedback to enhance tactile sensitivity, and motion scaling to improve motion control accuracy. Because the slave arm is not cooperatively moved by a human hand, its shape has fewer constraints and can therefore offer complex motion with low bulk. The disadvantages are that these systems are less user friendly compared with a comanipulated device and may require a longer learning curve.

The MMS-2 is a robot composed of a micromanipulator bearing multiple tools similar to the standard instruments used in otological surgery and a macromanipulator holding the first device.[15] Thus, the macromanipulator acts as a holder for the smaller and more accurate device. It is the micromanipulator that has been evaluated clinically. Its accuracy has been validated and compared with the accuracy of the surgeon's hand for completion of footplate fenestration. It was reported that the use of the robot would reduce the maximum force applied and force tremor on the footplate with increased accuracy. These benefits were obtained in both novice and experienced surgeon groups.[16] A novel application of a robot-based device was also proposed by the authors as a measuring tool to assess the choice of piston prosthesis by measuring the displacement of the tip of a tool from the footplate to the incus.[17]

The RobOtol system (Collin Ltd, Bagneux, France) is a multitasking robot-based platform dedicated to middle ear surgery and cochlear implantation. Otosclerosis is one of its target applications; the device specifications were initially defined by the constraints of the stapedotomy procedure.[18] It is composed of a cart bearing an effector arm, a controller, and a human interface instrument (**Fig. 1**). The device is placed on the opposite side of the operating table relative to the surgeon's position (Video 1).

This device can be used as a single arm or in dual form with 2 arms to perform the robot-based gesture with 2 tools even though a collision detection algorithm between the 2 arms has not been implemented yet. Because the device is teleoperated, it relies on visual control provided to the surgeon. The surgical field can be visualized either

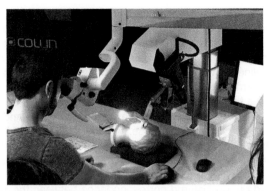

Fig. 1. The RobOtol system (2016 version) is a robot-based assistant for middle ear surgery and cochlear implantation. The current version has CE marking approval. It is composed of a cart, a human–machine interface screen, and the effector arm. It is presented here in a training session with a microscope configuration exposure. (*Courtesy of* Collin Medical, Bagneux, France)

with a surgical microscope or an endoscope (**Fig. 2**). In the microscope configuration, the surgical field is seen with binocular exposure in more than 90% of the arm positions because the arm is thin and light, and because the tools can be held far from the tip. As with any endoscope holder, the robot-based assistance offers stability of

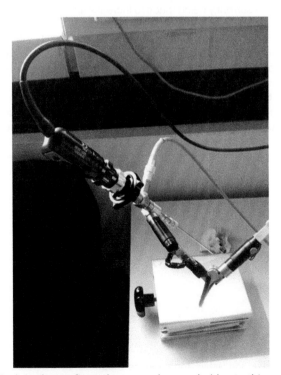

Fig. 2. The RobOtol can be configured as an endoscope holder. In this version of the arm, the motor in charge of the seventh degree of freedom, actuating tools such as microforceps or microscissors, has been removed. (*Courtesy of* Collin Medical, Bagneux, France)

surgical view, and the possibility to combine its use with a manual procedure with 2 tools, thus removing the limitation of 1-handed surgery. The RobOtol has an attachment port that can carry passive (micropick, sickle, microhook, suction, etc) and active tools (micro scissors, microforceps; **Fig. 3**). Active tools can be actuated with a motor placed collinearly with the last axis of the arm. However, this motor has to be removed if the arm is used as an endoscope holder. Two command interfaces are available to drive the device. The first is a space mouse (3D connexion, Boston, MA, **Fig. 4**, left). It can be oriented along 6 axes (3 translations and 3 rotations) and is configured in a velocity command mode. Various speeds of displacement can be selected from the human–machine interface tactile screen. The second interface is the Phantom Omni (Rock Hill, SC, see **Fig. 4**, right). With this interface, the surgeon needs to orientate the stylet from the interface and the robot follows its displacement. Command is based on a registered correspondence between the local frame of the stylet and the robot tool frame (position-to-position command mode). A downscale ratio from the command interface input to the arm can be used to ease command of the robot with greater accuracy.

The RobOtol was evaluated in multiple surgical scenarios in temporal bone specimens. Thus, robot-guided approaches and tasks could be achieved for ventilation tube placement (**Fig. 5**A) or laser sectioning of the stapedial tendon (**Fig. 5**B), crura, or stapedotomy and piston placement and crimping (Video 2). The preferred command mode depends on the surgeon's preference.[19] Neither of the 2 modes demonstrated superiority above the other for duration of the task or success at the first trial.

Initially, the specifications and design of the RobOtol focused on otosclerosis surgery, but modifications are currently being made to increase its capacity to perform other procedures, such as cochlear implantation or cerebellopontine angle tumor resection. The goal is to confer to the device a multitask role. Because most health care systems are facing economic constraints even in OECD countries, a robot-based device that has multiple applications has more chance of commercial success. The RobOtol obtained the "Conformité Européenne" marking (CE marking) in June 2016.

Another aspect that has been taken into consideration is how the RobOtol could be used for planned surgery or educational purposes. Indeed, the design of the system requires to take into consideration ergonomics and user friendliness, so as to

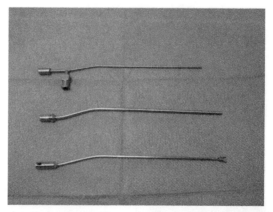

Fig. 3. Various passive and active tools can be mounted on the RobOtol system via an attachment port. Note the "bayonet" shape of the tool that allows maximal preservation of the visual field. (*Top*) Suction. (*Middle*) Smooth pointer. (*Bottom*) Microforceps. (*Courtesy of* Collin Medical, Bagneux, France)

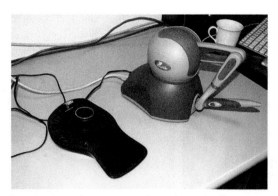

Fig. 4. The RobOtol can be driven by 2 command interfaces. (*Left*) Spacemouse, 3Dconnexion. (*Right*) Phantom Omni 3D, SensAble. (*Courtesy of* 3D Connexion, Waltham, MA; 3D Systems, Rock Hill, SC)

reduce the learning curve as much as possible. However, teaching and training with the system are still mandatory before one can consider using the robot for clinical applications. For this reason, a simulator was programmed to assist surgeons before their first hands-on surgery. A finite element virtual mechanical model of the ossicular chain (**Fig. 6**A) was built and validated for low- and high-frequency motions by analyzing its robustness by static force pressure simulations and middle ear transfer function.[20] A training simulator was designed based on this finite element model (**Fig. 6**B). It could be used to evaluate multiple arm surgery and technical modification of the otosclerosis procedure such as incus holding during piston placement to ease this complex step.[21] Combining a virtual scene based on preoperative imaging (virtual frame) and the operating field (patient frame) can allow planning of some surgical steps. Thus, if a complex but short task has to be performed (eg, stapedotomy, piston placement, or crimping), the simulator allows multiple tries to be performed in the virtual world. The surgeon then chooses his best attempt and validates the motion path that is then performed by the robot in the real world. This "immediate intraoperative planning" has been called the ghost mode for the RobOtol system (**Fig. 7**). This feature could redefine the way surgery is performed for complex tasks with intraoperative pauses to obtain good gestures systematically at the first attempt.

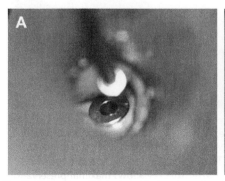
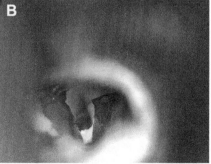

Fig. 5. Examples of robot-guided approaches for ventilation tube placement (*A*) and posterior tendon and crura laser ablation (*B*).

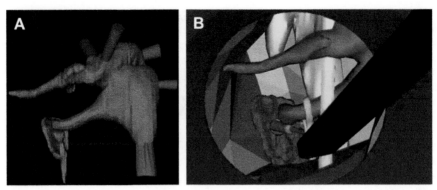

Fig. 6. (*A*) A 3-dimensional finite element ossicular chain model was built and implemented into an otosclerosis training and planning simulator. (*B*) This tool can be used to familiarize the surgeon with robot manipulation and evaluate new tools of command mode virtually before ex silico evaluation. Here, an otosclerosis piston prosthesis is placed with a microforceps on the incus.

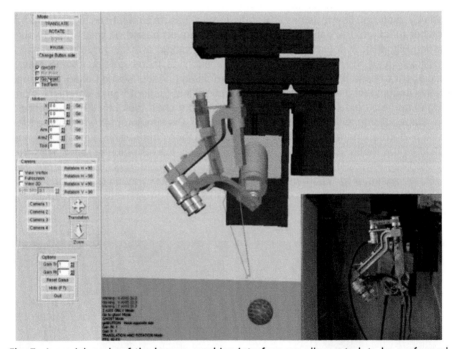

Fig. 7. A special mode of the human–machine interface can allow a task to be performed repeatedly in the virtual environment of the robot. When the surgeon is satisfied with the task performed by the robot in the virtual world, he can validate the command by pressing the "go target" button on the interface. The robot then performs in the surgical field the task that has just been done in the virtual world. This could allow an "immediate intraoperative planning" for short but difficult tasks (note here that the anatomic environment is not represented and replaced by a sphere).

Another approach that has been proposed is to use the concept of "soft robots" to develop a device that could be given distal dexterity through a flexible tool to reach recesses from the middle ear cleft.[22] Such a design offers the advantage of increasing workspace accessibility without drilling of the external auditory canal. It could, for example, guarantee access to the oval windows without the need for scutum lowering during the otosclerosis procedure and consequently reduce the risk of chorda tympani injury.

Semiautonomous Systems

The critical step in the otosclerosis procedure is footplate fenestration. The thickness and hardness of the bone are difficult to evaluate by the surgeon, even with preoperative imaging. This step is usually carried out at high magnification, and as a result, depth perception can be diminished. This shortcoming makes this task even more difficult. Improper use of mechanical tools (micropick, microhook, microdrill) can result in a floating footplate, a fracture, or even bone fragments sinking into the vestibule. Improper use of the laser can result in overheating of inner ear fluids and saccule damage, or even a facial nerve lesion in the case of laser misalignment.

To enhance the safety of this step, it has been proposed to perform cochlea opening with a robot-based device that could be controlled by a force sensor to guide the drilling. This confers 2 major benefits compared with the manual technique. First, a force sensor can be much more sensitive than the human hand, all the more so when the hand is covered with 1 or 2 pairs of gloves. Second, the delay between drill penetration into the inner ear and its shut down and withdrawal can be much shorter with a machine and can even be anticipated. Based on these considerations, the Smart Microdrill was designed and validated in a clinical application.[23] It consists of an intelligent drilling tool able to detect the passage of the drill from bone into soft tissue. The drill is placed in the vicinity of the footplate by the surgeon. The robot then automatically performs the bony fenestration while respecting the endosteum. Real-time measurement of the drill motor torque and axial force applied to the footplate with a force sensor enables the robot to stop the drill once the fenestration has been performed.

SUMMARY

Although cochlear implantation is the catalyst for robot-based innovation in hearing rehabilitation surgery, the recent growth of actors in the research robot-based surgery field and the growing interest of industrial partners might be the premise for evolution for otosclerosis rehabilitation. Robots for otosclerosis surgery are not restricted to laboratory prototypes anymore. Robot-based assistance has the promise of increased surgical accuracy and a higher quality of gesture. The technical challenge has already been answered, but before robots can be used as a matter of routine in every operating room, 2 major hurdles still remain to be reached and passed. First, the robot-based technique has to prove that it will reduce the rate of complications and/or improve surgical outcomes in clinical trials compared with the conventional technique. Second, a positive medicoeconomic balance has to be demonstrated to convince institutions to invest in these technologies. There is no doubt that the arrival of new competitors will stimulate the field and may also reduce the cost of the devices.

SUPPLEMENTARY DATA

Supplementary data related to this article can be found online at https://doi.org/10.1016/j.otc.2017.11.016.

REFERENCES

1. Caldart AU, Terruel I, Enge DJ Jr, et al. Stapes surgery in residency: the UFPR clinical hospital experience. Braz J Otorhinolaryngol 2007;73(5):647–53.
2. Lial PI, Soares VY, Viana LM, et al. Stapedotomy in a residency training program. Int Tinnitus J 2013;18(2):163–7.
3. Perkins RC. Laser stapedotomy for otosclerosis. Laryngoscope 1980;90(2): 228–40.
4. Nguyen Y, Bozorg Grayeli A, Belazzougui R, et al. Diode laser in otosclerosis surgery: first clinical results. Otol Neurotol 2008;29(4):441–6.
5. Canu G, Lauretani F, Russo FY, et al. Early functional results using the nitibond prosthesis in stapes surgery. Acta Otolaryngol 2017;137(3):259–64.
6. Nguyen Y, Mamelle E, De Seta D, et al. Modifications to a 3D-printed temporal bone model for augmented stapes fixation surgery teaching. Eur Arch Otorhinolaryngol 2017. Available at: http://link.springer.com/10.1007/s00405-017-4572-1. Accessed April 27, 2017.
7. Riviere CN, Reich SG, Thakor NV. Adaptive Fourier modeling for quantification of tremor. J Neurosci Methods 1997;74(1):77–87.
8. Taylor R, Jensen P, Whitcomb L, et al. A steady-hand robotic system for microsurgical augmentation. Int J Robot Res 1999;18(12):1201–10.
9. Mitchell B, Koo J, Iordachita I, et al. Development and application of a new steady-hand manipulator for retinal surgery. In Proceedings 2007 IEEE International Conference on Robotics and Automation. Roma, Italy, April 10–14, 2007. p. 623–9. Available at: http://ieeexplore.ieee.org/document/4209160/. Accessed February 7, 2018.
10. Wilkening P, Chien W, Gonenc B, et al. Evaluation of virtual fixtures for robot-assisted cochlear implant insertion. In 5th IEEE RAS/EMBS International Conference on Biomedical Robotics and Biomechatronics. Sao Paulo, Brazil, August 12–15, 2014. p. 332–8. Available at: http://ieeexplore.ieee.org/document/6913798/. Accessed February 7, 2018.
11. Berkelman PJ, Rothbaum DL, Roy J, et al. Performance evaluation of a cooperative manipulation microsurgical assistant robot applied to stapedotomy. In: Niessen WJ, Viergever MA, editors. Medical image computing and computer-assisted intervention – MICCAI 2001. MICCAI 2001. Lecture notes in computer sciencevol. 2208. Berlin: Springer; 2001. p. 1426–9.
12. Rothbaum DL, Roy J, Hager GD, et al. Task performance in stapedotomy: comparison between surgeons of different experience levels. Otolaryngol Head Neck Surg 2003;128(1):71–7.
13. Vendrametto T, McAfee JS, Hirsch BE, et al. Robot assisted stapedotomy ex vivo with an active handheld instrument. Conf Proc IEEE Eng Med Biol Soc 2015;2015: 4879–82.
14. Montes Grande G, Knisely AJ, Becker BC, et al. Handheld micromanipulator for robot-assisted stapes footplate surgery. In 2012 Annual International Conference of the IEEE Engineering in Medicine and Biology Society. San Diego, CA, August 28, 2012–Sept 1, 2012. p. 1422–5. Available at: http://ieeexplore.ieee.org/document/6346206/. Accessed February 7, 2018.
15. Entsfellner K, Schuermann J, Coy JA, et al. A modular micro-macro robot system for instrument guiding in middle ear surgery. In 2015 IEEE International Conference on Robotics and Biomimetics (ROBIO). Dec 6–9, 2015. p. 374–9. Available at: http://ieeexplore.ieee.org/document/7418796/. Accessed February 7, 2018.

16. Maier T, Strauss G, Scholz M, et al. A new evaluation and training system for micro-telemanipulation at the middle ear. In 2012 Annual International Conference of the IEEE Engineering in Medicine and Biology Society. San Diego, CA, August 28, 2012–Sept 1, 2012. p. 932–5. Available at: http://ieeexplore.ieee.org/document/6346085/.
17. Maier T, Strauss G, Bauer F, et al. Distance measurement in middle ear surgery using a telemanipulator. Med Image Comput Comput Assist Interv 2011;14(Pt 1):41–8.
18. Miroir M, Szewczyk J, Nguyen Y, et al. Design of a robotic system for minimally invasive surgery of the middle ear. In 2008 2nd IEEE RAS & EMBS International Conference on Biomedical Robotics and Biomechatronics. Scottsdale, AZ, October 19–22, 2008. p. 747–52. Available at: http://ieeexplore.ieee.org/document/4762795/. Accessed February 7, 2018.
19. Kazmitcheff G, Miroir M, Nguyen Y, et al. Evaluation of command modes of an assistance robot for middle ear surgery. In 2011 IEEE/RSJ International Conference on Intelligent Robots and Systems. San Francisco, CA, September 25–30, 2011. p. 2532–8. Available at: http://ieeexplore.ieee.org/document/6094634/. Accessed February 7, 2018.
20. Kazmitcheff G, Miroir M, Nguyen Y, et al. Validation method of a middle ear mechanical model to develop a surgical simulator. Audiol Neurootol 2014;19(2):73–84.
21. Kazmitcheff G, Duriez C, Miroir M, et al. Registration of a validated mechanical atlas of middle ear for surgical simulation. Med Image Comput Comput Assist Interv 2013;16(Pt 3):331–8.
22. Yasin R, O'Connell BP, Yu H, et al. Steerable robot-assisted micromanipulation in the middle ear: preliminary feasibility evaluation. Otol Neurotol 2017;38(2):290–5.
23. Coulson CJ, Assadi MZ, Taylor RP, et al. A smart micro-drill for cochleostomy formation: a comparison of cochlear disturbances with manual drilling and a human trial. Cochlear Implants Int 2013;14(2):98–106.

Controversies in the Evaluation and Management of Otosclerosis

John T. McElveen Jr, MD[a],*, J. Walter Kutz Jr, MD[b]

KEYWORDS

- Otosclerosis • Stapedectomy • Stapedotomy • Bisphosphonates • Lasers
- Implantable hearing devices • Middle ear actuators • Barotrauma

KEY POINTS

- Although genetic loci have been identified and the measles virus implicated in the development of otosclerosis, the exact mechanism of the bone remodeling associated with otosclerosis remains uncertain.
- Systemic treatments to prevent the progression of cochlear otosclerosis have been limited; however, new-generation bisphosphonates may be more effective, but not without risks.
- Proper preoperative evaluation minimizes the likelihood of stapes surgery on patients with a dehiscent superior semicircular canal or concomitant Meniere's disease.
- Although stapedotomy in children with juvenile-onset otosclerosis is effective, it is not without risk. Consequently, in children with unilateral disease, delaying surgery until adulthood may be preferred.
- Innovations in technology, such as middle ear actuators, may provide patients with far-advanced otosclerosis an alternative to traditional stapedotomy or cochlear implantation.

HISTORICAL PERSPECTIVE

Dating back to the times of Kessel[1] and Politzer,[2] controversies have surrounded the etiology and management of the entity that Politzer[2] first termed, *otosclerosis*. What was originally believed to be a condition attributed to "chronic interstitial middle ear catarrh" with secondary stapes fixation was discovered by Politzer[2] to be a primary disease of the labyrinthine capsule, which he referred to as "otosclerosis." Despite his publication of histologic evidence of otosclerosis in 16 cases of stapes fixation, it took almost half a century for Politzer's views to gain universal acceptance. Even today, controversy still surrounds the precise etiology of otosclerosis. Based on

Disclosure Statement: The authors have nothing to disclose.

[a] Carolina Ear & Hearing Clinic, PC, Carolina Ear Research Institute, 5900 Six Forks Road, Suite #200, Raleigh, NC 27609, USA; [b] Department of Otolaryngology, University of Texas Southwestern Medical Center, 5323 Harry Hines Boulevard, Dallas, TX 75390-9035, USA
* Corresponding author.
E-mail address: mcelveencehc@aol.com

Otolaryngol Clin N Am 51 (2018) 487–499
https://doi.org/10.1016/j.otc.2017.11.017
0030-6665/18/© 2017 Elsevier Inc. All rights reserved.

Fowler's[3] study in identical twins showing almost a 100% concordance rate of otosclerosis and the more recent identification of 10 genetic loci (OTSC1–10) associated with otosclerosis, most investigators concur that otosclerosis is an inherited disease that is transmitted in an autosomal dominant pattern with an incomplete penetrance rate of 20% to 40%.[3–5] The exact cause of the abnormal bone remodeling that produces the otosclerotic foci remains uncertain; however, ultrastructural and immunohistochemical evidence of measles-like structures and antigenicity in active otosclerotic lesions published by McKenna and colleagues[6,7] has implicated the measles virus in the formation of the otosclerotic foci. In addition, measles ribonucleic acid has been demonstrated in fresh footplate specimens as well as archival ones. This hypothesis may be further strengthened by the decline in otosclerosis after introduction of the measles vaccination.[8] Research is ongoing to clarify the role of the measles virus in the development of otosclerosis.

The controversies surrounding the etiology of otosclerosis pale in comparison to the controversies that have been associated with its management. Kessel,[1] who is considered the "Father of Stapes Surgery," was under the mistaken opinion that the hearing loss associated with otosclerosis was caused by increased pressure in the inner ear fluids. He theorized that by removing the stapes, he could relieve that pressure. Prior to testing his hypothesis in humans, he removed the columella, which is the stapes equivalent, in 2 pigeons. As he described it, clear fluid drained from their ears for 8 days until a membrane formed to seal the oval window. According to Kessel,[1] the pigeons did not experience any vertigo or hearing loss. Based on these "pre-clinical animal observations," he performed stapes mobilizations and stapes removal in humans. He reported "some improvement in hearing and no serious complications."[1] Obviously, his perceptions were not consistent with the perceptions of other clinicians. In many cases, the hearing improvement lasted only for a period of days to weeks, and there was always the risk of labyrinthitis and rarely meningitis. Consequently, stapes surgery fell into disrepute and was vehemently criticized by the leading otologists, Politzer, Siebenmann, and Moure, who in 1899 at the Sixth International Congress of Otology declared, "Stapes surgery is useless, often mutilating, and dangerous." They went on to say, "The question of surgical therapy for otosclerosis was interred with great pomp at the 1894 International Conference in Rome. There is no reason to revive it."[9,10]

Fortunately, more than 50 years later, Dr John Shea[11] revived stapes surgery. But even this revival was not without controversy. It was only with the assistance of Dr Howard P. House,[12] that Dr Shea was able to present his stapedectomy technique before the Triological Society in Montreal, Canada. At 11:00 AM on Thursday, May 17, 1956, Dr House was scheduled to moderate the panel, "Symposium - The Operation for the Mobilization of the Stapes in Otosclerotic Deafness." Just before the panel was to begin, Dr Shea told Dr House about his first patient who had successfully undergone a stapedectomy. Knowing that something like this would be extremely controversial, Dr House told Dr Shea that he would call on him as the last discussant from the audience. Dr Shea took the opportunity to approach the podium and present his stapedectomy experience to the membership of the Triological Society. Before Dr Shea could be unduly criticized by the audience, Dr House explained that unfortunately the time for the symposium had expired and brought down his gavel, ending the session.[12]

CURRENT CONTROVERSIES
Evaluation

With this historical perspective as a backdrop, the current controversies as they relate to the evaluation and management of otosclerosis are reviewed.

Patients undergoing stapedotomy are some of the most grateful otologic patients. The hearing results are, by and large, superior to those of other ossiculoplasty procedures, and complications are uncommon. Selecting the appropriate patients and the evaluation of those patients preoperatively, however, remain matters of controversy.

Few clinicians would argue the patient whose audiogram is represented in **Fig. 1** is a suitable candidate for stapedotomy. If this patient were a child, however, would he or she still be a suitable candidate for stapedotomy? One of the earliest articles advocating stapes surgery in children was written by House and colleagues[13] in 1980, reporting results of stapedectomy in 14 children with juvenile-onset otosclerosis. They recommended deferring any surgical treatment until a child was 5 years old, and then only if the child suffered from binaural disease and was not having problems with serous or recurrent otitis media. They also emphasized that the hearing loss should be greater than or equal to 35 dB. Otherwise, they recommended deferring surgical treatment. Currently, operating on children at a relatively young age for juvenile-onset otosclerosis remains controversial. First, the decision is made by the child's parents and, although the risks of complications are small, the consequences are not insubstantial. In a meta-analysis by Asik and colleagues[14] of children treated for juvenile otosclerosis, 80.2% of the children closed their air-bone gap to within 10 dB postoperatively, but 8 of the 229 (3.5%) children suffered sensorineural hearing loss (SNHL). Of the 8 children suffering a SNHL after surgery, 4 children suffered a profound hearing loss in the operated ear. This compares to a less than 1% SNHL in adult stapes surgery.[15] Regardless of whether or not the surgeon is an advocate for operating on patients with juvenile-onset otosclerosis, it is imperative that the parents and child be counseled regarding the slightly increased risk reported in the Asik and colleagues[14] meta-analysis.

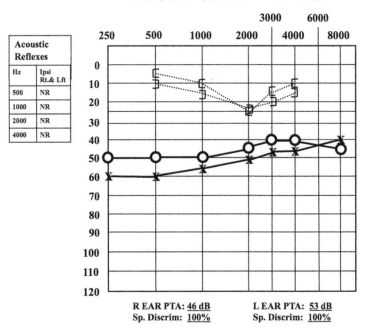

Fig. 1. Audiogram of a child with bilateral juvenile-onset otosclerosis.

Some European surgeons routinely obtain preoperative CT scans on both pediatric and adult patients with suspected otosclerosis, citing their ability to identify inner ear abnormalities and predict surgical outcomes and surgical risks based on the extent and location of the disease. In a study by Marx and colleagues,[16] the preoperative high-resolution CT scan findings in 200 patients correlated with surgical outcomes. The investigators found that overclosure of the bone line greater than 10 dB occurred in 20% of patients with isolated fenestral otosclerosis compared with 2.85% in patients with extensive otosclerosis.

Some counter that even though the surgical results may not be as good in patients with multifocal otosclerotic foci, these findings would not deter a surgeon from operating on a particular patient. In addition, the incidence of inner ear abnormalities, such as an enlarged vestibular aqueduct in conjunction with otosclerosis in adults, is rare.[17] Furthermore, patients with stapes gushers may have completely normal-appearing CT scans.[18] Lastly, the radiation exposure and costs associated with routine preoperative CT scans in the otosclerotic patient must be taken into consideration. In a systematic clinical review of Australians having undergone CT scans, there was a proportional increase in risk of all cancers by 9.38 per 100,000 person years with all CT in patients 0 to 19 years of age.[19] When specifically focused on CT scans of the brain and temporal bone, the current best evidence suggests brain malignancy arises in 1 per 4000 brain CT scans whereas the risk of thyroid cancer is 4 to 8 per 1,000,000 with temporal bone CT scans.[20,21] Although the risk of CT-related malignancy remains extremely low, it does exist.

The cost of a CT scan in Europe is relatively inexpensive; however, CT scans of the temporal bone in the United States have an average cost of $1250.[22] All these factors need to be taken into consideration when considering preoperative imaging.

Although there may be controversy with respect to preoperative imaging as it relates to patients with otosclerosis, it is universally accepted that all patients with otosclerosis should have a preoperative auditory assessment that includes tuning fork testing and diagnostic audiometry with speech discrimination and acoustic reflex testing. Acoustic reflex testing minimizes the likelihood of performing stapes surgery on patients whose conductive hearing loss is due to a dehiscence of the superior semicircular canal and not stapes fixation (**Fig. 2**). Most patients with otosclerosis have a classic conductive hearing loss in the low frequencies with a Carhart notch (decrease

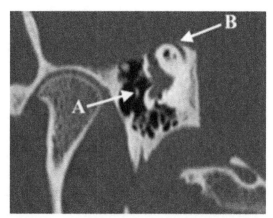

Fig. 2. Patient with (*A*) stapes prosthesis and (*B*) superior semicircular canal dehiscence. (*Courtesy of* Michael J. McKenna, MD, Massachusetts Eye and Ear, Boston, MA.)

in the bone line at approximately 2000 Hz); however, some patients may have a history of fluctuating hearing loss and vertigo in conjunction with otosclerosis. Is there a role for stapedotomy in patients with fluctuating hearing loss? In a series of 490 consecutive patients with otosclerosis, McCabe[23] diagnosed endolymphatic hydrops in 21(4%) patients. He recommended delaying surgery until the patient was asymptomatic of hydrops for "6 months or longer." In a subsequent study by Issa and colleagues,[24] they contended that having a disease-free interval did not result in the saccule "dropping away from the footplate." Based on a study of 8 temporal bones, 7 with Meniere's disease and 1 with Meniere's disease and otosclerosis, they believed that stapedectomy does not increase the risk of SNHL for patients with otosclerosis and Meniere's disease who have bone conduction levels of 35 dB or better at 500 Hz and no high-frequency hearing loss. Despite these findings, most surgeons would be hesitant to perform a stapedotomy on a patient with a history of concomitant Meniere's disease for fear they may place the prosthesis through a dilated saccule (**Fig. 3**).

Management

Intraoperative management
The universally accepted surgical treatment of stapedial otosclerosis with serviceable hearing is stapedotomy. There remain controversies, however, regarding the surgical approach and technique involved in performing the procedure. Some surgeons prefer straight local anesthesia or local anesthesia with sedation to assess the hearing and vestibular response intraoperatively, whereas other surgeons, particularly at teaching institutions, prefer a general anesthetic, citing patient comfort, lack of time constraints, and resident involvement. In 2008, Vital and colleagues[25] compared the incidence of a profound hearing loss between 160 operations under general anesthesia and 108 operations under local anesthesia and found a higher incidence of profound hearing loss in the general group (1.8%) compared with the local group (0%). In a more recent systematic review comparing local versus general anesthesia in 417 procedures, however, the investigators concluded that there was no statistical difference in the postoperative air-bone gap, worsening of SNHL, or postoperative vertigo.[26]

Although either method of anesthesia may be equally acceptable with primary stapes surgery, local anesthesia or local anesthesia with sedation has a distinct

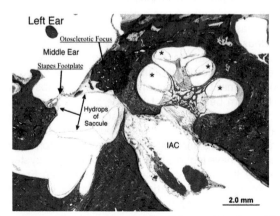

Fig. 3. Histologic section of left ear in a patient with otosclerosis and hydrops. Note the location of the saccule relative to the stapes footplate. The asterisks are scala media with hydrops. (*Courtesy of* Michael J. McKenna, MD, Massachusetts Eye and Ear, Boston, MA.)

advantage with revision stapes surgery. Should a patient experience vertigo while the surgeon is manipulating or removing the previously placed prosthesis, this may be indicative of adhesions between the prosthesis and the underlying saccule. Without a patient's feedback, the surgeon may continue to manipulate or remove the prosthesis, putting the patient's hearing at risk.

The surgical approach for stapes surgery has evolved over the years. Some surgeons prefer the classic transcanal approach, whereas others advocate the use of an endaural approach to improve exposure. More recently, the endoscopic approach has been used to perform a variety of middle ear procedures, including stapedotomy. The endoscopic advocates cite improved visualization and clarity, less need for curetting the scutum, and decreased chorda tympani manipulation.[27,28] The proponents of the traditional endaural and transcanal approaches point out the limitations of the endoscopic approach, which include lack of depth perception, potential for chorda tympani thermal injury, difficulty using the microdrill, and having to place the prosthesis with 1 hand. Despite these concerns, the audiologic results are comparable according to recent reports.[27,28]

Whereas Shea[11] originally removed the entire footplate, a more limited removal of the footplate is currently preferred by most surgeons performing stapes surgery. In some cases of isolated anterior footplate fixation, the laser stapedotomy minus prosthesis (STAMP) technique has been used.[29] In this technique, the anterior crus is separated from the footplate using a laser and the footplate divided in its midportion. This allows free movement of the posterior portion of the stapes despite anterior footplate fixation. Although in 1 study the laser STAMP technique resulted in better high-frequency responses compared with small fenestra stapedotomy, it was associated with a higher rate of refixation, requiring revision surgery. In addition, this technique can only be used in select cases of otosclerosis with limited anterior fixation and favorable anatomy.[30]

The small fenestra stapedotomy is the most frequently used approach. In a study by Fisch[31] comparing stapedectomy and stapedotomy, he concluded that stapedotomy is the procedure of choice because it achieved better hearing results than stapedectomy and was less traumatic to the inner ear. Despite the universal acceptance of the stapedotomy technique, there are variations of opinion on how best to create the fenestra and what size of fenestra to create. To create the fenestra, some surgeons advocate the use of the diamond microdrill; others prefer the laser, citing its lack of mechanical trauma; whereas others use a combination of laser and microdrill.

A variety of lasers has been used in stapes surgery. These include argon, Er-YAG, potassium-titanyl-phosphate (KTP), 532-nm diode, and CO_2 laser systems. In a study looking at the attenuation in seawater as a function of laser wavelength, the argon and KTP lasers traveled 229 ft before half of the energy was absorbed. The Er-YAG laser energy traveled 0.0007 mm before half of the energy was absorbed. The CO_2 laser beam traveled 0.007 mm before half of the energy was absorbed.[32] Advocates of the CO_2 lasers point out the increased energy absorption by the perilymph resulting in decrease penetration of energy into the vestibule. The CO_2 laser beam, however, is not visible to the human eye and originally required a micromanipulator. Advances in fiber-optic technology have led to a fiber-optic CO_2 delivery system with a separate aiming beam. Despite the theoretic advantages of using an Er-YAG or CO_2 laser, based on their beams' maximal absorption by perilymph, a recent article by Kamalski and colleagues[33] showed no difference in hearing outcomes or complications when comparing KTP, Er-YAG, and CO_2 lasers.

Regardless of which technique is used to create the fenestra, there remains debate regarding the optimal diameter of the fenestra, method of sealing the fenestra, type of prosthesis used, and technique to determine the appropriate prosthesis length. Temporal bone studies by Wegner and colleagues[34] demonstrated that the use of 0.6-mm and 0.8-mm diameter pistons resulted in better hearing outcomes compared with smaller diameter pistons. In the temporal bone study, the 0.6-mm piston predicted an air-bone gap of 8-dB to 12-dB and the 0.4-mm piston predicted an air bone gap of 15 dB to 20 dB.[35] Sennaroglu and colleagues[36] advocates a 0.8-mm diameter prosthesis over a 0.6-mm citing better hearing outcomes. Despite these results, clinical studies by Fisch[31] looking at long-term hearing results comparing the 0.4-mm and 0.6-mm pistons demonstrated parity on long-term follow-up. Fisch also commented on the relative ease of use with the smaller diameter piston, particularly as it related to the modified stapedotomy technique used by Fisch (the fenestra is created and the piston is placed prior to removing the suprastructure).

Once the fenestra has been created, the surgeon must make the determination on whether or not to seal the fenestra. Some surgeons advocate covering the fenestra with a connective tissue graft or vein graft prior to prosthesis placement to prevent the loss of perilymphatic fluids. Others clinicians advocate placing connective tissue around the piston after placement in the fenestra. Others do not place any soft tissue around the fenestra, instead allowing blood to pool around the piston at the fenestra. Although theoretically limiting perilymph loss with placement of a tissue seal should be attempted, there is no available evidence that demonstrates an increased incidence of SNHL or perilymph fistula without placement of a tissue seal.

A plethora of stapes prostheses are currently available, with some requiring manual crimping, some that crimp with heat activation, and others that require no crimping. Regardless of which prosthesis is selected, it is important that there is minimal pressure exerted on the long process of the incus and that the connection to the incus is firm to prevent vibration. To date, there is not 1 type of prosthesis that has been shown clearly superior to the others, and selection of the prosthesis is primarily surgeon dependent.

In addition to the debate regarding the optimal diameter of the piston, the method of determining prosthesis length may vary. Some surgeons measure from the top of the long process of the incus and subtract 0.25 mm from their measurement whereas others measure from the undersurface of the incus and add 0.25 mm to their measurement. Other surgeons do not measure at all and use a standard-length prosthesis for all procedures. Optimally, the measurement should result in the selection of a prosthesis that extends into the vestibular 0.25 mm to 0.5 mm.[37] This allows sufficient distance between the piston and the underlying saccule. Failure to measure may result in a prosthesis that extends too deeply into the vestibule, resulting in vertigo and hearing loss (**Fig. 4**).

Postoperative management

Just as there are variations in surgical technique with respect to stapes surgery, there are also variations in postoperative management. Once considered an inpatient-type procedure, stapedotomy in the United States has evolved into an outpatient, or 23 hr stay, procedure. Outside the United States, many centers believe it is important to hospitalize their patients after surgery. Although stapes surgery is considered clean otologic surgery, and the Cochrane report did not find any evidence supporting perioperative antibiotic therapy,[38] most centers continue to treat their patients with prophylactic antibiotics because the risks associated with poststapedotomy infection include deafness and labyrinthitis.[39] In addition, intraoperative and postoperative corticosteroids may be used to minimize the chance of serous labyrinthitis. Clinical studies supporting this are lacking, however. In a study from Germany, the use of

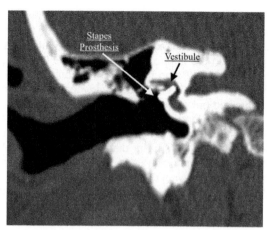

Fig. 4. CT scan demonstrating stapes prosthesis extending deeply into the vestibule.

steroids seemed to exacerbate the vestibular symptoms and had no effect on the change in bone conduction.[40]

Diving and flying after stapes surgery

Barotrauma in a patient who has undergone stapes surgery may result in sudden hearing loss or vertigo. If vertigo occurs while scuba diving or flying an aircraft, the situation may become life threatening. Because of these concerns, patients who had undergone a stapedectomy procedure were initially not allowed to scuba dive, skydive, or resume duties as a pilot. Harrill and colleagues[41] sent a questionnaire regarding postoperative barorestrictions after stapes surgery to members of the American Otological Society and the American Neurotology Society and found that 54.3% of surgeons who performed a stapedectomy or stapedotomy recommended a permanent restriction from scuba diving. In a comment after the Harrill article, Dr Joseph Farmer Jr, MD, FACS,[41] past President of the Undersea and Hyperbaric Medical Society, recommended against scuba diving after stapes surgery. Thiringer and Arriaga[42] reported on 16 US Air Force aircrew who had undergone a stapedotomy and allowed to return to flight duty after undergoing otologic testing to assess fitness to return to duty. All prostheses were variations of piston-type prosthesis, and the oval window seal was recorded in 4 patients and included vein, fascia, fat, and Gelfoam. None of the 26 aircrew experienced any symptoms while flying related to their stapedotomy procedure. Katzav and colleagues[43] reported 9 stapedotomy procedures in 6 high-performance airplane pilots in the Israeli Air Force who returned to flight duty as soon as 3 months after surgery without any vestibular symptoms. All the patients had a vein graft placed in conjunction with a bucket-handle prosthesis. House and colleagues[44] identified 22 patients who returned to scuba diving after undergoing a stapedectomy; 4 of the 22 patients had symptoms of otalgia (3), tinnitus (1), and transient vertigo on decent (1). Another patient developed sudden SNHL and vertigo 3 months after scuba diving. His ear was explored and a perilymph fistula was identified and successfully repaired. The perilymph fistula was not believed related to scuba diving because of the interval between diving and the onset of symptoms. This patient continued to dive without problems after the perilymph fistula repair. The investigators concluded that there is not an increased risk of barotrauma in scuba diving after stapedectomy if adequate eustachian tube function is present. Despite these reports condoning scuba diving and high-performance flying after stapes surgery, it is important for surgeons to address the potential risks of baro-trauma with any patient undergoing stapes surgery. In addition, sealing the oval win-dow with a tissue graft may provide an extra measure of safety in those patients at high risk of barotrauma.

Alternative management options

Patients suffering from long-term otosclerosis may develop far-advanced otosclerosis with air conduction thresholds greater than or equal to 85 dB and nonmeasurable bone conduction thresholds (because of the technical limitations of the audiometer). As originally advocated by House and Sheehy,[45] the traditional recommendation for these patients who were unable to benefit from hearing aids was stapes surgery. This approach is still recommended as a first line of treatment. With the development of implantable hearing devices, however, such as the direct acoustic cochlear implant (DACI) (Codacs, Cochlear Corporation, Ltd, Sydney, Australia), is this still the best initial treatment of these patients with far-advanced otosclerosis? The DACI is a fixed middle ear actuator system in which a stapedotomy is performed and the prosthesis is connected to an actuator that is anchored to the cortical skull (**Fig. 5**). Although the DACI system is not currently available in the United States, it is being implanted in Europe. In a study published by Lenarz and colleagues,[46] the sound field thresholds improved by an average of 48 dB, and the word recognition scores improved by 30% to 78%. In a comparative study, 25 DACI systems were compared with

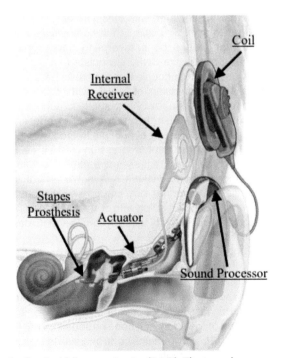

Fig. 5. Diagram of a fixed middle ear actuator (DACI). The sound processor converts acoustic energy into a digital signal that is transmitted through the skin to the internal receiver. The internal receiver converts the digital code into an analog signal. The actuator then converts the analog signal into mechanical vibrations of an artificial incus. The stapes prosthesis, which is attached to the artificial incus, transmits the vibrations to the inner ear. (*Courtesy of* Peter C. Weber, MD, Boston, MA.)

54 cochlear implants with comparable preoperative bone conduction thresholds. Speech in noise results in patients with the DACI system were 80% compared with 25% in patients who underwent a cochlear implant.[47]

In the United States, implantation of the DACI is currently not an option. Consequently, for those patients with far-advanced otosclerosis who no longer benefit from hearing aids, surgeons must decide between doing a stapedotomy or going directly to cochlear implantation. This decision is made even more difficult because a patient's preoperative speech discrimination scores may be underestimated. In Shea and colleagues'[48] far-advanced otosclerosis study, speech discrimination improved by 15%, and in the Lippy and colleagues[49] study, patients' speech discrimination continued to improve to reach an additional 32.7% after 2 years. In light of these data, most otologists currently recommend initially attempting a stapedotomy because it may be effective and considerably cheaper than cochlear implantation. In addition, based on studies by Calmels and colleagues[50] and Kabbara and colleagues,[51] a prior stapedotomy did not interfere with subsequent cochlear implantation outcomes. In Calmels and colleagues' study, the 4 patients who underwent prior stapedotomy had postoperative speech discrimination scores ranging from 70% to 95%, with a mean of 80%.[50]

Optimally, if the progression of the sensorineural component of the otosclerotic process could be limited with a pharmaceutical agent, there would be no need for cochlear amplifiers (DACIs) or cochlear implants. Histopathologic studies, demonstrating the involvement of the endosteal layer of the otic capsule, suggest that the SNHL (cochlear otosclerosis) associated with otosclerosis is the result of connective tissue deposition, referred to as hyalinization, in the spiral ligament.[52,53] A variety of pharmaceutical agents that reduce bone resorption have been prescribed as a possible treatment of the progressive SNHL associated with otosclerosis. Sodium fluoride has been widely used to treat cochlear otosclerosis based on studies showing a modest reduction in the progression of SNHL with minimal side effects.[54–56] Currently, however, third-generation bisphosphonates, such as risedronate and zoledronate, are available that demonstrate much more powerful antiresorptive properties. In a limited retrospective pilot study of patients treated with the third-generation bisphosphonates, there was no significant progression of SNHL (ie, stabilization) at an average follow-up of 13 months. Despite these encouraging results, the risks associated with systemic bisphosphonates include headache, arthralgia, renal damage, hypocalcemia, atrial fibrillation, osteonecrosis of the jaw, atypical femoral fractures, erosive esophagitis, ulceration, and bleeding with oral administration.[57] Consequently, controversy still surrounds the selection of these systemic agents based on their effectiveness and potential risks.

SUMMARY

Controversies have been associated with otosclerosis since the times of Kessel and Politzer. Although the hearing loss is no longer attributed to chronic interstitial middle ear catarrh, the exact cause of the abnormal bone remodeling that Politzer described as "dystrophy of the temporal bone" remains controversial. In addition, although stapedotomy has been universally accepted as the surgical treatment of most patients with stapedial otosclerosis, there remains a disparity of opinion regarding the role of preoperative imaging, the surgical technique used, and the implant selected. Although most agree that the controversies associated with otosclerosis delayed the development of its surgical treatment, few would argue with the ultimate outcome.

REFERENCES

1. Kessel. Über das Mobilisieren des Steigbugles durch Ausschneiden des Trommelfells, Hammers und Ambosses bei Undurchgängigkeit der Tuba. Arch Ohrenheil 1878;13:69–88.
2. Politzer A. Ueber primäre Erkrankung der knöchernen Labyrinthkapsel. Zeitschr Ohrenheil 1893;25:309–27.
3. Fowler EP. Otosclerosis in identical twins. A study of 40 pairs. Arch Otolaryngol 1960;83:324–8.
4. Morrison AW. Genetic factors in otosclerosis. Ann R Coll Surgeons Engl 1967;41: 202–37.
5. Bittermann AJ, Wegner I, Noordman BJ, et al. An introduction of genetics in otosclerosis: a systematic review. Otolaryngol Head Neck Surg 2014;150:34–9.
6. McKenna MJ, Mills BG. Immunohistochemical evidence of measles virus antigens in active otosclerosis. Otolaryngol Head Neck Surg 1989;101:415–21.
7. McKenna MJ, Kristiansen AG, Haines J. Polymerase chain reaction amplification of a measles virus sequence from human temporal bone sections with active otosclerosis. Am J Otol 1996;17:827–30.
8. Arnold W, Busch R, Arnold A, et al. The influence of measles vaccination on the incidence of otosclerosis in Germany. Eur Arch Otorhinolaryngol 2007;264:741–8.
9. Siebenmann F. Sur le traitement chirurgical de la sclerose otique. Congr Inter Med Sec Otol 1900;13:170.
10. Politzer A. Geschichte der otosclerose. Geschichte der Ohrenheilkunde, vol. 2. Stuttgart, Germany: Enke Verlag; 1913. p. 171–5.
11. Shea JJ Jr. Fenestration of the oval window. Ann Otol Rhinol Laryngol 1958;67: 932–51.
12. House HP. Symposium - The operation for the mobilization of the stapes in otosclerotic deafness. Paper presented at: The American Laryngological, Rhinological and Otological Society. Montreal, Canada, May 17, 1956.
13. House JW, Sheehy JL, Antunez JC. Stapedectomy in children. Laryngoscope 1980;90(11 Pt 1):1804–9.
14. Asik B, Binar M, Serdar M, et al. A meta-analysis of surgical success rates in congenital stapes fixation and juvenile otosclerosis. The Laryngoscope 2016; 126:191–8.
15. Vincent R, Sperling NM, Oates J, et al. Surgical findings and long-term hearing results in 3,050 stapedotomies for primary otosclerosis: a prospective study with the otology-neurotology database. Otol Neurotol 2006;27(8 Suppl 2):S25–47.
16. Marx M, Lagleyre S, Escude B, et al. Correlations between CT scan findings and hearing thresholds in otosclerosis. Acta Otolaryngol 2011;131:351–7.
17. Wieczorek SS, Anderson ME Jr, Harris DA, et al. Enlarged vestibular aqueduct syndrome mimicking otosclerosis in adults. Am J Otolaryngol 2013;34:619–25.
18. Krouchi L, Callonnec F, Bouchetemble P, et al. Preoperative computed tomography scan may fail to predict perilymphatic gusher. Ann Otol Rhinol Laryngol 2013; 122:374–7.
19. Mathews JD, Forsythe AV, Brady Z, et al. Cancer risk in 680,000 people exposed to computed tomography scans in childhood or adolescence: data linkage study of 11 million Australians. BMJ 2013;346:f2360.
20. Mazonakis M, Tzedakis A, Damilakis J, et al. Thyroid dose from common head and neck CT examinations in children: is there an excess risk for thyroid cancer induction? Eur Radiol 2007;17:1352–7.

21. Pearce MS, Salotti JA, Little MP, et al. Radiation exposure from CT scans in childhood and subsequent risk of leukaemia and brain tumours: a retrospective cohort study. Lancet 2012;380:499–505.

22. CT Ear Cost and Procedure Information. Available at: https://www.newchoicehealth.com/procedures/ct-ear. Accessed March 7, 2017.

23. McCabe BF. Otosclerosis and vertigo. Trans Pac Coast Otoophthalmol Soc Annu Meet 1966;47:37–42.

24. Issa TK, Bahgat MA, Linthicum FH Jr, et al. The effect of stapedectomy on hearing of patients with otosclerosis and Meniere's disease. Am J Otol 1983;4:323–6.

25. Vital V, Konstantinidis I, Vital I, et al. Minimizing the dead ear in otosclerosis surgery. Auris Nasus Larynx 2008;35:475–9.

26. Wegner I, Bittermann AJ, Zinsmeester MM, et al. Local versus general anesthesia in stapes surgery for otosclerosis: a systematic review of the evidence. Otolaryngol Head Neck Surg 2013;149:360–5.

27. Hunter JB, Rivas A. Outcomes following endoscopic stapes surgery. Otolaryngol Clin North Am 2016;49:1215–25.

28. Hunter JB, Zuniga MG, Leite J, et al. Surgical and audiologic outcomes in endoscopic stapes surgery across 4 institutions. Otolaryngol Head Neck Surg 2016; 154:1093–8.

29. Silverstein H. Laser stapedotomy minus prosthesis (laser STAMP): a minimally invasive procedure. Am J Otol 1998;19:277–82.

30. Acar GO, Kivekas I, Hanna BM, et al. Comparison of stapedotomy minus prosthesis, circumferential stapes mobilization, and small fenestra stapedotomy for stapes fixation. Otol Neurotol 2014;35:e123–9.

31. Fisch U. Stapedotomy versus stapedectomy. Am J Otol 1982;4(2):112–7.

32. Lesinksi G. Lasers in otology. In: Guyla AJ, ML, Poe D, editors. Glasscock-Shambaugh's Surgery of the Ear. 6th edition. Shelton (CT): People's Medical Publishing House; 2010. p. 331–48.

33. Kamalski DM, Wegner I, Tange RA, et al. Outcomes of different laser types in laser-assisted stapedotomy: a systematic review. Otol Neurotol 2014;35:1046–51.

34. Wegner I, Eldaebes MM, Landry TG, et al. The effect of piston diameter in stapedotomy for otosclerosis: a temporal bone model. Otol Neurotol 2016;37: 1497–502.

35. Rosowski JJ, Merchant SN. Mechanical and acoustic analysis of middle ear reconstruction. Am J Otol 1995;16:486–97.

36. Sennaroglu L, Unal OF, Sennaroglu G, et al. Effect of teflon piston diameter on hearing result after stapedotomy. Otolaryngol Head Neck Surg 2001;124:279–81.

37. Pauw BK, Pollak AM, Fisch U. Utricle, saccule, and cochlear duct in relation to stapedotomy. A histologic human temporal bone study. Ann Otol Rhinol Laryngol 1991;100:966–70.

38. Verschuur HP, de Wever WW, van Benthem PP. Antibiotic prophylaxis in clean and clean-contaminated ear surgery. Cochrane Database Syst Rev 2004;(3):CD003996.

39. Ottoline AC, Tomita S, Marques Mda P, et al. Antibiotic prophylaxis in otolaryngologic surgery. Int Arch Otorhinolaryngol 2013;17:85–91.

40. Riechelmann H, Tholen M, Keck T, et al. Perioperative glucocorticoid treatment does not influence early post-laser stapedotomy hearing thresholds. Am J Otol 2000;21:809–12.

41. Harrill WC, Jenkins HA, Coker NJ. Barotrauma after stapes surgery: a survey of recommended restrictions and clinical experiences. Am J Otol 1996;17:835–45 [discussion: 845–6].

42. Thiringer JK, Arriaga MA. Stapedectomy in military aircrew. Otolaryngol Head Neck Surg 1998;118:9–14.
43. Katzav J, Lippy WH, Shamiss A, et al. Stapedectomy in combat pilots. Am J Otol 1996;17:847–9.
44. House JW, Toh EH, Perez A. Diving after stapedectomy: clinical experience and recommendations. Otolaryngol Head Neck Surg 2001;125:356–60.
45. House HP, Sheehy JL. Stapes surgery: selection of the patient. Ann Otol Rhinol Laryngol 1961;70:1062–8.
46. Lenarz T, Zwartenkot JW, Stieger C, et al. Multicenter study with a direct acoustic cochlear implant. Otol Neurotol 2013;34:1215–25.
47. Kludt E, Buchner A, Schwab B, et al. Indication of direct acoustical cochlea stimulation in comparison to cochlear implants. Hear Res 2016;340:185–90.
48. Shea PF, Ge X, Shea JJ Jr. Stapedectomy for far-advanced otosclerosis. Am J Otol 1999;20:425–9.
49. Lippy WH, Burkey JM, Arkis PN. Word recognition score changes after stapedectomy for far advanced otosclerosis. Am J Otol 1998;19:56–8.
50. Calmels MN, Viana C, Wanna G, et al. Very far-advanced otosclerosis: stapedotomy or cochlear implantation. Acta Otolaryngol 2007;127:574–8.
51. Kabbara B, Gauche C, Calmels MN, et al. Decisive criteria between stapedotomy and cochlear implantation in patients with far advanced otosclerosis. Otol Neurotol 2015;36:e73–8.
52. Parahy C, Linthicum FH Jr. Otosclerosis: relationship of spiral ligament hyalinization to sensorineural hearing loss. The Laryngoscope 1983;93:717–20.
53. Kwok OT, Nadol JB Jr. Correlation of otosclerotic foci and degenerative changes in the organ of Corti and spiral ganglion. Am J Otolaryngol 1989;10:1–12.
54. Bretlau P, Salomon G, Johnsen NJ. Otospongiosis and sodium fluoride. A clinical double-blind, placebo-controlled study on sodium fluoride treatment in otospongiosis. Am J Otol 1989;10:20–2.
55. Shambaugh GE Jr, Scott A. Sodium fluoride for arrest of otosclerosis; theoretical considerations. Arch Otolaryngol 1964;80:263–70.
56. Causse JR, Causse JB. Clinical studies on fluoride in otospongiosis. Am J Otol 1985;6:51–5.
57. Quesnel AM, Seton M, Merchant SN, et al. Third-generation bisphosphonates for treatment of sensorineural hearing loss in otosclerosis. Otol Neurotol 2012;33:1308–14.

Moving?

Make sure your subscription moves with you!

To notify us of your new address, find your **Clinics Account Number** (located on your mailing label above your name), and contact customer service at:

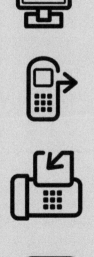

Email: journalscustomerservice-usa@elsevier.com

800-654-2452 (subscribers in the U.S. & Canada)
314-447-8871 (subscribers outside of the U.S. & Canada)

Fax number: 314-447-8029

Elsevier Health Sciences Division
Subscription Customer Service
3251 Riverport Lane
Maryland Heights, MO 63043

Printed and bound by CPI Group (UK) Ltd, Croydon, CR0 4YY

07/10/2024

01040500-0006